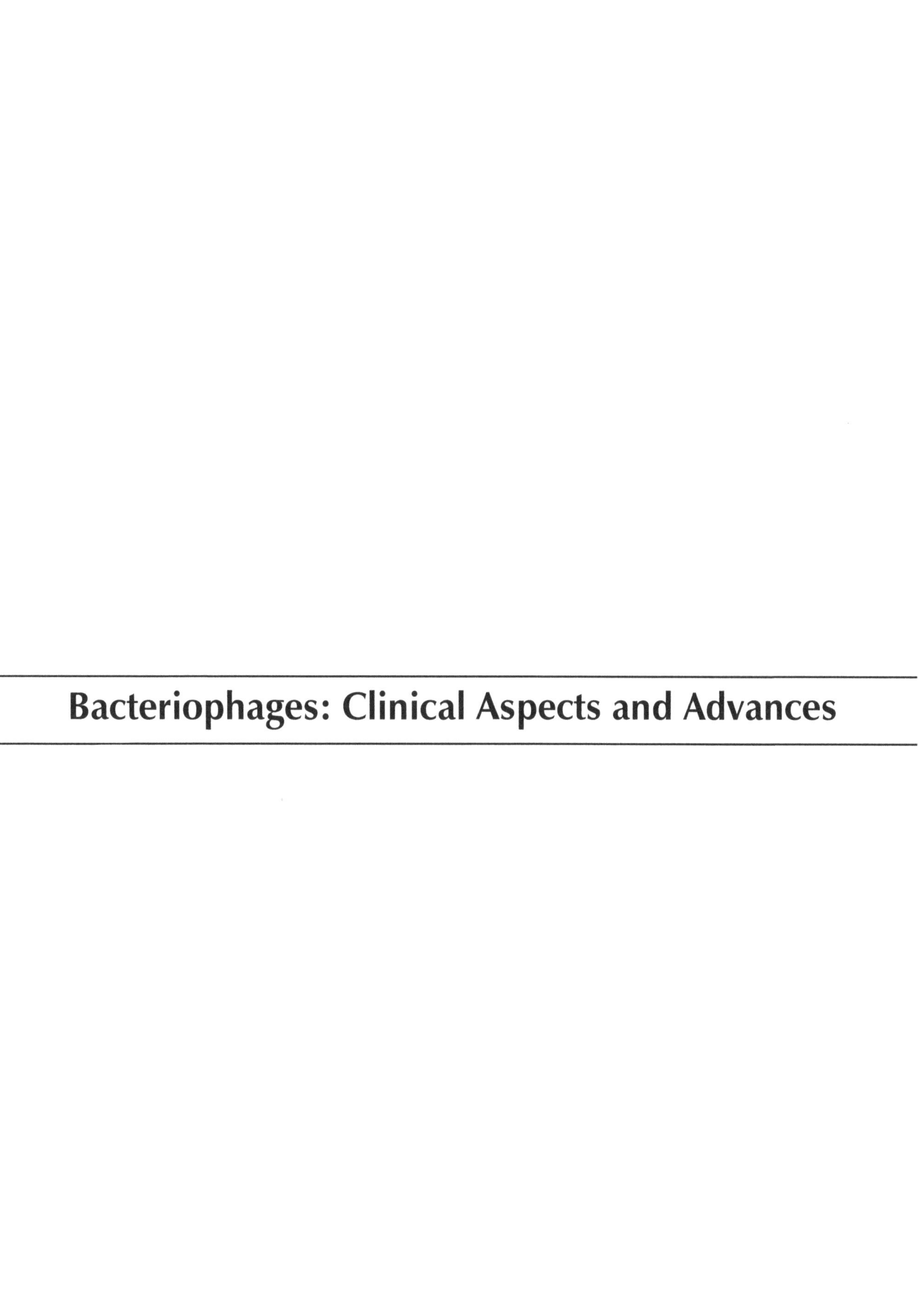

Bacteriophages: Clinical Aspects and Advances

Bacteriophages: Clinical Aspects and Advances

Editor: Rebecca Chesterton

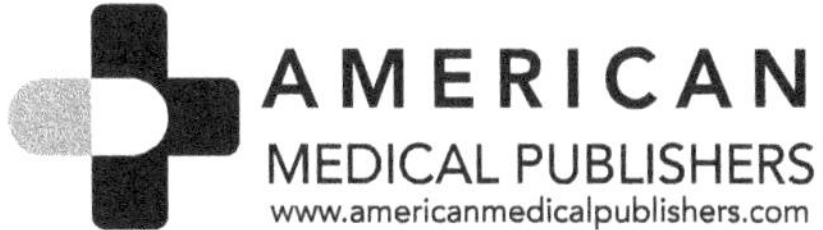

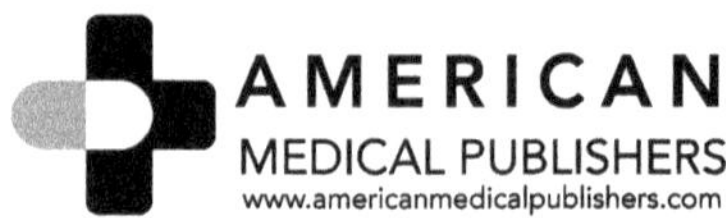

Cataloging-in-Publication Data

Bacteriophages : clinical aspects and advances / edited by Rebecca Chesterton.
p. cm.
Includes bibliographical references and index.
ISBN 978-1-63927-594-6
1. Bacteriophages. 2. Bacteriophages--Health aspects.
3. Bacteriophages--Therapeutic use. I. Chesterton, Rebecca.
QR342 .B333 2023
579.26--dc23

American Medical Publishers,
41 Flatbush Avenue,
1st Floor, New York,
NY 11217, USA

ISBN 978-1-63927-594-6 (Hardback)

Contents

Preface

Bacteriophages are a type of virus which infect and replicate inside archaea and bacteria. They are made up of proteins which encapsulate either the RNA or DNA genome, and may have simple or complex structures. Their genomes can contain as few as four genes like MS2 or may contain hundreds of genes. Phages reproduce inside the bacterium, after their genome is injected into its cytoplasm. They are the most usual and distinct entities found in the biosphere. These viruses are ubiquitous in nature and can be discovered anywhere near bacteria. They can be used as a therapy against multi-drug-resistant strains for a variety of bacteria. Phages also interact with the immune system both directly and indirectly. They directly impact the bacterial clearance and innate immunity, and indirectly interact through bacterial expression of phage-encoded proteins. This book unravels the recent studies on bacteriophages. Those in search of information to further their knowledge will be greatly assisted by it.

Various studies have approached the subject by analyzing it with a single perspective, but the present book provides diverse methodologies and techniques to address this field. This book contains theories and applications needed for understanding the subject from different perspectives. The aim is to keep the readers informed about the progresses in the field; therefore, the contributions were carefully examined to compile novel researches by specialists from across the globe.

Indeed, the job of the editor is the most crucial and challenging in compiling all chapters into a single book. In the end, I would extend my sincere thanks to the chapter authors for their profound work. I am also thankful for the support provided by my family and colleagues during the compilation of this book.

Editor

Origin and Evolution of *Studiervirinae* Bacteriophages Infecting *Pectobacterium*: Horizontal Transfer Assists Adaptation to New Niches

Peter V. Evseev [1], Anna A. Lukianova [1,2], Mikhail M. Shneider [1], Aleksei A. Korzhenkov [3], Eugenia N. Bugaeva [1,4], Anastasia P. Kabanova [1,4], Kirill K. Miroshnikov [5], Eugene E. Kulikov [5], Stepan V. Toshchakov [5], Alexander N. Ignatov [4] and Konstantin A. Miroshnikov [1,*]

1 Shemyakin–Ovchinnikov Institute of Bioorganic Chemistry, Russian Academy of Sciences, 117997 Moscow, Russia; petevseev@gmail.com (P.V.E.); a.al.lukianova@gmail.com (A.A.L.); mm_shn@mail.ru (M.M.S.); bygaeva.genia@gmail.com (E.N.B.); asiasay@yandex.ru (A.P.K.)
2 Department of Biology, Lomonosov Moscow State University, 119991 Moscow, Russia
3 Federal Research Center "Kurchatov Institute", 123182 Moscow, Russia; oscypek@yandex.ru
4 Research Center "PhytoEngineering" Ltd., Rogachevo, 141880 Moscow Region, Russia; an.ignatov@gmail.com
5 Winogradsky Institute of Microbiology, Federal Research Center "Fundamentals of Biotechnology", Russian Academy of Sciences, 117312 Moscow, Russia; infon18@gmail.com (K.K.M.); eumenius@gmail.com (E.E.K.); stepan.toshchakov@gmail.com (S.V.T.)
* Correspondence: kmi@ibch.ru

Abstract: Black leg and soft rot are devastating diseases causing up to 50% loss of potential potato yield. The search for, and characterization of, bacterial viruses (bacteriophages) suitable for the control of these diseases is currently a sought-after task for agricultural microbiology. Isolated lytic *Pectobacterium* bacteriophages Q19, PP47 and PP81 possess a similar broad host range but differ in their genomic properties. The genomic features of characterized phages have been described and compared to other *Studiervirinae* bacteriophages. Thorough phylogenetic analysis has clarified the taxonomy of the phages and their positioning relative to other genera of the *Autographiviridae* family. *Pectobacterium* phage Q19 seems to represent a new genus not described previously. The genomes of the phages are generally similar to the genome of phage T7 of the *Teseptimavirus* genus but possess a number of specific features. Examination of the structure of the genes and proteins of the phages, including the tail spike protein, underlines the important role of horizontal gene exchange in the evolution of these phages, assisting their adaptation to *Pectobacterium* hosts. The results provide the basis for the development of bacteriophage-based biocontrol of potato soft rot as an alternative to the use of antibiotics.

Keywords: phage; *Autographiviridae*; *Pectobacterium*; tail spike; horizontal transfer; evolution; phage therapy

1. Introduction

The potato (*Solanum tuberosum L.*) is one of the most essential food crops and is cultivated all over the world. Black leg and soft rot in potatoes inflict great losses in the production of this crop [1]. These diseases are caused by "soft rot *Pectobacteriaceae*" (SRP), which includes species of genera *Pectobacterium* and *Dickeya* [2,3]. The cells of SRP are mostly spread by contaminated seed material and can survive on other crops, wild and weedy plants, in irrigation water and on farm equipment [2,4]. The use of efficient antibacterial compounds in agriculture is restricted or limited, so there is a lack of effective methods to control soft rot [1]. The use of bacteriophages (phages) specific to the bacteria causing plant diseases is considered to be a promising strategy [5–8]. A number of successful experiments in the prevention and control of potato soft rot by applying *Pectobacterium* and *Dickeya* phages in vitro, in planta [9,10] and in the field [11,12] have been reported. However, besides traditional hurdles on production and regulation of phage-based preparations, the construction of SRP-directed phage cocktails has problems with basic requirements. The consensus of opinion on candidate phages is that they should be lytic, specific to the target bacteria, and have a reasonably broad range. Different phages should be included in the composition to reduce the formation of phage-resistant mutants of bacteria [13,14].

Recent studies have revealed the great diversity of SRP, reflected in the fact that there are currently over 30 species of *Pectobacterium* and *Dickeya* [15,16], most of them adapted to the conditions of all environments and climatic zones used for the production of potatoes.

The taxonomy of bacteriophages (and viruses in general) has also undergone recent revolutionary changes [17,18]. The order *Caudovirales* (dsDNA tailed viruses, the largest group of known bacteriophages) has been elevated to the *Uroviricota* phylum level. Correspondingly, existing and newly formed lower level taxa of phages have been elevated and separated (https://talk.ictvonline.org/taxonomy/). For instance, short-tailed phages resembling a model phage T7 are currently represented as the *Autographiviridae* family, which has nine subfamilies and 63 genera. Thus, morphologically indistinguishable phages with a similar architecture of the genome can be categorised as belonging to different genera or even subfamilies. The question of specificity and genetic diversity of SRP phages deserves a very careful investigation.

In this work, we present a comprehensive characterisation of three related lytic bacteriophages isolated in the Moscow region within a five-year period. The study describes the biological and genomic properties of *Pectobacterium* phages PP47, PP81, and Q19 with respect to their suitability for phage control applications.

The results of a comparative phylogeny of phages belonging to the subfamily *Studiervirinae* and infecting *Pectobacterium* spp., and a bioinformatic analysis of adsorption apparatus and the whole phage genome, suggest hypotheses for possible mechanisms of adaptation of these *Pectobacterium* phages to the host.

2. Materials and Methods

2.1. Bacterial Strains and Growth Conditions

Characterised propagation strains *Pectobacterium brasiliense* F157 (PB38), NCBI accession number NZ_PJDL00000000.1 and other strains and field isolates listed in Table S1 were grown at 28 °C in LB broth or LB agar plates (1.5% agar) for 24–48 h. The strains were kept in 20% glycerol at −80 °C for long-term storage.

2.2. Bacteriophage Isolation and Purification

Bacteriophages were isolated from samples collected in the Moscow region. The sources were washing water in a potato warehouse (geographical coordinates 56°25′28″ N, 37°9′15″ E) in 2014 for PP47, a sample of rotten potatoes from a dump (56°25′33″ N, 37°34′13″ E) in 2015 for PP81 and urban wastewater (55°40′27″ N, 37°57′49″ E) in 2018 for Q19. The presence of the phages in the sample was analysed using a soft agar overlay protocol [19]. Phages were propagated using *P. brasiliense* strain F157. Cell cultures grown at 28 °C to OD_{600} ~0.5 were infected with corresponding bacteriophages at a multiplicity of infection (MOI) of 0.01 and incubated for a further 4 h with moderate agitation. Cell debris were removed by centrifugation at 10,000× *g* for 20 min at 4 °C. The supernatant was passed through a 0.22 μm membrane filter. The phages were concentrated by centrifugation at 22,000× *g* for 40 min at 4 °C. The resulting pellet was resuspended in a phage buffer to a concentration ~10^9 pfu/mL and stored at 4 °C until used.

2.3. Host Range of Bacteriophages

Forty strains representing different species of *Pectobacterium* and *Dickeya*, as well as soil bacteria usually accompanying soft rot infections (Table S1), were used to assess the infection range of phages.

500 µL of liquid culture of each strain was mixed with 4 mL of 0.7% soft LB agar and overlaid onto LB plates containing 1.5% agar. 20 µL of PP47, PP81 and Q19 suspensions (10^9 pfu/mL) were spotted onto the lawns and the plates were incubated overnight at 28 °C. Bacterial susceptibility was determined by the clarification of phage application spots. Lytic ability was verified using the titration by overlay method, with the corresponding bacterial strain.

2.4. Biological Activity of Bacteriophages

Adsorption and one-step-growth curve tests were processed according to [9]. Bacterial strains were grown to the mid-exponential phase and infected by individual phages at MOI = 0.01. Aliquots were taken at specified intervals, diluted using a phage buffer and centrifuged at 10,000× *g* for 1 min. The titers of unadsorbed and reversibly adsorbed phages were determined by serial dilution.

The long-term effects of the phages on bacterial growth were measured by monitoring the OD_{600} for 12 h post-infection with each phage. Bacterial cells in mid-exponential phase (10^9 cfu/mL) were mixed with the solution of phages at an MOI of 1 and diluted with LB broth. The OD_{600} of the reaction mixtures were monitored with a microplate reader (Victor, Thermo Scientific) at 28 °C over 3 h.

2.5. Electron Microscopy

The morphology of phages PP47, PP81 and Q19 was analysed by transmission electron microscopy (TEM). Phage suspension (~10^9 pfu/mL) was purified by ultracentrifugation in a CsCl gradient (rotor SW28, Beckman, 22,000× *g* for 40 min at 4 °C), dialysed against the phage buffer, placed on individual copper grids, negatively stained with 1% uranyl acetate and examined using an FEI Tecnai G2 microscope at 100kV acceleration voltage. The dimensions were averaged among ~20 individually measured particles.

2.6. Phage Genome Sequencing and Annotation

Phage DNA was extracted using the phenol-chloroform method and fragmented with a Bioruptor sonicator (Diagenode). Paired-end libraries were constructed using a Nebnext Ultra DNA library prep kit (New England Biolabs) and sequenced on the Illumina MiSeq™ platform (Illumina) using paired 150 bp reads. After filtering using CLC Genomics Workbench 8.5 (Qiagen), overlapping paired-end library reads were merged with the SeqPrep tool (https://github.com/jstjohn/SeqPrep). Reads were assembled using CLC Genomic workbench v. 7.5. The phage genome was annotated by predicting and validating open reading frames (ORFs) using Prodigal 2.6.1 [20] and Prokka [21] pipelines. Identified ORFs were manually curated to ensure fidelity. Functions were assigned to ORFs using a BLAST search on a custom phage protein database compiled from annotated phage GenBank sequences, InterPro server (https://www.ebi.ac.uk/interpro/entry/InterPro) and HHpred server (https://toolkit.tuebingen.mpg.de) with Pfam-A_v32.0, NCBI_Consreved_Domain_v.3.16, SMART_v6.0, PRK_6.9, PDB, SCOPe70_2.07, ECOD_ECOD_F70_20190225 and COG_KOG_v1.0 databases. Custom BLAST databases were compiled using the BLAST tool (https://blast.ncbi.nlm.nih.gov/). tRNA coding regions were searched using tRNAscan-SE [22] and ARAGORN [23]. The resulting genome map was visualised in Geneious Prime, version 2020.2.3 (https://www.geneious.com). The intergenic genome regions of the phages were searched for promoters with PhagePromoter [24] in the Galaxy framework (https://galaxy.bio.di.uminho.pt/) with threshold 0.65.

2.7. Phylogenetic Analysis

Phage reference genomes were downloaded from NCBI GenBank (ftp://ftp.ncbi.nlm.nih.gov/genbank). Where necessary, the genomes were annotated using Prokka [21], with a custom phage protein database compiled from annotated phage GenBank sequences. A search for homologous sequences was conducted using a BLAST search and sequences found were checked for the presence of annotated homologous genes in NCBI genomes. Genes were extracted from GenBank annotations. For some unannotated sequences, ORFs were found using Glimmer [25]. ORFs were validated and corrected by comparison with known homologous genes. Protein alignments were made with MAFFT (L-INS-i algorithm, BLOSUM62 scoring matrix, 1.53 gap open penalty, 0.123 offset value) [26]. The alignments were trimmed manually and with trimAL [27] with gappyout settings. Best protein models were found with MEGAX 10.0.5 [28]. Trees were constructed using the maximum likelihood (ML) method with an RAxML program [29] and a WAG+G protein model, and the robustness of the trees was assessed by bootstrapping (1000) and with MrBayes [30,31].

2.8. Whole-Genome and Proteome Analysis

Average nucleotide identity (ANI) was computed using the OrthoANIu tool [32], employing USEARCH (http://www.drive5.com/usearch/) over BLAST (https://www.ezbiocloud.net/tools/orthoaniu) with default settings. Core protein extraction was performed with BPGA software [33]. Searches for homologous sequences were conducted with BLAST on custom databases based on Genbank sequences and on the nr/nt NCBI database. The VIRIDIC server (http://rhea.icbm.uni-oldenburg.de/VIRIDIC/) was employed for calculating phage intergenomic similarities (BLASTN parameters '-word_size 7-reward 2-penalty-3-gapopen 5-gapextend 2') [34].

2.9. D Homology Modelling, Alignment and Visualisation

Protein remote homology detection, 3D structure prediction and template-based homology prediction were made using the Phyre2 protein fold recognition server (http://www.sbg.bio.ic.ac.uk/~phyre2) [35], HHpred (https://toolkit.tuebingen.mpg.de/tools/hhpred). The obtained structures were aligned and visualised with UCSF Chimera [36].

3. Results

3.1. General Properties of Pectobacterium Bacteriophages PP47, PP81 and Q19

Pectobacterium brasiliense (syn: *P. carotovorum* subsp. *brasiliense*) [37,38] is one of the major concerns in relation to the soft rot pathogenesis of potatoes in Central European Russia, and has been since the early 2010s [39,40]. *P. brasilense* has a certain heterogeneity in terms of its genomic and physiological properties [41,42]. Several genetically distinct strains of it were isolated in Russia [39,43], and they are used as components of enrichment culture to isolate SRP-specific bacteriophages. On the lawn of the isolation strain F157, bacteriophages formed clear plaques with a diameter of 2–3 mm for PP47 and P81, and 3-5 mm for Q19 (LB/1.5% w/v bottom agar, 0.5% w/v top agar, 28 °C).

Infectivity assays of all three phages, in standard conditions and on the same bacterial host, showed certain differences in their infection cycle. All phages demonstrated fast adsorption, in 3–5 min, and fast lysis of the host culture. Phage PP81 had a notably longer latent period and a smaller burst size (64 progeny phages/cell vs 87 for Q19 and 163 for PP47) (Figure 1).

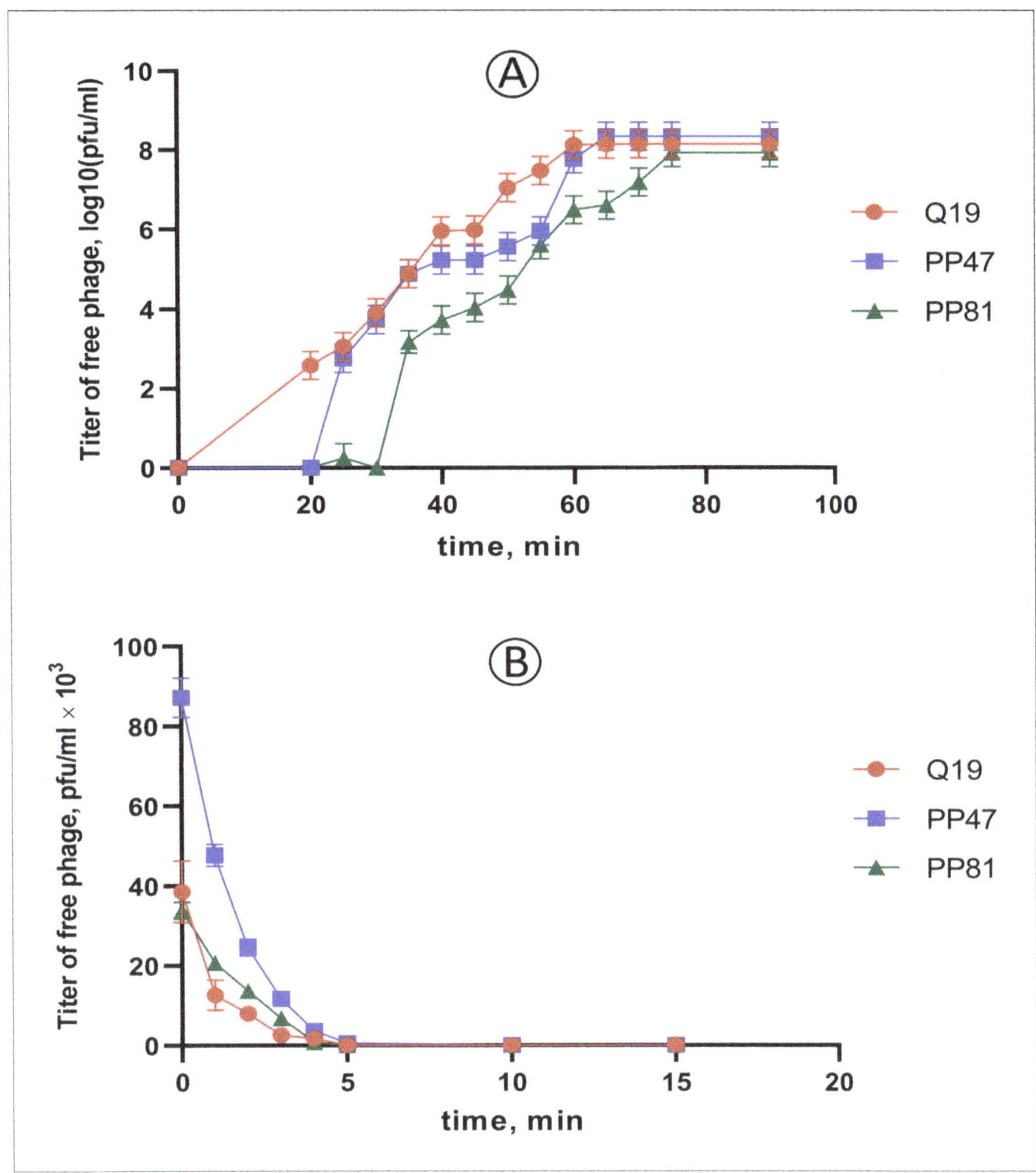

Figure 1. (**A**) One-step growth curve of phages Q19 (red), PP47 (blue) and PP81 (green) using *P. brasiliense* F157 as host strain in MOI = 0.01. (**B**) Adsorption of phages Q19 (red), PP47 (blue) and PP81 (green) at the surface of *P. brasiliense* F157 in MOI = 0.001.

Phages PP47, PP81 and Q19 demonstrated a fairly similar host range. All three phages infected *P. brasiliense* strains F157 and F126, while *P. brasiliense* F128 was susceptible to Q19 only, and strain F152 was resistant to all phages. All three phages infected *P. polaris* strain F109, most tested strains of *P. versatile* and some insufficiently attributed pectolytic isolates. All tested strains of *P. carotovorum*, *P. parmentieri* and *P. aquaticum*, and all *Dickeya* spp. used in the experiment, seemed to be resistant to PP47, PP81 and Q19 (Table S1). Therefore, in compliance with the definition of a phage suitable for phage therapy [44], the host range of the studied phages can be considered to be broad.

The morphology of Q19, PP47 and PP81, as revealed by TEM, was typical for *Autographiviridae* phages [17,45]. The virions corresponded to Podoviral morphotype C1, with an icosahedral capsid about 60 nm in diameter and a short tail about 10 nm long. Small appendages corresponding to the phage adsorption apparatus can be seen around the tail (Figure 2).

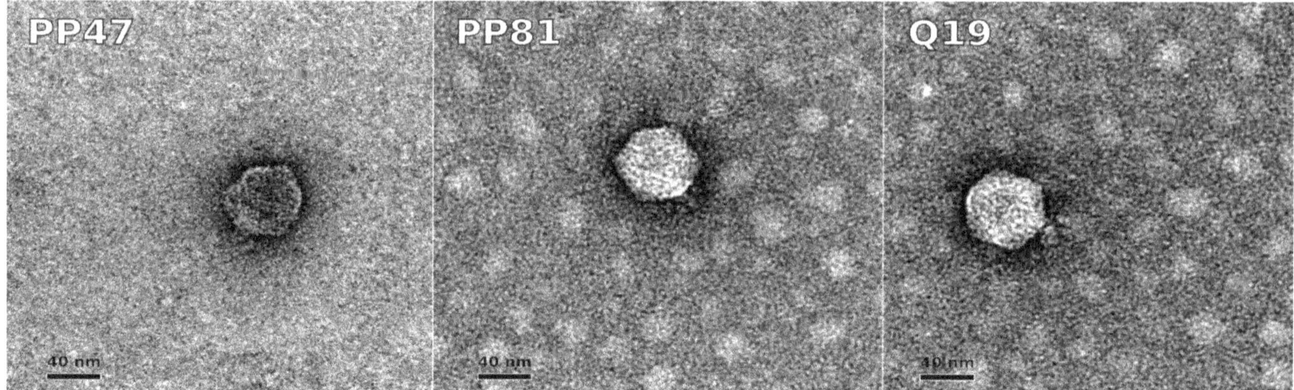

Figure 2. Transmission electron microscopy of bacteriophages PP47, PP81, and Q19. Staining was with 1% uranyl acetate. The scale bar is 40 nm.

3.2. Taxonomy

Intergenomic comparisons were made through calculations of average nucleotide identity using orthoANIu and whole-genome similarity by VIRIDIC, using all Genbank complete genome sequences of *Autographiviridae* phages. The latter algorithm was demonstrated to correspond to the primary classification technique used by the International Committee on Taxonomy of Viruses (ICTV), but to a higher degree [34]. The ANI calculations show a significant similarity between phages PP47 and PP81 (about 98%, Tables S2 and S3) and a lesser similarity with Q19 and all other phages (about 92%, compared to *Klebsiella* virus KP32 genome, the closest to Q19), (Table S4). These data correspond to the results of VIRIDIC analysis (Figure 3), testifying to the affiliation of PP47 and PP81 with the genus *Pektosvirus* of the *Studiervirinae* subfamily, and the affiliation of Q19 with an as yet unassigned genus. The ANI and VIRIDIC calculations point to *Pectobacterium* phages MA6 and MA1A as other members of the *Pektosvirus* genus and to the closeness of their genomes (their intergenomic similarity being higher than 95% of the species threshold). The intergenomic similarity of phages PP47 and PP81 is also higher than the species threshold. Thus, PP47 and PP81 can be considered to be strains of the same species, as well as phages MA6 and MA1A.

The proteomic tree made with ViPTree by BIONJ clustering of similar predicted protein sequences belonging to 447 phage genomes of *Podoviridae* and *Autographiviridae* families (Figure S1), and manually curated to correspond to the latest taxonomy (Figure 4), attributes the *Pectobacterium* phage Q19 to the *Studiervirinae* subfamily and also groups phages PP47, PP81, PPWS4, MA6 and MA1A together. The tree suggests the *Escherichia* phage SRT7 as a possible closest relative of *Pektosvirus* phages, and *Pectobacterium* phages Jarilo and DU_PP_II as possible closest relatives of phage Q19.

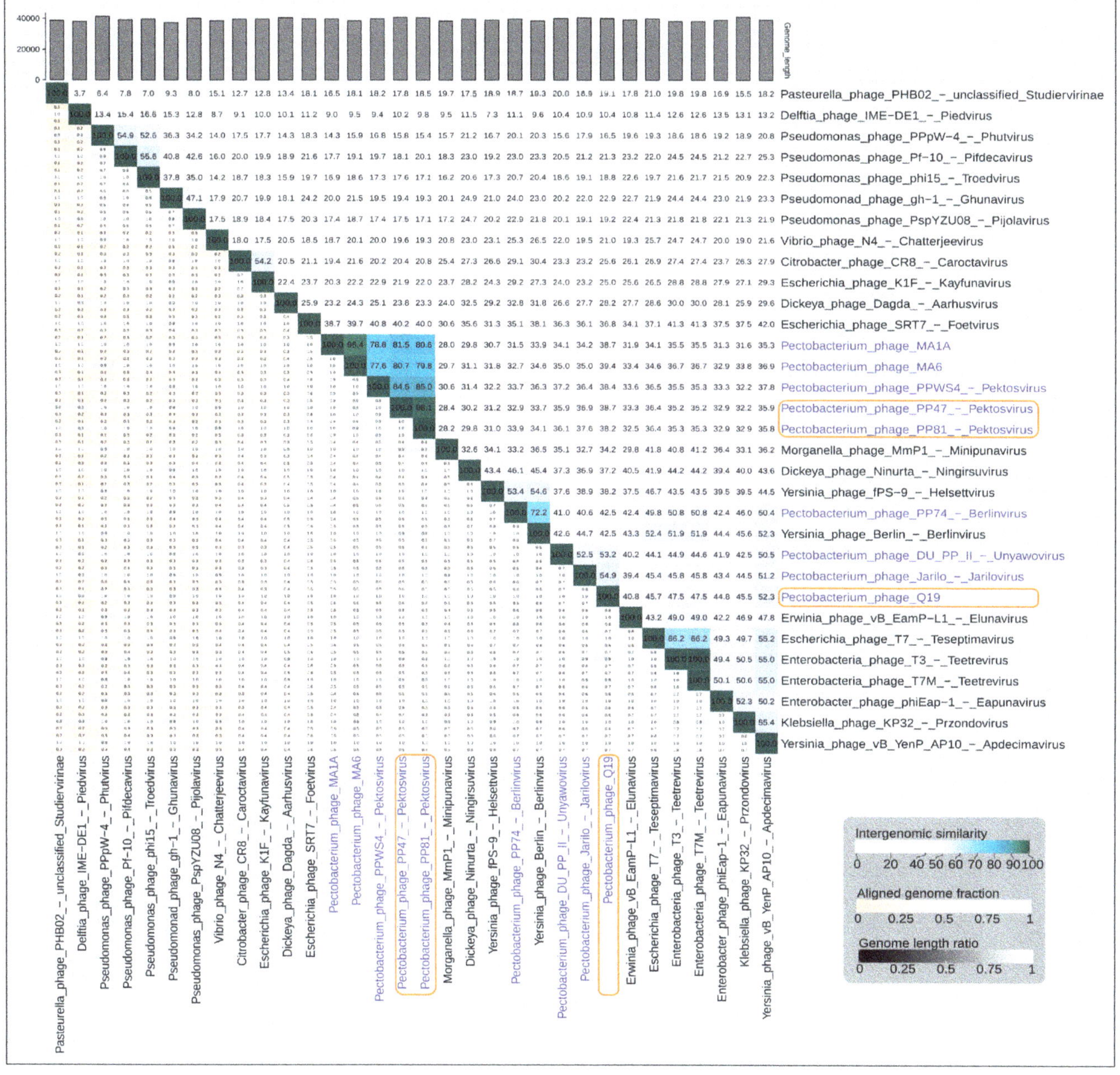

Figure 3. VIRIDIC generated heatmap of 30 *Studiervirinae* phages and a representative of the *Piedvirus* genus, which is closely related to *Studiervirinae*. The heatmap incorporates intergenomic similarity values (right half) and alignment indicators (left half and top annotation). In the right half, the colour coding allows a rapid visualisation of the clustering of the phage genomes based on intergenomic similarity. The numbers represent the similarity values for each genome pair, rounded to the first decimal. In the left half, three indicator values are represented for each genome pair, from top to bottom: aligned fraction genome 1 (for the genome found in this row), genome length ratio (for the two genomes in this pair) and aligned fraction genome 2 (for the genome found in this column). *Pectobacterium* phages PP47, PP81, PPWS4, MA6 and MA1A are clustered with an intergenomic similarity higher than the genus threshold of 70%. *Pectobacterium* phage Q19 has an intergenomic similarity that is lower than 70% compared to any other phage.

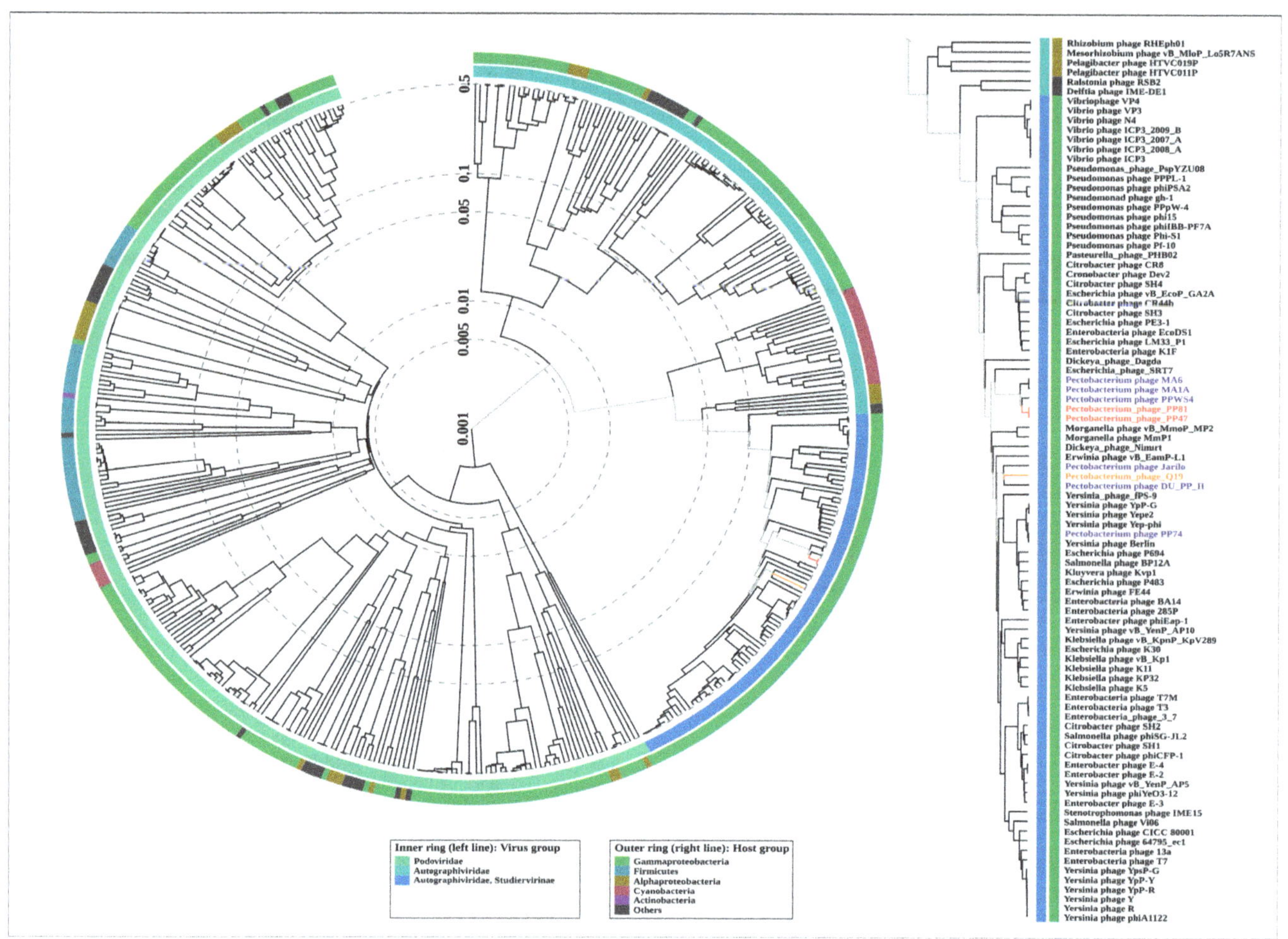

Figure 4. Circular proteomic tree of 447 *Podovoridae* and *Autographiviridae* phage genomes, and the *Studiervirinae* part of the tree (right) constructed using ViPTree. The branches representing *Pectobacterium* phages PP47 and PP81 are coloured red, and the branch representing *Pectobacterium* phage Q19 is coloured orange.

The phage genomes possess a number of features which may compromise the accurate deduction of their evolutionary history [46]. These include a high level of recombination [47,48], mosaicism of the genome [49,50] and high rate of point mutations, at least for a number of proteins [51,52]. To confirm preliminary taxonomic conclusions, the phylogeny was carried out using concatenated sequences of five conserved proteins, namely DNA polymerase, a large subunit of terminase, a head-tail connector protein, a major capsid protein and a single-strand DNA binding protein. The Bayesian tree obtained for 31 phages, including 29 *Studiervirinae* phages, recognised by ICTV as master species, *Pectobacterium* phage PP74 and *Delphia* phage IME-DE1 employed as an outgroup, proposes an evolutionary history that is somewhat different to that shown in a proteomic tree (Figure 5). This tree, nevertheless, also groups phages PP47, PP81, PPWS4, M6 and MA1A as a distinct clade, and points to *Escherichia* phage SRT7 representing the genus *Foetvirus* as a sister group. In agreement with the proteomic tree and genome similarity measurements, the concatenated protein phylogeny testifies to *Pectobacteium* phages Jarilo and DU_PP_II being close relatives of phage Q19.

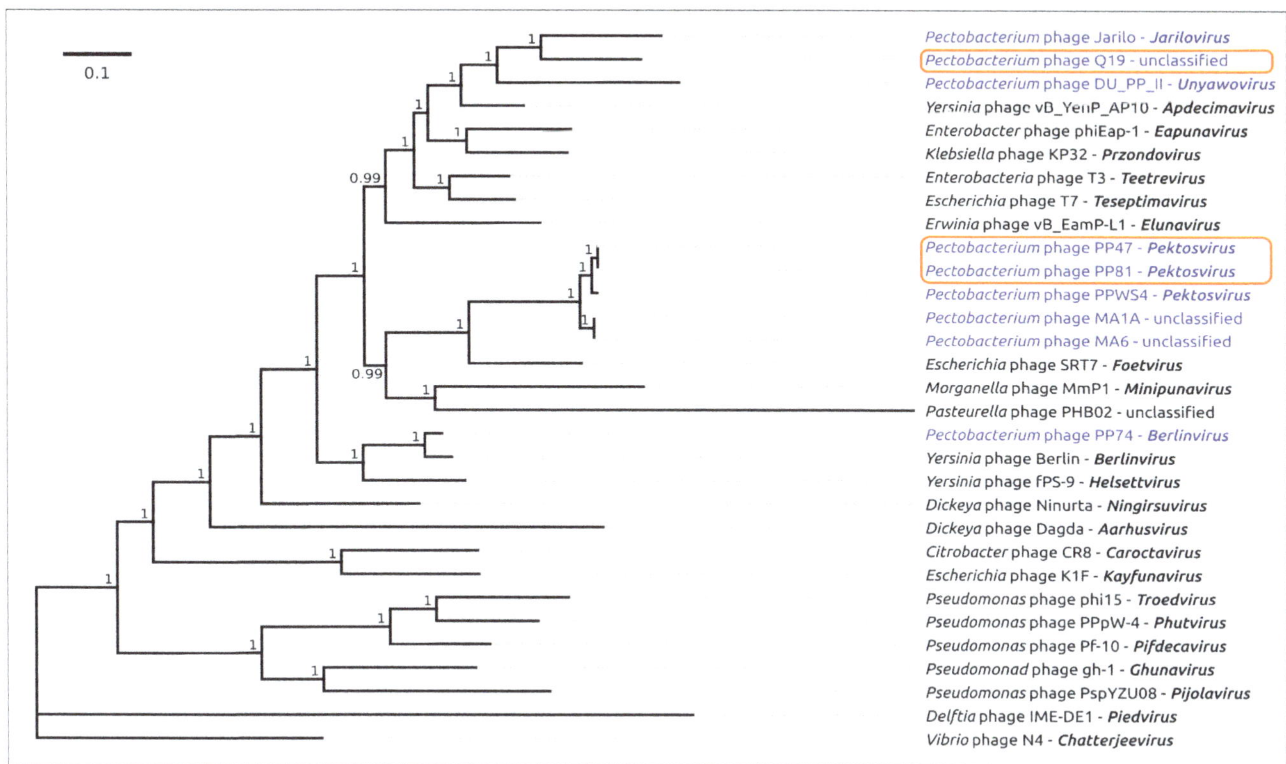

Figure 5. Phylogenetic tree obtained with MrBayes, based on concatenated sequences of DNA polymerase, a large subunit of terminase, a head-tail connector protein, a major capsid protein and a single-strand DNA binding protein extracted from the genomes of 29 phages, recognised by International Committee on Taxonomy of Viruses (ICTV) as master species belonging to the *Studiervirinae* subfamily, *Pectobacterium* phage PP74 of the *Berlinvirus* genus and *Delphia* phage IME-DE1. Bayesian posterior probabilities are indicated above their branch. Taxonomic classification is taken from ICTV and is shown to the right of the organism name. The scale bar shows 0.1 estimated substitutions per site and the tree was rooted to *Delphia* phage IME-DE1; of 2,000,000 generations, every 200 generations were sampled, with an average standard deviation of split frequencies of 0.0027.

Terminase and major capsid protein (MCP) are the two most conserved proteins encoded in bacteriophage genomes, and they are often used for phage taxonomy purposes [53]. The analysis of the results of a BLAST search on the protein sequences of *Autographiviridae* indicated that terminase can be a better choice for evaluation of the phage evolutionary history than MCP at a large scale, since this protein seems to be more conservative. For the construction of the phylogeny, use was made of protein sequences extracted from 100 genomes comprising the representatives of almost all subfamilies of *Autographiviridae* and the genera not assigned to any subfamily. The tree (Figure 6) suggests early divergence of the ancestors of *Autographiviridae* into two large groups, one of which contains current *Molineuxvirinae*, *Colwellvirinae*, *Krylovirinae*, *Melnykvirinae*, *Okabevirinae* subfamilies and unassigned genera, with the other group containing the *Studiervirinae* subfamily and some unassigned genera. Interestingly, the second group also includes temperate *Pelagibacter* phages [54] and proposedly temperate cyanophages [55–57]. These phages can integrate their genomic DNA at tRNA sites, and the evolutionary branches of these phages are located closer to the root of the tree than those of the *Enterobacteria* phage. The topology of the *Studiervirinae* part of the terminase tree is congruent to the topology of the concatenated core proteins tree (Figure 5) and assumes the *Studiervirinae* bacteriophages infecting *Pectobacterium* have a multiple origin from different ancestral lines of phages.

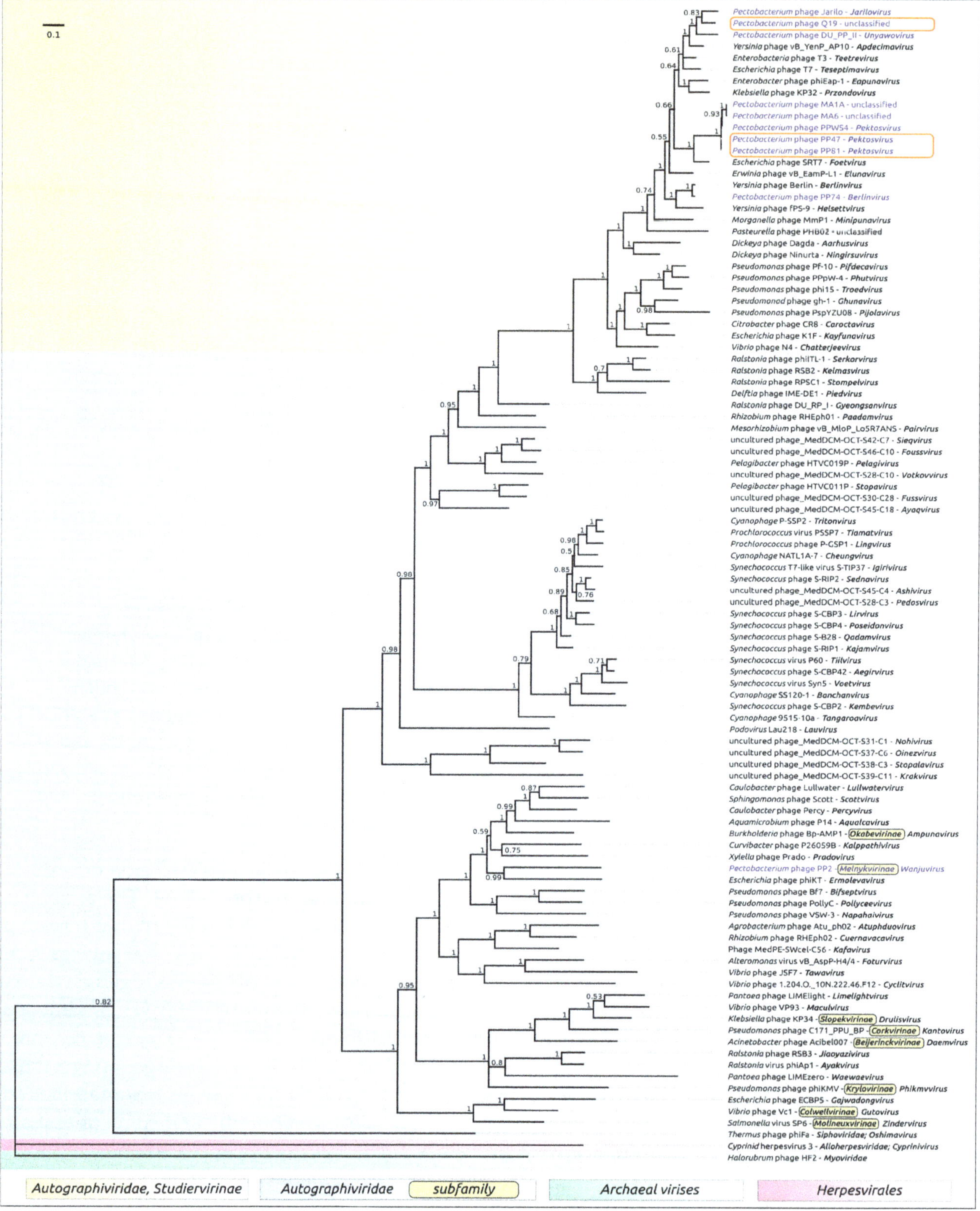

Figure 6. Phylogenetic tree obtained with MrBayes based on 100 terminase large subunit protein sequences. Bayesian posterior probabilities are indicated above their branch. Taxonomic classification is taken from ICTV and is shown to the right of the organism name. The scale bar shows 0.1 estimated substitutions per site and the tree was rooted to *Cyprinid* herpesvirus 3; of 2,000,000 generations, every 200 generations were sampled, with an average standard deviation of split frequencies of 0.012.

3.3. Proteome Analysis

The proteome studies were conducted with a BLAST search with predicted protein sequences on Genbank databases. Table S5 contains the data collected from the examination of the genomes with BLAST searches on Q19, PP47 and PP81 gene products with the Genbank phage database. This data may demonstrate the complex character of evolutionary relations between these *Pectobacterium* phages. The search revealed unique proteins at the level of species and genera. In addition, the results of the BLAST examination pointed to the presence of proteins unique to several taxonomically distant *Pectobacterium* phages or proteins, which have more similarities in primary sequence with phages from comparatively taxonomically distant groups infecting *Pectobacterium*, than to taxonomically closer phages infecting other hosts. The list of proteins typical for Pectobacterial phages includes putative RNA polymerase σ54 factor (Q19 gp2) possessing a structural similarity to *E. coli* σ54 factor (HHpred probability 94%), tail spike protein, tRNA-nucleotidyltransferase and minor capsid protein. tRNA-nucleotidyltransferase and tail spike protein sequences collected the largest number of homologs from *Pectobacterium* phages of other taxa (right column in Table S5).

Interestingly, the results of a BLAST search using the nr/nt NCBI database demonstrated a greater similarity between some *Pectobacteruim* phage proteins and their bacterial homologs than that between *Pectobacteruim* phage proteins and non-*Pectobacteruim* phage proteins. This might have been a consequence of horizontal transfer. A BLAST search of the Genbank bacterial database indicated the presence of bacterial homologs for 25 of the 50 predicted proteins of Q19 and for 26 of the 55 predicted proteins of PP47. The list of these homologs contained the proteins encoded in all three phage genome regions (early, middle and late).

3.4. Genomic Analysis

Pectobacterium phages PP47 (Genbank accession KY250035), PP81 (accession KY124276) and Q19 (accession MK290739) have linear dsDNA genomes of 40,995 bp, 40,751 bp and 40,227 bp, respectively. The GC content of Q19 genome was 49.7% and the GC content of PP47 and PP81 was 48.9%. This is slightly less that the CG content (51.8–52.0%) of bacterial hosts with sequenced genomes. The genomes of PP47, PP81 and Q19 encoded 55, 54 and 50 predicted gene products (gp), respectively. The genomes were flanked with terminal repeats with a size of 151 bp (PP47, PP81) and 222 bp (Q19). The BLAST comparison of genes indicated that the genomes of PP47 and PP81 are very similar—the only difference in gene content is an extra gene*22* in PP47, encoding a hypothetical protein. The homologs of gp22 were present in related *Pectobacterium* phages MA6 and MA1A but were not found in other phages. The Q19 phage genome appears to be more distinct from PP47 and PP81. Genomic maps of the phages are shown on Figure 7.

Generally, the genome organisation of phages PP47, PP81 and Q19 is typical for *sensu lato* T7-like phages, now comprising the subfamily *Studiervirinae* within the family *Autographiviridae*. Unidirectional open reading frames can be divided into three major functional regions, relating to host conversion, DNA metabolism and particle formation. The location of predicted promoters is close for genomes of phages PP47/81 and Q19 (Figure 7) and is similar to the corresponding promoter site arrangement in the genome of the model phage T7 [58].

The structural blocks of all three phages are very similar and encode 12 proteins with predicted function and high similarity among *Studiervirinae* phages. The only exception is a putative minor capsid protein encoded downstream of a major capsid protein gene. It has no homologs in T7 but is similar to predicted minor capsid proteins in some *Studiervirinae* phages, including *Citrobacter* phage CR8 and *Klebsiella* phage KP32, belonging to genera *Caroctavirus* and *Przondovirus*, respectively.

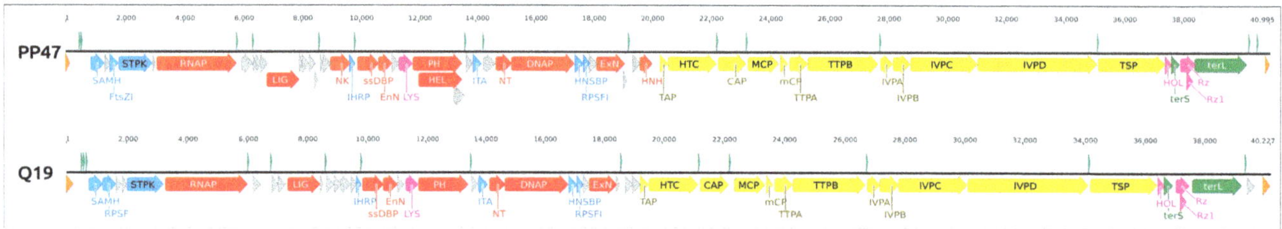

Figure 7. Genetic map of phages PP47 and Q19. The colors of different functional modules are as follows: yellow, morphogenesis; red, replication, transcription and nucleic acids processing; green, packaging; purple, lysis proteins; blue, regulation of host defense and metabolic processes; orange, terminal repeats; grey, hypothetical proteins. Putative transcriptional promoters, predicted with Phage Promoters, are shown above each sequence (presented as a black line) and colored cyan. Numbers above the sequences show the position in genomes. Genes' names are as follows: SAMH, S-adenosyl-L-methionine hydrolase; RPSF, RNA polymerase σ54 factor; FtsZI, cell division FtsZ inhibitor; STPK, seryl-threonyl protein kinase; RNAP, DNA-directed RNA polymerase; LIG, DNA ligase; NK, nucleotide kinase; IHRP, inhibitor of host bacterial RNA polymerase; ssDBP, ssDNA-binding protein CDS; EnN, endonuclease I; LYS, lysozyme, N-acetylmuramoyl-L-alanine amidase; PH, DNA primase/helicase; HEL, DNA helicase; ITA, inhibitor of toxin/antitoxin system; NT, nucleotidyltransferase; DNAP, DNA polymerase; HNSBP, H-NS and tRNA binding protein CDS; RPSFI, host RNA polymerase σ70 factor inhibitor; ExN, 5′-3′ exonuclease; HNH, HNH endonuclease; TAP, tail assembly protein; HTC, head-tail connector protein; CAP, capsid assembly protein; MCP, major capsid protein; mCP, minor capsid protein; TTPA, tail tubular protein A; TTPB, tail tubular protein B; IVPA, internal virion protein A; IVPB, internal virion protein B; IVPC, internal virion protein C; IVPD, internal virion protein D; TSP, tail spike protein, SGNH hydrolase domain-containing protein; HOL, class II holin; terS, terminase small subunit; Rz, Rz lysis protein; Rz1, Rz1 lysis protein; terL, terminase large subunit.

The products of early genes are often produced immediately after infection and protect the bacteriophage DNA from bacterial defense mechanisms or adapt the host-cell metabolism to establish an efficient infection cycle [59]. These genes are most diverse within the subfamily, and the composition of the first block of genes differs for PP47/PP81 and Q19. All three phages encoded S-adenosyl-L-methionine hydrolase (first predicted gene in the genomes, gp1), homologous hypothetical proteins (gp2 in PP47/PP81 and gp3 in Q19) and serine/threonine kinase (gp4 in PP47/PP81 and gp5 in Q19). The difference in the composition of the products of early genes is the presence of a predicted cell division inhibitor FtsZ (gp3 in PP47/PP81) [60] which has no obvious homologs in the Q19 predicted proteome. Conversely, the genome of Q19 (but not PP47/PP81) encodes a putative RNA polymerase σ factor that has structural homology with bacterial σ54 enhancer-dependent σ54 transcription factor [27], revealed by HMM-HMM search with HHpred (PDB entry: 5ui5; Probability: 94.35%; E-value: 0.67; Score: 37.59). One other hypothetical protein, gp4, encoded in the early gene block of Q19, also has no phage homologs or similar structural proteins.

The middle (nucleic acid metabolism) genome regions of PP47, PP81 and Q19 are closely related. The hallmark of the *Studiervirinae* subfamily, a single subunit, DNA-dependent RNA-polymerase located in the left-most part of this region, is very conservative in all three phages. The gene for nucleotide kinase (PP47/PP81 gp18) homologous to the T7 gene 1.7 product is an enzyme distant from all other nucleotide kinases and is able to phosphorylate both dTMP and dGMP independent of divalent cations [61]. This gene was missing in Q19, as was a putative HNH endonuclease (PP47 gp38 and PP81 gp37) located at the end of the middle genome region.

Several small hypothetical proteins were present in PP47/81 and missing in Q19, or vice versa. Putative CCA-nucleotidyltransferases (tRNA nucleotidyltransferases) of PP47 (gp28) and PP81 (gp29) share 99% of amino acid identity, while the Q19 gp24 with the same function has only 48% amino acid identity with CCA-nucleotidyltransferases of PP47/81. These gene products have no direct analogues in type phage T7 and are encoded in a few *Studiervirinae* phages. However, many *Autographiviridae* phages infecting *Pectobacterium*, even attributed to different subfamilies and genera, do have CCA-nucleotidyltransferases in their predicted proteome. This feature is discussed below, as a possible hallmark of Pectobacterial *Autographiviridae*.

The genome comparison map made with TBLASTX comprising *Pectobacterium* phages Q19, PP47 and PP81, and phages Jarilo, *Klebsiella* phage KP32 and *Escherichia* phage T7 as representatives of different genera of *Studiervirinae*, confirms the similarity of the genomes in the regions encoding replication, structural packaging and lysis blocks (Figure 8). Non-homologous parts of the genomes are located mainly in the early gene block, hypothetical proteins of the middle region and tail spike/tail fiber proteins.

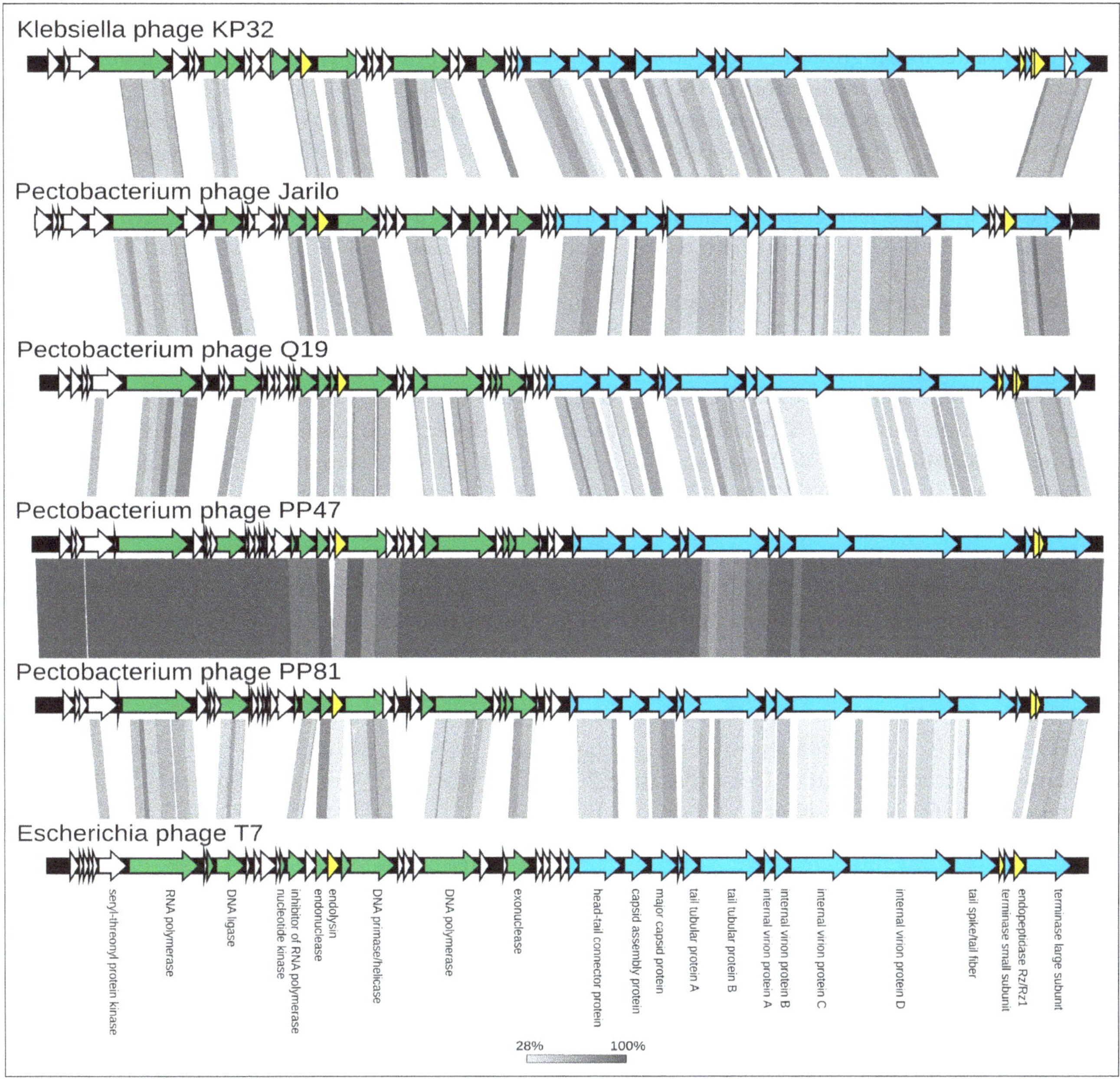

Figure 8. Genome sequence comparison among six *Studiervirinae* viral genomes exhibiting co-linearity detected by TBLASTX. The percentage of sequence similarity is indicated by the intensity of the grey color. Vertical blocks between analyzed sequences indicate regions with at least 28% similarity. Nucleic acid-processing genes are colored green, morphogenesis and packaging genes are colored blue and lysis genes are colored yellow. The most significant differences are observed for tail proteins and a number of hypothetical proteins of early and middle regions.

3.5. Tail Spike Proteins

Bacteriophage tail spike and tail fibre proteins play an important role in the phage, serving as receptor-binding proteins (RBP). Besides the function of receptor recognition, they can participate in binding and degrading lipopolysaccharides or polysaccharide capsules [51,62,63]. Some tail spikes are known to depolymerize surface polysaccharides of the host, while others show no enzymatic activity and others can deacetylate surface polysaccharides leaving the backbone of the polysaccharide intact [43,64]. The composition and structure of these RBPs are related to the host spectrum [51,65].

The bacteriophage *E. coli* T7 tail fibre is a protrusion which is about 16 nm long and 2 nm in diameter, consisting of a homo-trimer of the viral protein gp17. This protein is responsible for initial reversible host cell recognition. The following irreversible interaction with the bacterial membrane is probably mediated by one or more of the tail-tube proteins [66,67]. The tail fibers of phage T7 possess a modular structure and share a conserved N-terminal domain of ~140 residues that anchor the tail fibre to the phage particle. Tail fibre proteins of T7-like phages are examples of a horizontal transfer of the C-terminal receptor-binding (RBP) domain [68]. The tail spike protein of *Enterobacteria* phage K1F, belonging to the *Autographiviridae* family, also possesses a modular structure with a C-terminal chaperone protein mediating homodimerization and proper folding of the catalytic endo-N trimer [69].

Tail spikes of phages PP47, PP81 and Q19, as predicted by HMM-HMM and a BLAST homologs search, contain two identifiable parts. The N-terminal part (residues 1-159 in Q19) is structurally similar to the T7 fibre. The central part (residues 163-589 in Q19) structurally resembles the SGNH hydrolase domain and supposedly possesses deacetylation activity. This SGNH hydrolase domain is structurally similar to the gp63.1 tail spike protein of N4-like phage *Escherichia* phage vB_EcoP_G7C (HHpred Probability: 99.85%; E-value: 5.7×10^{-18}; Score: 210.69), which is responsible for host cell recognition and attachment. G7C gp63.1 deacetylates the O-antigen of *E. coli* 4s lipopolysaccharide [64]. G7C gp63.1 is attached to the phage tail via gp66, which also participates in host cell binding. The homology modelling and structure comparison identifies the presence of the SGNH domain and the structural similarity of the central domains of these three phages' tail spikes. The modelled structures demonstrate the presence of the SGNH hydrolase hallmark of a three-layer alpha/beta/alpha structure, where the β-sheets are composed of five parallel strands and contain catalytic residues Ser, Gly, Asn and His, which are conservative for SGNH hydrolases (shown in Figure S2) [70–72]. Homology recognition server Phyre2 (http://www.sbg.bio.ic.ac.uk/phyre2/) pointed to the structure of SGNH esterase (CEX) from a commensal gut bacterium as being the closest known structure (PBD structure 6hfz, confidence 100% for more than 70% of residues of C-domain) (Figure 9). A biological understanding of the removal of acetyl groups from β-mannan by esterase (CEX) is a key step toward efficient utilisation of this glycan [73].

The BLAST examination using the Genbank phage database indicated closer similarities of TSP from PP47, PP81, MA6, MA1A and PPWS4 to each other, than to other *Studievirinae* phages of *Pectobacterium* hosts. Moreover, the central part of the primary sequences of PP47, PP81 and Q19 tail spikes resemble proteins from *Pectobacterium* phages that are comparatively distant from PP47/PP81 and Q19, and that belong to *Corkvirinae*, *Melnykvirinae* and *Molineuxvirinae*. Interestingly, the tail spikes/fibre protein sequences from some phages, which were closer to *Pektosvirus* and Q19 in evolutionary terms, such as *Pectobacterium* phages Jarilo and DU_PP_II, demonstrated less similarity than those *Pectobacterium* phages belonging to *Corkvirinae*, *Melnykvirinae* and *Molineuxvirinae*. The homology modelling, the comparison of primary and secondary structure, indicated a discontinuous variation in tail spike/fibre proteins in the evolution of *Pectobacterium Autographiviridae* phages (Figure S3).

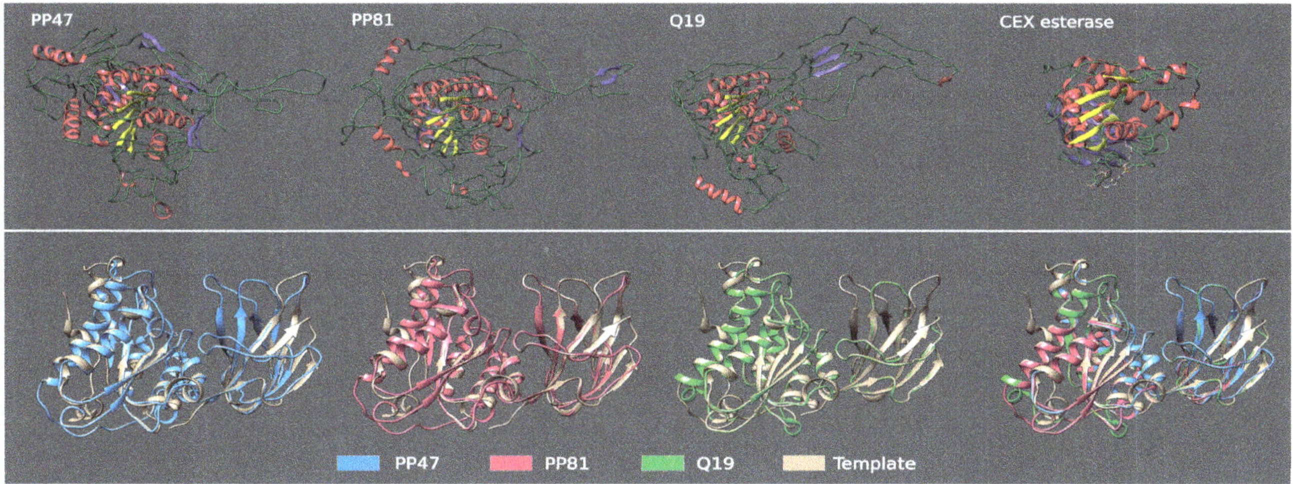

Figure 9. Upper picture: 3D homology modelling of tail spike proteins of *Pectobacterium* phages Q19, PP47 and PP81, and PDB structure of SGNH domain of bacterial esterase (CEX) active on acetylated mannans PDB structure 6hfz. Lower picture: 3D-alignment of modelled Q19, PP47 and PP81 tail spike SGNH domains, with SGNH domain of bacterial esterase (CEX) as a template. In the upper picture, the five parallel β-sheets intrinsic for all SGNH are colored yellow; the other β-sheets are colored blue, α-helices are colored red and coils are colored green.

To understand the nature of the evolution of *Studiervirinae Pectobacterium* phage tail spikes, BLAST searches of protein sequences of N-part and SGNH-like domains obtained from HHpred alignment on nr/nt and Genbank bacterial databases were conducted. The searches revealed homologous sequences in the genomes of several pathogenic *Pectobacterium* strains, including strains of *P. brasiliense* and *P. versatile*, as well as in a number of other bacteria. It has been demonstrated experimentally that *P. brasiliense* and *P. versatile* serve as natural hosts for phages PP47, PP81 and Q19. The phylogenetic trees constructed with these sequences demonstrate the different evolutionary history of the T7-like N-part domain and the G7C-like SGNH domain (Figures 10 and 11), suggesting the possible role of horizontal transfer in the formation of PP47, PP81 and Q19 tail spikes. *Pectobacterium* hosts of the ancestors of the phages could participate in the transfer.

Interestingly, the location of the genes of SGNH-domain proteins, homologous to Q19 and PP47/81 tail spike proteins, in the genomes of phages of other *Autographiviridae* subfamilies is different. The genomes of *Pectobacterium* phages PP1 and POP72 of the *Molineuxvirinae* subfamily contained comparatively short 969 bp tail fibre protein genes at the end of the structural blocks and 1803 bp SGNH-domain proteins at the end of the genomes (Figure 12A). Meanwhile, the position of both tail spike protein (TSP) genes and tail fibre protein (TFP) genes is conserved in the genomes of all *Pectobacterium Studiervirinae* phages, between the genes of internal virion protein D and holin. The genome of *Pectobacterium* phage PP74 [12] includes two genes of TFP. The 100 aa-long C-end segment of the first TFP shares significant homology with the N-part of the second TFP. HMM-HMM analysis demonstrated that TFP1 resembles the first half of T7 TFP, and TFP2 the second half. Tail fibre proteins of *Pectobacterium* phages Jarilo and DU_PP_II also seem to resemble the T7 TFP in terms of structure (HHpred probability 100%). Thus, two typical structures of tail spike/fibre proteins can be distinguished for *Pectobacterium Studiervirinae* phages—T7-like tail fibre proteins for phages Jarilo, DU_PP_II and, possibly, PP74, and tail spike proteins with T7-like N-domain and SGNH-hydrolase containing C-domain for phages Q19, PP47, PP81, PPWS4, MA6 and MA1A.

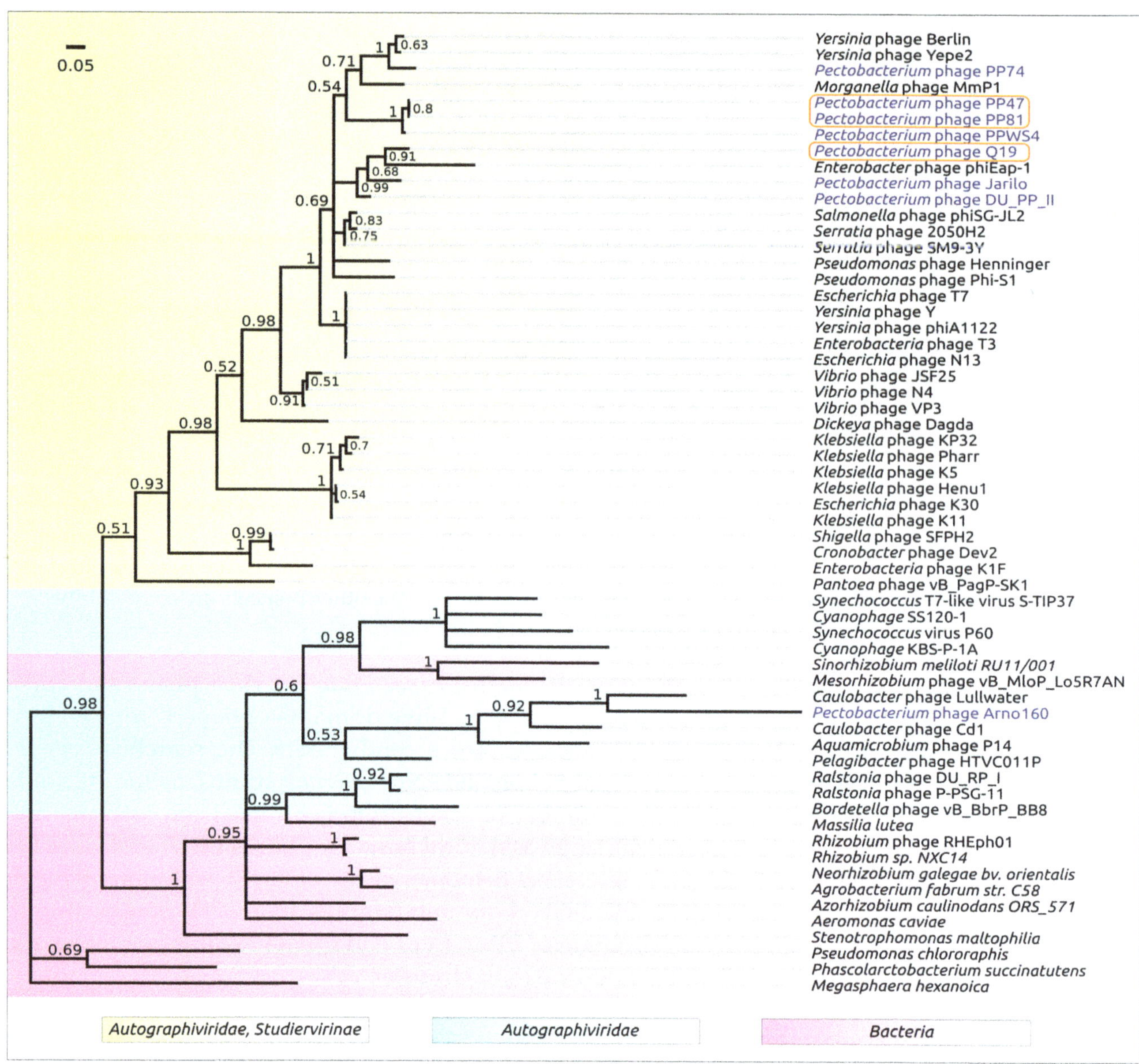

Figure 10. Phylogenetic tree obtained with MrBayes, based on amino acid sequences of the N-domain of tail fibre/tail spike proteins and homologous sequences obtained by a BLAST search of Genbank phage and bacterial databases. Bayesian posterior probabilities are indicated above their branch. The scale bar shows 0.05 estimated substitutions per site and the tree was rooted to *Megasphaera hexanoica*; of 2,000,000 generations, 200 generations were sampled, with an average standard deviation of split frequencies of 0.011.

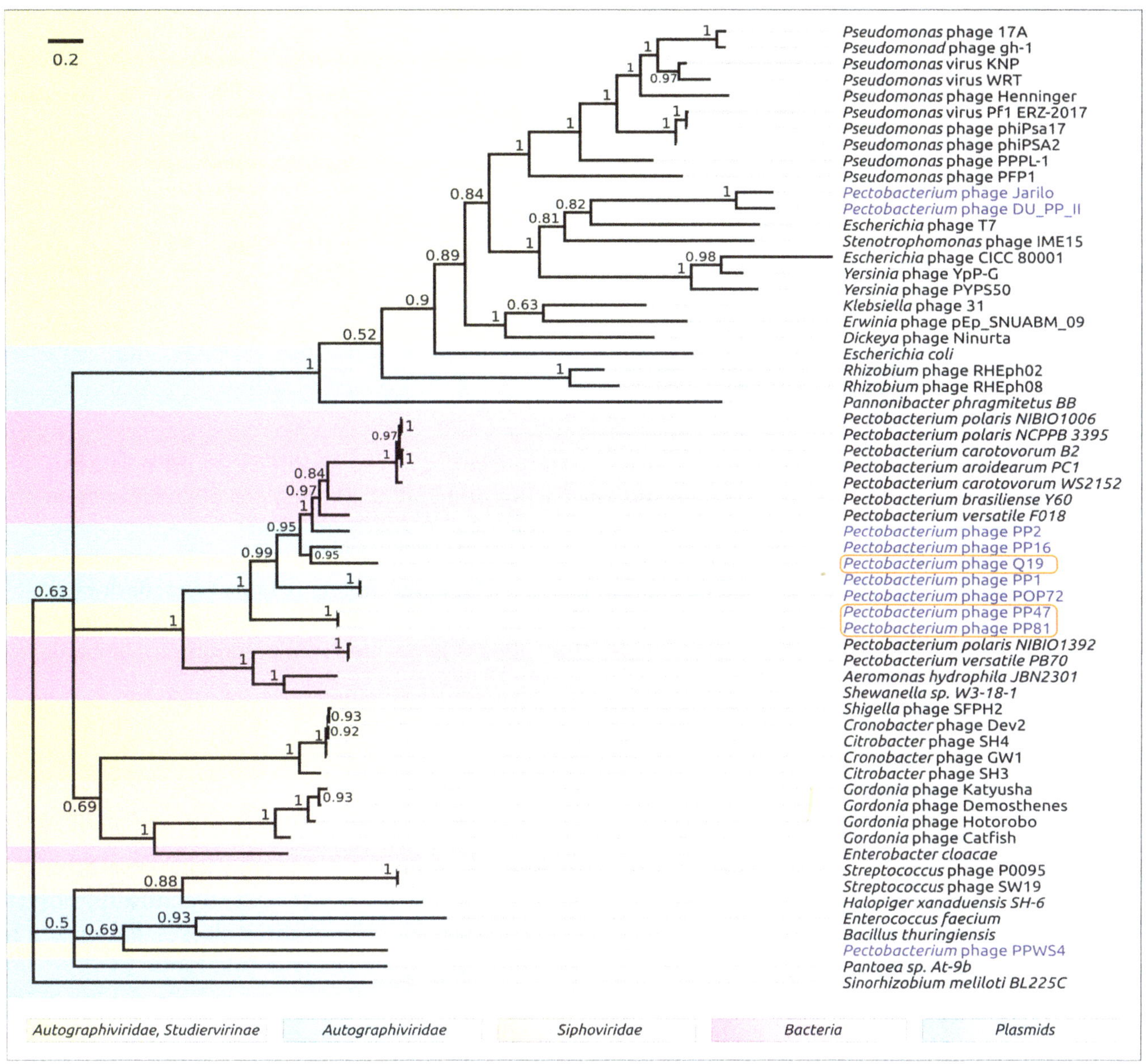

Figure 11. Phylogenetic tree obtained with MrBayes, based on amino acid sequences of the central domain of tail fibre/tail spike proteins and homologous sequences obtained by a BLAST search of Genbank phage and bacterial databases. Bayesian posterior probabilities are indicated above their branch. The scale bar shows 0.2 estimated substitutions per site and the tree was rooted to *Sinorhizobium meliloti BL225C* plasmid; of 2,000,000 generations, 200 generations were sampled, with an average standard deviation of split frequencies of 0.0062.

The SGNH-domain proteins found in *Pectobacterium* bacteria are located within conserved regions, which also include recombination protein RecR and conjugal transfer protein TraB genes possibly involved in the recombination processes (Figure 12B).

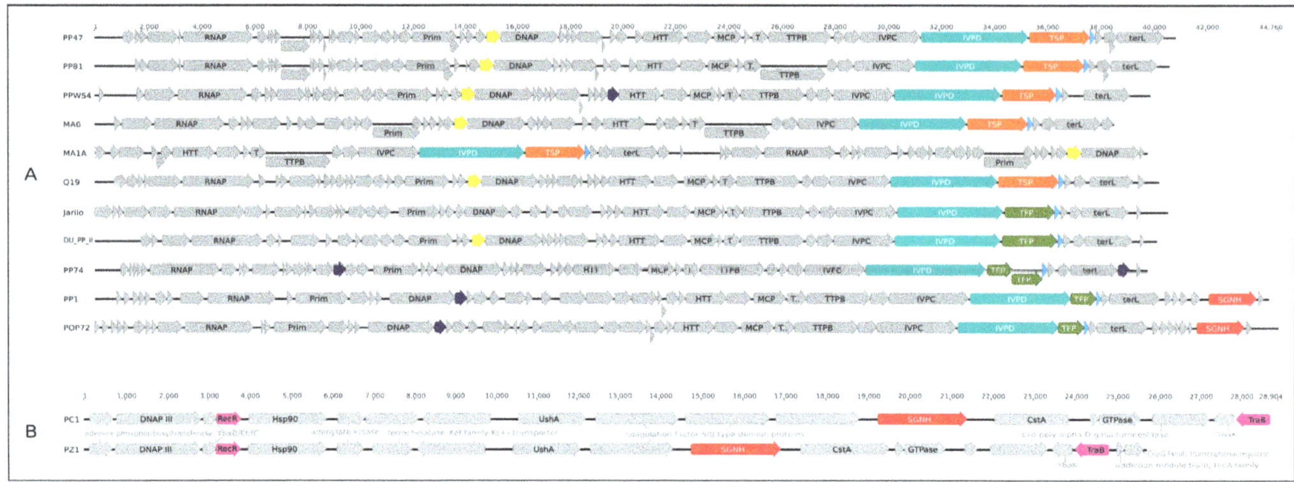

Figure 12. (**A**) Simplified genetic maps of *Pectobacterium Studiervirinae* phages PP47, PP81, PPWS4, MA6, MA1A, Q19, Jarilo, DU_PP_II and PP74, and phages PP1 and POP72. (**B**) Regions of *Pectobacterium aroidearum* PC1 and *Pectobacterium polaris* PZ1 containing the genes of SGNH-domain proteins, homologous to Q19 and PP47/81 tail spike proteins. The colors of different genes are as follows: orange, tail spike protein; green, tail fibre protein; cyan, tail tubular protein B; blue, holin; dark-blue, HNH endonuclease; yellow, nucleotidyltransferase; purple, recombination protein RecR and conjugal transfer protein TraB; grey, other genes. Putative functions of genes are given according to Genbank annotations and BLAST search (Tables S6–S8).

3.6. *tRNA-Nucleotidyltransferase*

tRNA-nucleotidyltransferase (CCA-nucleotidyltransferase) is an ancient enzyme with an unusual mechanism of polymerisation, adding nucleotide triplet CCA to the 3′-end of tRNAs [74]. tRNA-nycleotidyltransferases, together with similar (by primary sequence and structurally) poly(A) polymerases, comprise a single large superfamily and can be divided into three classes, exhibiting no strong homology to one another: archaeal CCA-adding enzymes, bacterial and eukaryotic CCA-adding enzymes and bacterial poly(A) polymerases [75].

Analysis of annotations of Genbank genomes shows that tRNA-nucleotidyltransferase genes have been found in many bacteriophages, including 18 *Studiervirinae* phages, but, as found by BLAST search, the real number of phage genomes containing CCA-nycleotidyltransferase is higher because of a lack of annotation. Remarkably, a significant part of these phages infects *Pectobacterium* and evolutionary related plant pathogenic *Dickeya* species. It was also not possible to identify homologous genes in most of *Studiervirinae* and *Autographiviridae* genomes, nor did the analysis find proteins homologous to Q19, PP47 and PP81 putative tRNA-nycleotidyltransferases among bacteria and organisms of other kingdoms of life. However, HMM-HMM comparison demonstrated the high structural similarity of the models of these enzymes to bacterial and eukaryotic mitochondrial tRNA-nycleotidyltransferases. Interestingly, homologous modelling indicated a structural similarity between tRNA-nycleotidyltransferase from *Pectobacterium* phage PP47 and the tRNA-nycleotidyltransferase domain of a bacterial enzyme from *Pectobacerium aroidearum* PC1, in spite of the lack of any significant primary sequence similarity (Figure 13).

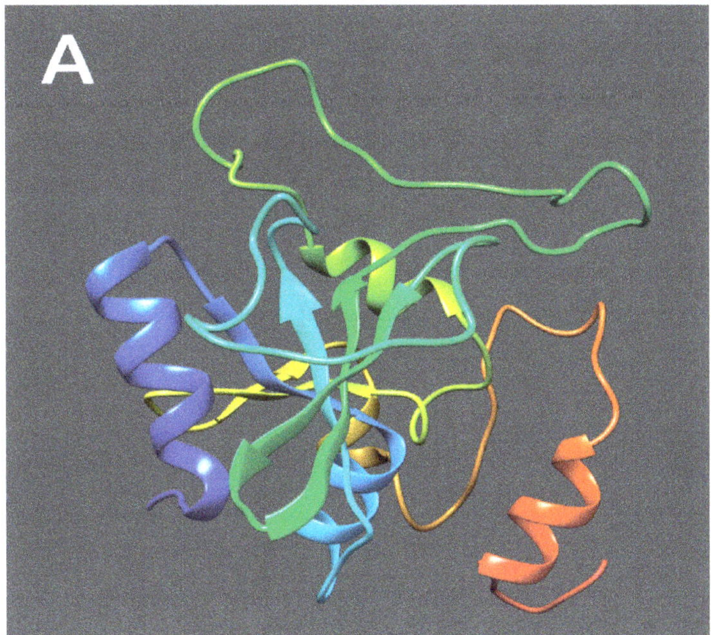

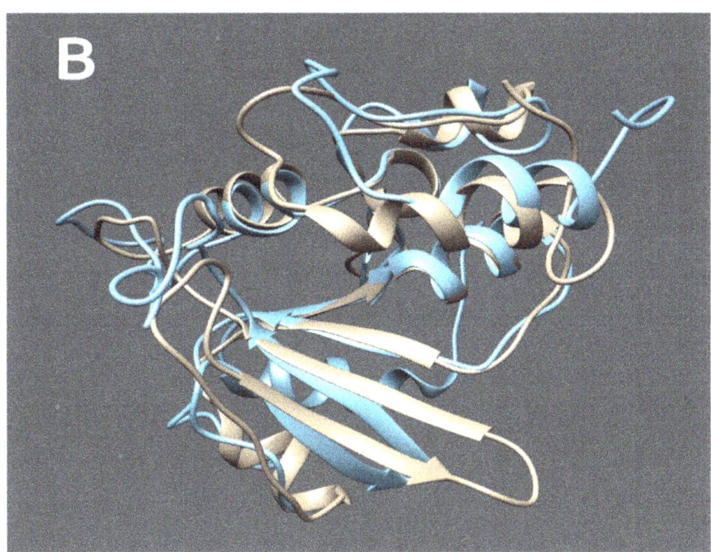

Figure 13. (**A**) 3D structure homology modelling of tRNA-nycleotidyltransferase from *Pectobacterium* phage PP47. The model is colored based on a rainbow gradient scheme, where the N-terminus of the polypeptide chain is colored blue and the C-terminus is colored red. (**B**) 3D-alignment of modelled tRNA-nycleotidyltransferase from *Pectobacterium* phage PP47 (colored blue) and *Pectobacerium aroidearum* PC1 (colored sand).

BLAST examination of Q19, PP47 and PP81 tRNA-nucleotidyltransferases demonstrated the sequence similarity of tRNA-nucleotidyltransferase of *Pectobacterium* phages belonging to various distant *Autographiviridae* taxa. The phylogenetic analysis performed with extracted, annotated and homologous proteins grouped the tRNA-nycleotidyltransferase sequences belonging to Q19, *Pektosvirus* and *Unyawovirus* of the *Studiervirinae* subfamily in one clade with *Corkvirinae*, *Melnykvirinae*, *Molineuxvirinae* and *Slopekvirinae*, and separately from other *Studiervirinae* sequences (Figure 14).

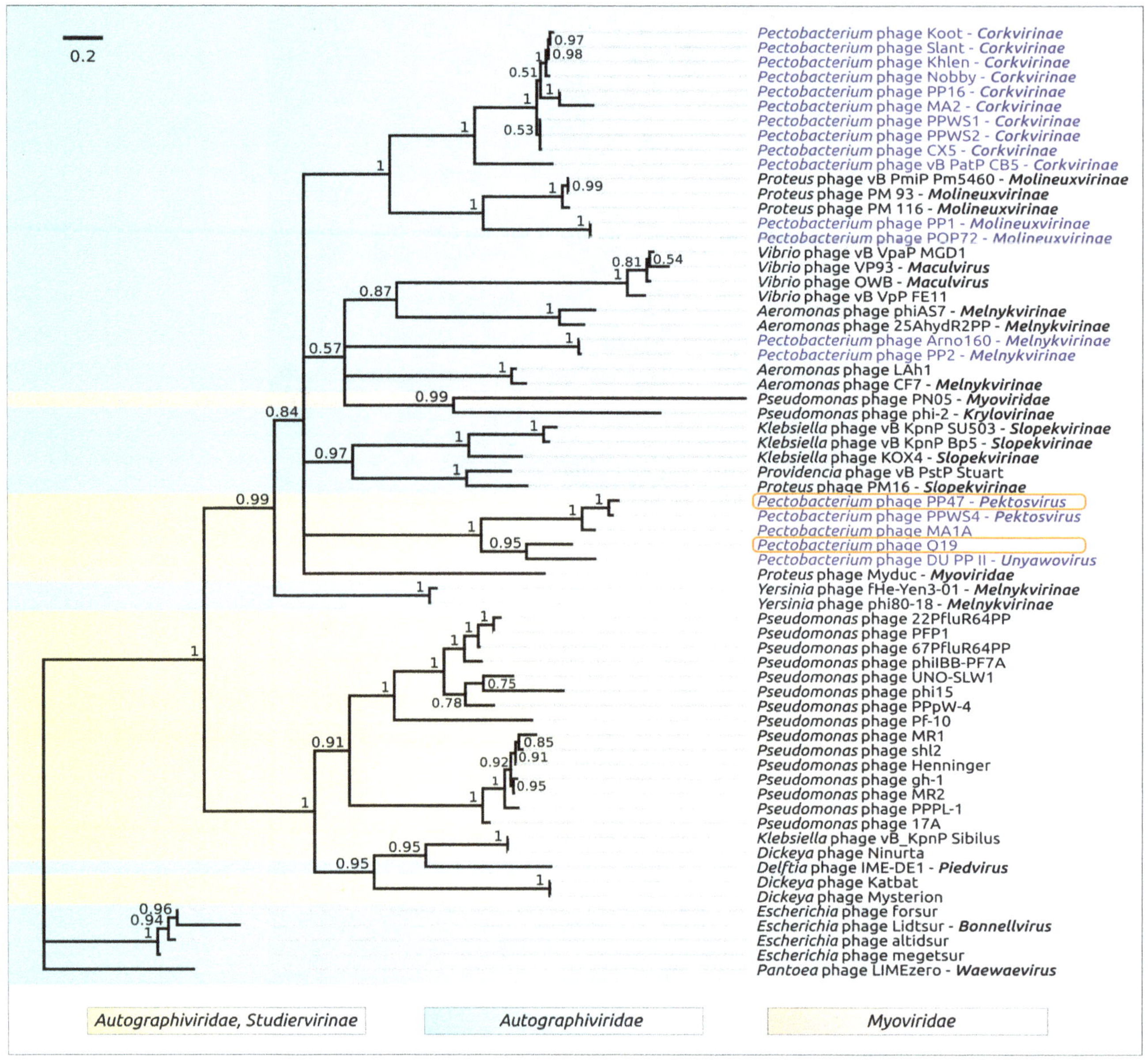

Figure 14. Phylogenetic tree obtained with MrBayes, based on amino acid sequences of tRNA-nucleotidyltransferase and homologous sequences obtained by a BLAST search of Genbank phage databases. Bayesian posterior probabilities are indicated above their branch. The scale bar shows 0.2 estimated substitutions per site and the tree was rooted to *Pantoea* phage LIMEzero; of 2,000,000 generations, every 200 generations were sampled, with an average standard deviation of split frequencies of 0.0071.

4. Discussion

4.1. Origin, Phylogeny and Taxonomy

The whole-genome comparisons, including VIRIDIC and ANI, as well as phylogenetic studies, indicate that *Pectobacterium* bacteriophages of the *Studiervirinae* subfamily have a complex origin, comprising several independent lines of descent. From this point of view, they share a common feature of phages, noted by Hans-Wolfgang Ackermann: "Bacteriophages are polyphyletic, arose repeatedly in different hosts" [76]. At the moment, they include the genera of *Pektosvirus* (line 1), *"Q19-virus"*, *Jarilovirus*, *Unyawovirus* (line 2) and *Pectobacterium* phage PP74 (*Berlinvirus*) (line 3). *"Q19-virus"*, *Jarilovirus* and *Unyawovirus* seem to form a monophyletic group, and *Yersinia* phage vB_YenP_AP10 of the *Apdecimavirus* genus appears to be their closest related classified phage. Phages PP47 and PP81, together with *Pectobacterim* phages PPWS4, MA6 and MA1A, form the genus of *Pektosvirus*. *Escherichia* phage SRT of the *Foetvirus* genus appears to be the closest known relative of *Pektosvirus* phages and shares with them the last common ancestor.

According to ICTV rules, phages PP47 and PP81 seem to be two strains of the same species, since their intergenomic similarity is higher than 95%. MA6 and MA1A *Pektosvirus* phages can be strains of the same species clonal group. Phage PP47 differs from PP81 in terms of proteome composition, although these phages are members of the same clonal group—the PP47 genome contains one more gene-encoding hypothetical protein that may affect the observed course of infection. Actually, PP47 and PP81 do have differences in behaviour, e.g., in infection cycle.

The origin of *Studiervirinae* is related to the early divergence of *Autographiviridae* into two large clades, one of which includes modern *Studiervirinae* phages, cyanophages, *Pelagibacter* phages and other groups, as may concluded from terminase (Figure 6) and proteome (Figure 4 and Figure S1) phylogeny.

4.2. Genome, Adsorption Apparatus and Horizontal Transfer

The genome organization of Q19, PP47, PP81 and other *Pectobacterium Studiervirinae* phages shares many common features with T7, T3 and other related phages, but also has specific variations, including the presence of unique genes at the level of both genera and species, the length and composition of terminal repeats and non-coding sequences, and small variations in GC-content.

While the genome organization and protein composition of *Pectobacterium Studiervirinae* phages have much in common with their phylogenetic relatives, the phages share similarities in a number of proteins with other taxonomically distant *Pectobacterium* phages. Probably, those proteins can be important in terms of specificity to the *Pectobacterium* host. An intriguing example of tRNA-nucleotidyltransferase found in 37 of 46 Pectobacterium phages belonging to different *Autographiviridae* subfamilies, and only in 60 of more than 500 remaining *Autographiviridae* phages, raises questions about the role of this enzyme in phage infection and the possibility to use this finding for practical purposes. The presence of tRNA-nucleotidyltransferase in the bacterial genome was shown to have importance for phage reproduction [77]. tRNA-nucleotidyltransferases participate in various processes in the cell and influence bacterial growth [78,79] and interact with other bacterial proteins [80]. The biological functions, origin and evolution of tRNA-nucleotidyltransferase and other specific genes of *Pectobacterium* phages can be studied in further research.

We suggest that at least some *Pectobacterium* phage specific proteins were acquired by horizontal transfer, which contributes significantly to phage evolution [52,81–84]. Bacteriophages can mediate the processes involved with horizontal transfer in bacteria [82,83,85] and bacteriophage-mediated horizontal transfer can override the mutations [84]. It has been shown that processes such as recombinations in phage genomes [52] and point mutations also drive phage evolution [86]. It would be interesting to study the possible effects of convergent evolution on *Pectobacterium* phage genes.

The adsorption apparatus has a special meaning for host specificity [87–91] and the mechanism of developing such specificity to certain hosts is a matter of fundamental and applied interest. Horizontal transfer of tail fibre (tail spike) protein modules appears to be an important instrument for adaptation to new hosts [68,89]. As has been shown by the homology search, and by the structural and phylogenetic analysis, of the current research, *Pectobacterium* tail spike proteins can be formed with the assistance of horizontal transfer and the involvement of *Pectobacterium* hosts. Further research into various aspects of the evolution of adsorption apparatus can facilitate phage therapy.

5. Conclusions

Pectobacterium bacteriophages of the *Studiervirinae* subfamily have a complex origin. There are three independently evolved lines that can be distinguished. One of monophyletic group includes *Pectobacterium* phages Q19, phage Jarilo of the *Jarilovirus* genus and DU_PP_II of the *Unyawovirus* genus. Another group comprises *Pectobacterium* phages PP81, PP47, PPWS4, M6A and MA1A of the

Pektosvirus genus and the third group is represented by *Pectobacterium* phage PP74 of the *Berlinvirus* genus. Phage Q19 represents a new genus not previously described. Phages PP47 and PP81, as well as phages M6A and MA1A, seem to represent clonal groups. Phages Q19, PP47 and PP81 infect a broad spectrum of related *Pectobacterium* hosts and possess a similar tail spike protein, which could be the consequence of exchange with other phages infecting *Pectobacterium* hosts with participation of bacterial hosts. Horizontal transfer can be the reason for the similarity of a number of genes of taxonomically distant *Pectobacterium* phages. Studying the processes of genome formation and, in particular, the adsorption apparatus can assist the search for, and design of, new phages for effective phage therapy.

Supplementary Materials:
Figure S1: Proteomic tree of 447 *Podovoridae* and *Autographiviridae* phage genomes constructed using ViPTree. Figure S2: Alignment of secondary structures of phage tail spike proteins and SGNH-hydrolase made with UCSF Chimera, and possible active centre and conserved residues (circled with red) found by comparison with published structures. Figure S3: 3D structures of tail spike and tail fibre proteins of *Pectobacterium* phages Q19, Jarilo, DU_PP_II, PP47, PP81 and PPWS4 obtained by homology modelling and MAFFT alignment of primary sequences of tail spike and tail fibre proteins, and distance matrix for the proteins. Jarilo and DU_PP_II are suggested to be the closest relatives of Q19, and phages PP47, PP81 and PPWS4 are the members of the *Pektosvirus* genus. The models are colored based on a rainbow gradient scheme, where the N-terminus of the polypeptide chain is coloured blue and the C-terminus is colored red. Table S1: Infectious range of *Pectobacterium* phages PP47, PP81 and Q19. Table S2: Average nucleotide identity (ANI) between *Pectobacterium* phage PP47 and all *Autographiviridae* phage genomes deposited in the NCBI GenBank (threshold 0.5). Table S3: Average nucleotide identity (ANI) between and all *Autographiviridae* phage genomes deposited in the NCBI GenBank (threshold 0.5). Table S4: Average nucleotide identity (ANI) between *Pectobacterium* phage Q19 and all *Autographiviridae* phage genomes deposited in the NCBI GenBank (threshold 0.5). Table S5: The results of the BLAST examination of Q19 and PP47 gene products using the Genbank phage database (Bit-score > 40). Table S6: Functional assignments of *Pectobacterium* phage PP47 genes. Table S7: Functional assignments of *Pectobacterium* phage PP81 genes. Table S8: Functional assignments of *Pectobacterium* phage Q19 genes.

Author Contributions: Conceptualization, P.V.E., A.N.I. and K.A.M.; methodology, P.V.E., A.A.L., M.M.S. and E.E.K.; validation, M.M.S., A.A.L., K.K.M. and K.A.M.; formal analysis, P.V.E., A.A.L., M.M.S. and K.A.M.; investigation, P.V.E., A.A.L., A.A.K., M.M.S., E.N.B., E.E.K., A.P.K. and S.V.T.; resources, A.N.I. and K.A.M.; data curation, P.V.E., A.A.L. and K.K.M.; writing—original draft preparation, P.V.E., A.A.L. and K.A.M.; writing—review and editing, A.N.I. and K.A.M.; visualization, P.V.E., A.A.L. and K.K.M.; supervision, K.A.M.; project administration, K.A.M.; funding acquisition, K.A.M. All authors have read and agreed to the published version of the manuscript.

References

1. Czajkowski, R.; Pérombelon, M.C.M.; Van Veen, J.A.; Van der Wolf, J.M. Control of blackleg and tuber soft rot of potato caused by Pectobacterium and Dickeya species: A review. *Plant. Pathol.* **2011**, *60*, 999–1013. [CrossRef]
2. Pérombelon, M.C.M. Potato diseases caused by soft rot erwinias: An overview of pathogenesis. *Plant. Pathol.* **2002**, *51*, 1–12.
3. Ma, B.; Hibbing, M.E.; Kim, H.-S.; Reedy, R.M.; Yedidia, I.; Breuer, J.J.; Breuer, J.J.; Glasner, J.D.; Perna, N.T.; Kelman, A.; et al. Host range and molecular phylogenies of the soft rot enterobacterial genera pectobacterium and dickeya. *Phytopathology* **2007**, *97*, 1150–1163. [CrossRef] [PubMed]
4. Motyka, A.; Zoledowska, S.; Sledz, W.; Lojkowska, E. Molecular methods as tools to control plant diseases caused by Dickeya and Pectobacterium spp: A minireview. *New Biotechnol.* **2017**, *39*, 181–189. [CrossRef] [PubMed]
5. Svircev, A.; Roach, D.; Castle, A. Framing the future with bacteriophages in agriculture. *Viruses* **2018**, 218. [CrossRef] [PubMed]
6. Sillankorva, S.M.; Oliveira, H.; Azeredo, J. Bacteriophages and their role in food safety. *Int. J. Microbiol.* **2012**, *2012*, 863945. [CrossRef] [PubMed]

7. Zaczek, M.; Weber-Dabrowska, B.; Górski, A. Phages in the global fruit and vegetable industry. *J. Appl. Microbiol.* **2015**, *118*, 537–556. [CrossRef] [PubMed]
8. Buttimer, C.; McAuliffe, O.; Ross, R.P.; Hill, C.; O'Mahony, J.; Coffey, A. Bacteriophages and Bacterial Plant Diseases. *Front. Microbiol.* **2017**, *8*, 34. [CrossRef] [PubMed]
9. Czajkowski, R.; Ozymko, Z.; Lojkowska, E. Isolation and characterization of novel soilborne lytic bacteriophages infecting Dickeya spp. biovar 3 ('D. solani'). *Plant. Pathol.* **2014**, *63*, 758–772. [CrossRef]
10. Carstens, A.B.; Djurhuus, A.M.; Kot, W.; Hansen, L.H. A novel six-phage cocktail reduces Pectobacterium atrosepticum soft rot infection in potato tubers under simulated storage conditions. *FEMS Microbiol. Lett.* **2019**, *366*, i97–i104. [CrossRef]
11. Adriaenssens, E.M.; van Vaerenbergh, J.; Vandenheuvel, D.; Dunon, V.; Ceyssens, P.J.; de Proft, M.; Kropinski, A.M.; Noben, J.P.; Maes, M.; Lavigne, R. T4-related bacteriophage LIMEstone isolates for the control of soft rot on potato caused by "Dickeya solani". *PLoS ONE* **2012**, *7*, e33227. [CrossRef] [PubMed]
12. Voronina, M.V.; Bugaeva, E.N.; Vasiliev, D.N.; Kabanova, A.P.; Barannik, A.P.; Shneider, M.M.; Kulikov, E.E.; Korzhenkov, A.A.; Toschakov, S.V.; Ignatov, A.N.; et al. Characterization of Pectobacterium carotovorum subsp. carotovorum Bacteriophage PP16 Prospective for Biocontrol of Potato Soft Rot. *Mikrobiologiia* **2019**, *13*, 458–469. [CrossRef]
13. Hyman, P.; Abedon, S.T. Bacteriophage host range and bacterial resistance. *Adv. Appl. Microbiol.* **2010**, *70*, 217–248. [CrossRef] [PubMed]
14. Chan, B.K.; Abedon, S.T.; Loc-Carrillo, C. Phage cocktails and the future of phage therapy. *Future Microbiol.* **2013**, *8*, 769–783. [CrossRef]
15. Adeolu, M.; Alnajar, S.; Naushad, S.; Gupta, R.S. Genome-based phylogeny and taxonomy of the 'Enterobacteriales': Proposal for enterobacterales ord. nov. divided into the families Enterobacteriaceae, Erwiniaceae fam. nov., Pectobacteriaceae fam. nov., Yersiniaceae fam. nov., Hafniaceae fam. nov., Morgane. *Int. J. Syst. Evol. Microbiol.* **2016**, *66*, 5575–5599. [CrossRef]
16. Zhang, Y.; Fan, Q.; Loria, R. A re-evaluation of the taxonomy of phytopathogenic genera Dickeya and Pectobacterium using whole-genome sequencing data. *Syst. Appl. Microbiol.* **2016**, *39*, 252–259. [CrossRef]
17. Adriaenssens, E.M.; Sullivan, M.B.; Knezevic, P.; van Zyl, L.J.; Sarkar, B.L.; Dutilh, B.E.; Alfenas-Zerbini, P.; Łobocka, M.; Tong, Y.; Brister, J.R.; et al. Taxonomy of prokaryotic viruses: 2018-2019 update from the ICTV Bacterial and Archaeal Viruses Subcommittee. *Arch. Virol.* **2020**. [CrossRef]
18. Walker, P.J.; Siddell, S.G.; Lefkowitz, E.J.; Mushegian, A.R.; Adriaenssens, E.M.; Dempsey, D.M.; Dutilh, B.E.; Harrach, B.; Harrison, R.L.; Hendrickson, R.C.; et al. Changes to virus taxonomy and the Statutes ratified by the International Committee on Taxonomy of Viruses (2020). *Arch. Virol.* **2020**. [CrossRef] [PubMed]
19. Clokie, M.R.J.; Kropinski, A.M. *Bacteriophages: Methods and Protocols Volume 1: Isolation, Characterization, and Interactions*; Humana Press: Leicester, UK, 2009; ISBN 9781588296825.
20. Hyatt, D.; Chen, G.-L.; Locascio, P.F.; Land, M.L.; Larimer, F.W.; Hauser, L.J. Prodigal: Prokaryotic gene recognition and translation initiation site identification. *BMC Bioinform.* **2010**, *11*, 119. [CrossRef] [PubMed]
21. Seemann, T. Prokka: Rapid prokaryotic genome annotation. *Bioinform.* **2014**, *30*, 2068–2069. [CrossRef]
22. Schattner, P.; Brooks, A.N.; Lowe, T.M. The tRNAscan-SE, snoscan and snoGPS web servers for the detection of tRNAs and snoRNAs. *Nucleic Acids Res.* **2005**, *33*. [CrossRef]
23. Laslett, D.; Canback, B. ARAGORN, a program to detect tRNA genes and tmRNA genes in nucleotide sequences. *Nucleic Acids Res.* **2004**, *32*, 11–16. [CrossRef]
24. Sampaio, M.; Rocha, M.; Oliveira, H.; DIas, O.; Valencia, A. Predicting promoters in phage genomes using PhagePromoter. *Bioinformatics* **2019**, *35*, 5301–5302. [CrossRef] [PubMed]
25. Delcher, A.L.; Harmon, D.; Kasif, S.; White, O.; Salzberg, S.L. Improved microbial gene identification with GLIMMER. *Nucleic Acids Res.* **1999**, *27*, 4636–4641. [CrossRef]
26. Katoh, K.; Misawa, K.; Kuma, K.K.; Miyata, T. MAFFT: A novel method for rapid multiple sequence alignment based on fast Fourier transform. *Nucleic Acids Res.* **2002**, *30*, 3059–3066. [CrossRef]
27. Rappas, M.; Bose, D.; Zhang, X. Bacterial enhancer-binding proteins: Unlocking σ54-dependent gene transcription. *Curr. Opin. Struct. Biol.* **2007**, *17*, 110–116. [CrossRef] [PubMed]
28. Kumar, S.; Tamura, K.; Nei, M. MEGA: Molecular Evolutionary Genetics Analysis software for microcomputers. *Bioinformatics* **1994**, *10*, 189–191. [CrossRef] [PubMed]

29. Stamatakis, A. RAxML version 8: A tool for phylogenetic analysis and post-analysis of large phylogenies. *Bioinformatics* **2014**, *30*, 1312–1313. [CrossRef] [PubMed]
30. Huelsenbeck, J.P.; Ronquist, F. MRBAYES: Bayesian inference of phylogenetic trees. *Bioinformatics* **2001**, *17*, 754–755. [CrossRef]
31. Ronquist, F.; Huelsenbeck, J.P. MrBayes 3: Bayesian phylogenetic inference under mixed models. *Bioinformatics* **2003**, *19*, 1572–1574. [CrossRef] [PubMed]
32. Lee, I.; Kim, Y.O.; Park, S.C.; Chun, J. OrthoANI: An improved algorithm and software for calculating average nucleotide identity. *Int. J. Syst. Evol. Microbiol.* **2016**, *66*, 1100–1103. [CrossRef] [PubMed]
33. Chaudhari, N.M.; Gupta, V.K.; Dutta, C. BPGA-an ultra-fast pan-genome analysis pipeline. *Sci. Rep.* **2016**, *6*, 24373. [CrossRef]
34. Moraru, C.; Varsani, A.; Kropinski, A.M. VIRIDIC-a novel tool to calculate the intergenomic 1 similarities of prokaryote-infecting viruses 2. *bioRxiv* **2020**. [CrossRef]
35. Kelley, L.A.; Mezulis, S.; Yates, C.M.; Wass, M.N.; Sternberg, M.J.E. The Phyre2 web portal for protein modeling, prediction and analysis. *Nat. Protoc.* **2015**, *10*, 845–858. [CrossRef] [PubMed]
36. Goddard, T.D.; Huang, C.C.; Meng, E.C.; Pettersen, E.F.; Couch, G.S.; Morris, J.H.; Ferrin, T.E. UCSF ChimeraX: Meeting modern challenges in visualization and analysis. *Protein Sci.* **2018**, *27*, 14–25. [CrossRef]
37. Duarte, V.; De Boer, S.H.; Ward, L.J.; De Oliveira, A.M.R. Characterization of atypical Erwinia carotovora strains causing blackleg of potato in Brazil. *J. Appl. Microbiol.* **2004**, *96*, 535–545. [CrossRef]
38. Portier, P.; Pédron, J.; Taghouti, G.; Fischer-Le Saux, M.; Caullireau, E.; Bertrand, C.; Laurent, A.; Chawki, K.; Oulgazi, S.; Moumni, M.; et al. Elevation of Pectobacterium carotovorum subsp. odoriferum to species level as Pectobacterium odoriferum sp. nov., proposal of Pectobacterium brasiliense sp. nov. and Pectobacterium actinidiae sp. nov., emended description of Pectobacterium carotovorum and description of Pectobacterium versatile sp. nov., isolated from streams and symptoms on diverse plants. *Int. J. Syst. Evol. Microbiol.* **2019**, *69*, 3207–3216. [CrossRef]
39. Voronina, M.V.; Kabanova, A.P.; Shneider, M.M.; Korzhenkov, A.A.; Toschakov, S.V.; Miroshnikov, K.K.; Miroshnikov, K.A.; Ignatov, A.N. First Report of *Pectobacterium carotovorum* subsp. *brasiliense* Causing Blackleg and Stem Rot Disease of Potato in Russia. *Plant. Dis.* **2019**, *103*, 364. [CrossRef]
40. Malko, A.; Frantsuzov, P.; Nikitin, M.; Statsyuk, N.; Dzhavakhiya, V.; Golikov, A.; Malko, A.; Frantsuzov, P.; Nikitin, M.; Statsyuk, N.; et al. Potato Pathogens in Russia's Regions: An Instrumental Survey with the Use of Real-Time PCR/RT-PCR in Matrix Format. *Pathogens* **2019**, *8*, 18. [CrossRef]
41. Lee, D.H.; Kim, J.B.; Lim, J.A.; Han, S.W.; Heu, S. Genetic diversity of Pectobacterium carotovorum subsp. brasiliensis isolated in Korea. *Plant. Pathol. J.* **2014**, *30*, 117–124. [CrossRef] [PubMed]
42. Li, X.; Ma, Y.; Liang, S.; Tian, Y.; Yin, S.; Xie, S.; Xie, H. Comparative genomics of 84 Pectobacterium genomes reveals the variations related to a pathogenic lifestyle. *BMC Genom.* **2018**, *19*, 889. [CrossRef]
43. Lukianova, A.A.; Shneider, M.M.; Evseev, P.V.; Shpirt, A.M.; Bugaeva, E.N.; Kabanova, A.P.; Obraztsova, E.A.; Miroshnikov, K.K.; Senchenkova, S.N.; Shashkov, A.S.; et al. Morphologically Different Pectobacterium brasiliense Bacteriophages PP99 and PP101: Deacetylation of O-Polysaccharide by the Tail Spike Protein of Phage PP99 Accompanies the Infection. *Front. Microbiol.* **2020**, *10*, 3147. [CrossRef] [PubMed]
44. Miedzybrodzki, R.; Borysowski, J.; Weber-Dabrowska, B.; Fortuna, W.; Letkiewicz, S.; Szufnarowski, K.; Pawełczyk, Z.; Rogóz, P.; Kłak, M.; Wojtasik, E.; et al. Clinical Aspects of Phage Therapy. *Adv. Virus Res.* **2012**, *83*, 73–121. [CrossRef]
45. Lavigne, R.; Seto, D.; Mahadevan, P.; Ackermann, H.W.; Kropinski, A.M. Unifying classical and molecular taxonomic classification: Analysis of the Podoviridae using BLASTP-based tools. *Res. Microbiol.* **2008**, *159*, 406–414. [CrossRef]
46. Lawrence, J.G.; Hatfull, G.F.; Hendrix, R.W. Imbroglios of viral taxonomy: Genetic exchange and failings of phenetic approaches. *J. Bacteriol.* **2002**, *184*, 4891–4905. [CrossRef]
47. Hillyar, C.R.T. Genetic recombination in bacteriophage lambda. *Biosci. Horiz.* **2012**, *5*. [CrossRef]
48. Dragos, A.; B, P.; Hasan, Z.; Lenz-Strube, M.; Kempen, P.J.; Maroti, G.; Kaspar, C.; Bischofs, I.B.; Kovacs, A.T. Phage recombination drives evolution of spore-forming Bacilli. *bioRxiv* **2020**. [CrossRef]
49. Susskind, M.M.; Botstein, D. Molecular genetics of bacteriophage P22. *Microbiol. Rev.* **1978**, *42*, 385–413. [CrossRef]

50. Casjens, S.R.; Thuman-Commike, P.A. Evolution of mosaically related tailed bacteriophage genomes seen through the lens of phage P22 virion assembly. *Virology* **2011**, *411*, 393–415. [CrossRef]
51. Latka, A.; Maciejewska, B.; Majkowska-Skrobek, G.; Briers, Y.; Drulis-Kawa, Z. Bacteriophage-encoded virion-associated enzymes to overcome the carbohydrate barriers during the infection process. *Appl. Microbiol. Biotechnol.* **2017**, *101*, 3103–3119. [CrossRef] [PubMed]
52. Cuevas, J.M.; Duffy, S.; Sanjuán, R. Point mutation rate of bacteriophage ΦX174. *Genetics* **2009**, *183*, 747–749. [CrossRef] [PubMed]
53. Smith, K.C.; Castro-Nallar, E.; Fisher, J.N.B.; Breakwell, D.P.; Grose, J.H.; Burnett, S.H. Phage cluster relationships identified through single gene analysis. *BMC Genom.* **2013**, *14*, 410. [CrossRef] [PubMed]
54. Zhao, Y.; Qin, F.; Zhang, R.; Giovannoni, S.J.; Zhang, Z.; Sun, J.; Du, S.; Rensing, C. Pelagiphages in the Podoviridae family integrate into host genomes. *Environ. Microbiol.* **2019**, *21*, 1989–2001. [CrossRef]
55. Labrie, S.J.; Frois-Moniz, K.; Osburne, M.S.; Kelly, L.; Roggensack, S.E.; Sullivan, M.B.; Gearin, G.; Zeng, Q.; Fitzgerald, M.; Henn, M.R.; et al. Genomes of marine cyanopodoviruses reveal multiple origins of diversity. *Environ. Microbiol.* **2013**, *15*, 1356–1376. [CrossRef]
56. Huang, S.; Zhang, S.; Jiao, N.; Chen, F. Comparative genomic and phylogenomic analyses reveal a conserved core genome shared by estuarine and oceanic cyanopodoviruses. *PLoS ONE* **2015**, *10*, e0142962. [CrossRef] [PubMed]
57. Mizuno, C.M.; Rodriguez-Valera, F.; Kimes, N.E.; Ghai, R. Expanding the Marine Virosphere Using Metagenomics. *PLoS Genet.* **2013**, *9*, e1003987. [CrossRef] [PubMed]
58. Chen, Z.; Schneider, T.D. Information theory based T7-like promoter models: Classification of bacteriophages and differential evolution of promoters and their polymerases. *Nucleic Acids Res.* **2005**, *33*, 6172–6187. [CrossRef]
59. Roucourt, B.; Lavigne, R. The role of interactions between phage and bacterial proteins within the infected cell: A diverse and puzzling interactome. *Environ. Microbiol.* **2009**, *11*, 2789–2805. [CrossRef] [PubMed]
60. Kiro, R.; Molshanski-Mor, S.; Yosef, I.; Milam, S.L.; Erickson, H.P.; Qimron, U. Gene product 0.4 increases bacteriophage T7 competitiveness by inhibiting host cell division. *Proc. Natl. Acad. Sci. USA* **2013**, *110*, 19549–19554. [CrossRef]
61. Tran, N.Q.; Tabor, S.; Amarasiriwardena, C.J.; Kulczyk, A.W.; Richardson, C.C. Characterization of a nucleotide kinase encoded by bacteriophage T7. *J. Biol. Chem.* **2012**, *287*, 29468–29478. [CrossRef]
62. Cuervo, A.; Pulido-Cid, M.; Chagoyen, M.; Arranz, R.; González-García, V.A.; Garcia-Doval, C.; Castón, J.R.; Valpuesta, J.M.; van Raaij, M.J.; Martín-Benito, J.; et al. Structural Characterization of the Bacteriophage T7 Tail Machinery. *J. Biol. Chem.* **2013**, *288*, 26290–26299. [CrossRef] [PubMed]
63. Holtzman, T.; Globus, R.; Molshanski-Mor, S.; Ben-Shem, A.; Yosef, I.; Qimron, U. A continuous evolution system for contracting the host range of bacteriophage T7. *Sci. Rep.* **2020**. [CrossRef] [PubMed]
64. Prokhorov, N.S.; Riccio, C.; Zdorovenko, E.L.; Shneider, M.M.; Browning, C.; Knirel, Y.A.; Leiman, P.G.; Letarov, A.V. Function of bacteriophage G7C esterase tailspike in host cell adsorption. *Mol. Microbiol.* **2017**, *105*, 385–398. [CrossRef] [PubMed]
65. Bradley, P.; Cowen, L.; Menke, M.; King, J.; Berger, B. BETAWRAP: Successful prediction of parallel β-helices from primary sequence reveals an association with many microbial pathogens. *Proc. Natl. Acad. Sci. USA* **2001**, *98*, 14819–14824. [CrossRef]
66. Steven, A.C.; Trus, B.L.; Maizel, J.V.; Unser, M.; Parry, D.A.D.; Wall, J.S.; Hainfeld, J.F.; Studier, F.W. Molecular substructure of a viral receptor-recognition protein. The gp17 tail-fiber of bacteriophage T7. *J. Mol. Biol.* **1988**, *200*, 351–365. [CrossRef]
67. Garcia-Doval, C.; Van Raaij, M.J. Structure of the receptor-binding carboxy-terminal domain of bacteriophage T7 tail fibers. *Proc. Natl. Acad. Sci. USA* **2012**, *109*, 9390–9395. [CrossRef]
68. Latka, A.; Leiman, P.G.; Drulis-Kawa, Z.; Briers, Y. Modeling the Architecture of Depolymerase-Containing Receptor Binding Proteins in Klebsiella Phages. *Front. Microbiol.* **2019**, *10*, 2649. [CrossRef]
69. Hallenbeck, P.C.; Vimr, E.R.; Yu, F.; Bassler, B.; Troy, F.A. Purification and properties of a bacteriophage-induced endo-N-acetylneuraminidase specific for poly-alpha-2,8-sialosyl carbohydrate units. *J. Biol. Chem.* **1987**, *262*, 3553–3561.

70. Mølgaard, A.; Kauppinen, S.; Larsen, S. Rhamnogalacturonan acetylesterase elucidates the structure and function of a new family of hydrolases. *Structure* **2000**, *8*, 373–383. [CrossRef]
71. Akoh, C.C.; Lee, G.C.; Liaw, Y.C.; Huang, T.H.; Shaw, J.F. GDSL family of serine esterases/lipases. *Prog. Lipid Res.* **2004**, *43*, 534–552. [CrossRef]
72. Wei, Y.; Schottel, J.L.; Derewenda, U.; Swenson, L.; Patkar, S.; Derewenda, Z.S. A novel variant of the catalytic triad in the streptomyces scabies esterase. *Nat. Struct. Biol.* **1995**, *2*, 218–223. [CrossRef] [PubMed]
73. Michalak, L.; La Rosa, S.L.; Leivers, S.; Lindstad, L.J.; Røhr, Å.K.; Aachmann, F.L.; Westereng, B. A pair of esterases from a commensal gut bacterium remove acetylations from all positions on complex β-mannans. *Proc. Natl. Acad. Sci. USA* **2020**, *117*, 7122–7130. [CrossRef] [PubMed]
74. Mörl, M.; Betat, H.; Rammelt, C. TRNA nucleotidyltransferases: Ancient catalysts with an unusual mechanism of polymerization. *Cell. Mol. Life Sci.* **2010**, *67*, 1447–1463.
75. Yue, D.; Maizels, N.; Weiner, A.M. CCA-adding enzymes and poly(A) polymerases are all members of the same nucleotidyltransferase superfamily: Characterization of the CCA-adding enzyme from the archaeal hyperthermophile Sulfolobus shibatae. *RNA* **1996**, *2*, 895–908. [PubMed]
76. Ackermann, H.W. Bacteriophage observations and evolution. *Res. Microbiol.* **2003**, *154*, 245–251. [CrossRef]
77. Morse, J.W.; Deutscher, M.P. A physiological role for tRNA nucleotidyltransferase during bacteriophage infection. *Biochem. Biophys. Res. Commun.* **1976**, *73*, 953–959. [CrossRef]
78. Wellner, K.; Pöhler, M.T.; Betat, H.; Mörl, M. Dual expression of CCA-adding enzyme and RNase T in Escherichia coli generates a distinct cca growth phenotype with diverse applications. *Nucleic Acids Res.* **2019**, *47*, 3631–3639. [CrossRef]
79. Whiteley, A.T.; Eaglesham, J.B.; de Oliveira Mann, C.C.; Morehouse, B.R.; Lowey, B.; Nieminen, E.A.; Danilchanka, O.; King, D.S.; Lee, A.S.Y.; Mekalanos, J.J.; et al. Bacterial cGAS-like enzymes synthesize diverse nucleotide signals. *Nature* **2019**, *567*, 194–199. [CrossRef]
80. Ye, Q.; Lau, R.K.; Mathews, I.T.; Birkholz, E.A.; Watrous, J.D.; Azimi, C.S.; Pogliano, J.; Jain, M.; Corbett, K.D. HORMA Domain Proteins and a Trip13-like ATPase Regulate Bacterial cGAS-like Enzymes to Mediate Bacteriophage Immunity. *Mol. Cell* **2020**, *77*, 709–722. [CrossRef]
81. Proux, C.; Van Sinderen, D.; Suarez, J.; Garcia, P.; Ladero, V.; Fitzgerald, G.F.; Desiere, F.; Brüssow, H. The dilemma of phage taxonomy illustrated by comparative genomics of Sfi21-like Siphoviridae in lactic acid bacteria. *J. Bacteriol.* **2002**, *184*, 6026–6036. [CrossRef]
82. Villa, T.G.; Feijoo-Siota, L.; Rama, J.R.; Sánchez-Pérez, A.; Viñas, M. Horizontal Gene Transfer Between Bacteriophages and Bacteria: Antibiotic Resistances and Toxin Production. In *Horizontal Gene Transfer*; Springer International Publishing: Cham, Switzerland, 2019; pp. 97–142.
83. Wang, G.H.; Sun, B.F.; Xiong, T.L.; Wang, Y.K.; Murfin, K.E.; Xiao, J.H.; Da Huang, W. Bacteriophage WO can mediate horizontal gene transfer in endosymbiotic Wolbachia genomes. *Front. Microbiol.* **2016**, *7*, 1867. [CrossRef]
84. Frazão, N.; Sousa, A.; Lässig, M.; Gordo, I. Horizontal gene transfer overrides mutation in Escherichia coli colonizing the mammalian gut. *Proc. Natl. Acad. Sci. USA* **2019**, *116*, 17906–17915. [CrossRef]
85. Varble, A.; Meaden, S.; Barrangou, R.; Westra, E.R.; Marraffini, L.A. Recombination between phages and CRISPR−cas loci facilitates horizontal gene transfer in staphylococci. *Nat. Microbiol.* **2019**, *4*, 956–963. [CrossRef] [PubMed]
86. Eggers, C.H.; Gray, C.M.; Preisig, A.M.; Glenn, D.M.; Pereira, J.; Ayers, R.W.; Alshahrani, M.; Acabbo, C.; Becker, M.R.; Bruenn, K.N.; et al. Phage-mediated horizontal gene transfer of both prophage and heterologous DNA by φBB-1, a bacteriophage of Borrelia burgdorferi. *Pathog. Dis.* **2016**, *74*, ftw107. [CrossRef]
87. Heller, K.J. Identification of the phage gene for host receptor specificity by analyzing hybrid phages of T5 and BF23. *Virology* **1984**, *139*, 11–21. [CrossRef]
88. Duplessis, M.; Moineau, S. Identification of a genetic determinant responsible for host specificity in Streptococcus thermophilus bacteriophages. *Mol. Microbiol.* **2001**, *41*, 325–336. [CrossRef]
89. Mahichi, F.; Synnott, A.J.; Yamamichi, K.; Osada, T.; Tanji, Y. Site-specific recombination of T2 phage using IP008 long tail fiber genes provides a targeted method for expanding host range while retaining lytic activity. *FEMS Microbiol. Lett.* **2009**, *295*, 211–217. [CrossRef]

90. Schwarzer, D.; Buettner, F.F.R.; Browning, C.; Nazarov, S.; Rabsch, W.; Bethe, A.; Oberbeck, A.; Bowman, V.D.; Stummeyer, K.; Muhlenhoff, M.; et al. A Multivalent Adsorption Apparatus Explains the Broad Host Range of Phage phi92: A Comprehensive Genomic and Structural Analysis. *J. Virol.* **2012**, *86*, 10384–10398. [CrossRef]
91. Le, S.; He, X.; Tan, Y.; Huang, G.; Zhang, L.; Lux, R.; Shi, W.; Hu, F. Mapping the Tail Fiber as the Receptor Binding Protein Responsible for Differential Host Specificity of Pseudomonas aeruginosa Bacteriophages PaP1 and JG004. *PLoS ONE* **2013**, *8*, e68562. [CrossRef] [PubMed]

2

Bacteriophage Therapy for Clinical Biofilm Infections: Parameters that Influence Treatment Protocols and Current Treatment Approaches

James B. Doub

Division of Infectious Diseases, University of Maryland School of Medicine, Baltimore, MD 21201, USA; jdoub@ihv.umaryland.edu

Abstract: Biofilm infections are extremely difficult to treat, which is secondary to the inability of conventional antibiotics to eradicate biofilms. Consequently, current definitive treatment of biofilm infections requires complete removal of the infected hardware. This causes significant morbidity and mortality to patients and therefore novel therapeutics are needed to cure these infections without removal of the infected hardware. Bacteriophages have intrinsic properties that could be advantageous in the treatment of clinical biofilm infections, but limited knowledge is known about the proper use of bacteriophage therapy in vivo. Currently titers and duration of bacteriophage therapy are the main parameters that are evaluated when devising bacteriophage protocols. Herein, several other important parameters are discussed which if standardized could allow for more effective and reproducible treatment protocols to be formulated. In addition, these parameters are correlated with the current clinical approaches being evaluated in the treatment of clinical biofilm infections.

Keywords: biofilm; bacteriophage therapy; prosthesis related infections; hardware infections; left ventricular assist devices

---

1. Introduction

When bacteria attach to surfaces they can form an extracellular matrix comprised of proteins, polysaccharides, extracellular DNA and water [1–5]. The extracellular matrix and the bacteria that reside within this matrix are what comprise biofilms. Contrary to planktonic bacteria that are free floating, biofilm bacteria are sessile. Bacteria in these sessile states have drastically different characteristics than planktonic bacteria causing conventional antibiotics to have limited ability to eradicate biofilms [1–5]. This stems from the reduced metabolic activity of biofilm bacteria and the architecture of biofilm itself [1]. The minimal inhibitory concentration of antibiotics to biofilm bacteria can be up to 1000 times that of planktonic bacteria [1]. Therefore to definitively cure these infections surgical removal of all the hardware (Figure 1) that harbor biofilms, in combination with prolonged systemic antibiotic therapy, is required. However, this causes significant morbidity and mortality to the patients who suffer from these infections. As a result, new antimicrobial methods are needed that can treat these biofilm infections without removal of the hardware. Bacteriophages might be such an adjuvant therapeutic.

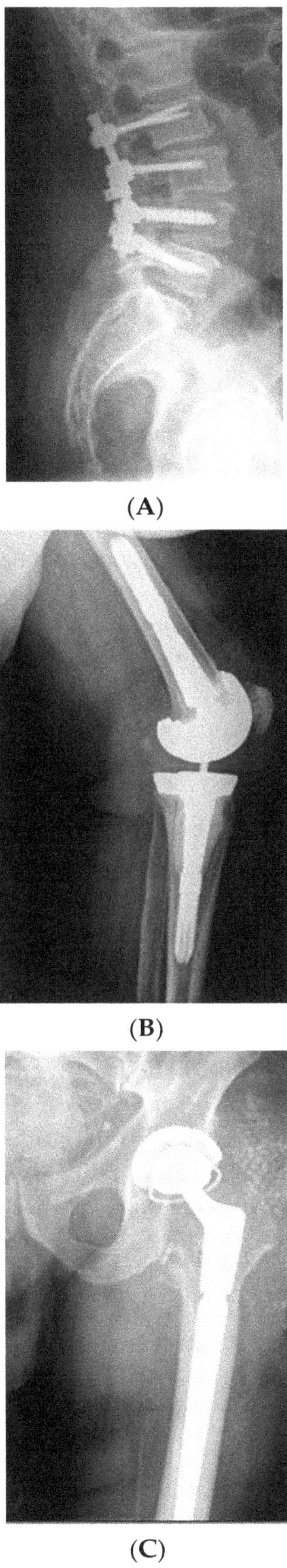

Figure 1. Examples of a few types of "hardware" that once infected require removal for definitive cure of these biofilm infections. (**A**) A lumbar posterior spinal rods and pedicle screw construct. (**B**) Total knee arthroplasty with long stem femoral and tibial components. (**C**) Total hip arthroplasty.

1.1. Bacteriophages

Bacteriophages are viruses with a very narrow spectrum of activity to only certain strains of a certain bacterial species. Infection of human cells has not been observed and therefore bacteriophages are attractive therapeutics to use in bacterial infections [6,7]. These viruses can either be lytic or lysogenic. Lytic bacteriophages hold the most promise in treating infections given their ability to lyse bacteria. Lysogenic bacteriophages incorporate into bacterial DNA and do not induce bacterial lysis until reactivated at a later time, making them not advantageous in the treatment of infections. In nature, the majority of bacteria live in sessile states associated with biofilms and through evolution bacteriophages have coevolved to be able to infect and lyse bacteria inside biofilms [6,7].

1.2. Bacteriophage Activity in Biofilms

In order to eradicate a clinical biofilm, an effective agent must be able to penetrate the biofilm and kill the bacteria that are present in various metabolic states while also degrading the biofilm extracellular matrix. Bacteriophages possess these abilities, but are not motile agents [6,7]. Therefore if bacteriophages can establish an infection within a biofilm, high rates of replication can occur given the high densities of biofilm bacteria in a structured space [8]. Bacteriophages even retain lytic activity against reduced metabolically active bacteria [9,10]. In the deepest regions of a biofilm, bacteria known as persister cells are semi-dormant [11]. All conventional therapeutics have limited activity to persister cells [11]. However, bacteriophages have the ability to infect persister cells and then lyse these bacteria once they become metabolically active again [12].

Bacteriophages also can enzymatically degrade the biofilm extracellular matrix thus allowing for dissemination within the biofilm. This occurs through use of endolysins and depolymerases [13,14]. Enodolysins are enzymes produced by bacteriophages to weaken the bacterial cell wall allowing for lysis to occur releasing their progeny [13]. Endolysins also have activity in degrading the extracellular matrix [13]. Depolymerases are enzymes attached to some bacteriophages that can also degrade the biofilm matrix in functionally different ways to endolysins [13]. Unique to bacteriophages is their ability to self-replicate and increase their own concentrations. This occurs when bacteriophage induced bacterial lysis causes release of progeny into the local environment to infect other bacterial cells. In the confined space of a biofilm this could be advantageous allowing for bacteriophages to infect biofilm bacteria and slowly degrade the biofilm [6]. However bacteriophages are not motile agents and finding biofilm bacteria may be an arduous undertaking if not directly applied to the biofilm.

Several preclinical animal studies support the use of bacteriophage therapy in clinical biofilm infections [15–23]. These studies show that local administrations of bacteriophages to the site of biofilm infections result in biofilm reduction [15–23]. In addition, these studies show that, without local administration of bacteriophage therapy, reduction in biofilms on hardware is not significantly reduced [19]. One of the most relevant preclinical studies was conducted by Morris et al. [19]. Rats were implanted with replica orthopedic prosthetics and then infected with *Staphylococcus aureus.* A total of 3 weeks later rats were given intraperitoneal bacteriophage therapy for 3 days. Results show synergistic activity of bacteriophage therapy with vancomycin in local infected tissues but no statistical reductions in biofilm burden on infected prosthetic material [19]. These findings support other preclinical testing that direct instilment of bacteriophage therapy to the site of biofilm infection is needed to achieve significant biofilm reduction. The intrinsic abilities of bacteriophages and results of animal studies support evaluation of bacteriophages in the treatment of clinical biofilm infections. However bacteriophages are not like conventional antibiotics and several parameters need to be understood before using this therapeutic in vivo.

2. Parameters that Impact Treatment Protocols

Unlike conventional antibiotics, bacteriophage therapy is not a one size fits all antimicrobial therapeutic. Rather a bacteriophage that has robust activity to a clinical isolate of a specific bacterial species may have widely different activity or no activity to another clinical isolate of the same bacterial species. Many other aspects of bacteriophage therapy are poorly understood and not standardized, making creation of treatment protocols an arduous undertaking. At the present time, standardization of protocols can only be achieved with respect to bacteriophage titers and duration of therapy. However, this limits bacteriophage therapy to be used similarly to conventional antibiotics and does not incorporate many other parameters that need to be considered to devise advantageous, reproducible treatment protocols. Herein several additional important parameters are discussed.

2.1. Current "Susceptibility" Testing

At the present time, bacteriophage therapy requires a clinical isolate to be tested against either a library of individual bacteriophages or to a set cocktail of bacteriophages to ensure susceptibility. Given the narrow spectrum of activity, even with the use of bacteriophage cocktails, susceptibility testing is warranted. There is no proverbial gold standard of susceptibility testing and no standardized "breakpoints" are available to determine if a bacteriophage has adequate activity to be used clinically. Therefore, it is vital to understand how in vitro susceptibility testing is conducted to be able to extrapolate these findings to in vivo use. Testing for phage susceptibility usually includes two methods.

(1) Bacterial growth inhibition or "Phagogram": This is conducted when a clinical bacterial isolate is grown in vitro and then inoculated into wells of a 96-microwell plate. The concentration of bacteria in each well is standardized. Then several different bacteriophages (or cocktails) that have potential activity are applied to the wells and monitored for 24 to 48 h to compare growth inhibition to positive controls (Figure 2). It should be noted that the multiplicity of infection (MOI) is usually 100:1. This means bacteriophages outnumber the bacteria 100 to 1. Bacteriophages that inhibit growth of bacteria for durations longer then the positive control are considered candidates. However, no standardized time durations have been established for what is considered long enough growth inhibition to be used in vivo.

(2) Formation of plaques: Once candidate bacteriophages are determined based on growth inhibition, the ability to form plaques on lawns of the bacterial isolate are then conducted. This usually is conducted with double agar overlay plaque assays.

Bacteriophages that form plaques and can inhibit bacterial growth are considered potential therapeutic options. Complicating this testing is that different MOIs can have drastically different growth inhibition durations. For instance an MOI of 100 might inhibit growth for 24 h while an MOI of 10 for the same bacteriophage might not inhibit growth at all. Figure 1 reinforces this for a *Staphylococcus epidermidis* clinical isolate in which PM448, PM472, PM421 have different growth inhibition durations for different MOIs of 100 and 10. This has ramifications when treating biofilm infections as reproducing the high MOI seen in vitro may not occur unless direct bacteriophage application is applied to biofilms. This can also have implications for resistance formation which will be discussed below.

Another important implication of this testing is the lack of standardization with respect to the duration of growth inhibition. A bacteriophage that inhibits growth for 48 h likely has different therapeutic potential compared to a different bacteriophage that only inhibits growth for 8 h. In correlation, different in vivo bacterial metabolic states may require different levels of growth inhibition. For instance, biofilm bacteria are less metabolically active then planktonic bacteria and therefore less in vitro growth inhibition might be needed compared to if bacteriophage therapy is being used to treat a planktonic infection. No standardized growth inhibition duration has been proposed, thereby exposing treatment protocols to potential reproducibility issues. To improve reproducibility, it may be important to standardize what is considered adequate growth inhibition depending on how a bacteriophage therapy is going to be used (intravenously vs. directly applied to biofilms). It should also be mentioned that "susceptibility" testing is usually only conducted against planktonic bacteria. Routine testing for a bacteriophage's ability to remove in vitro biofilms is usually not conducted.

However, in the treatment of biofilm infections, determining the ability of a candidate bacteriophage (or cocktail) to reduce in vitro biofilms should be considered as an additional susceptibility testing step once adequate growth inhibition and formation of plaques has been proven.

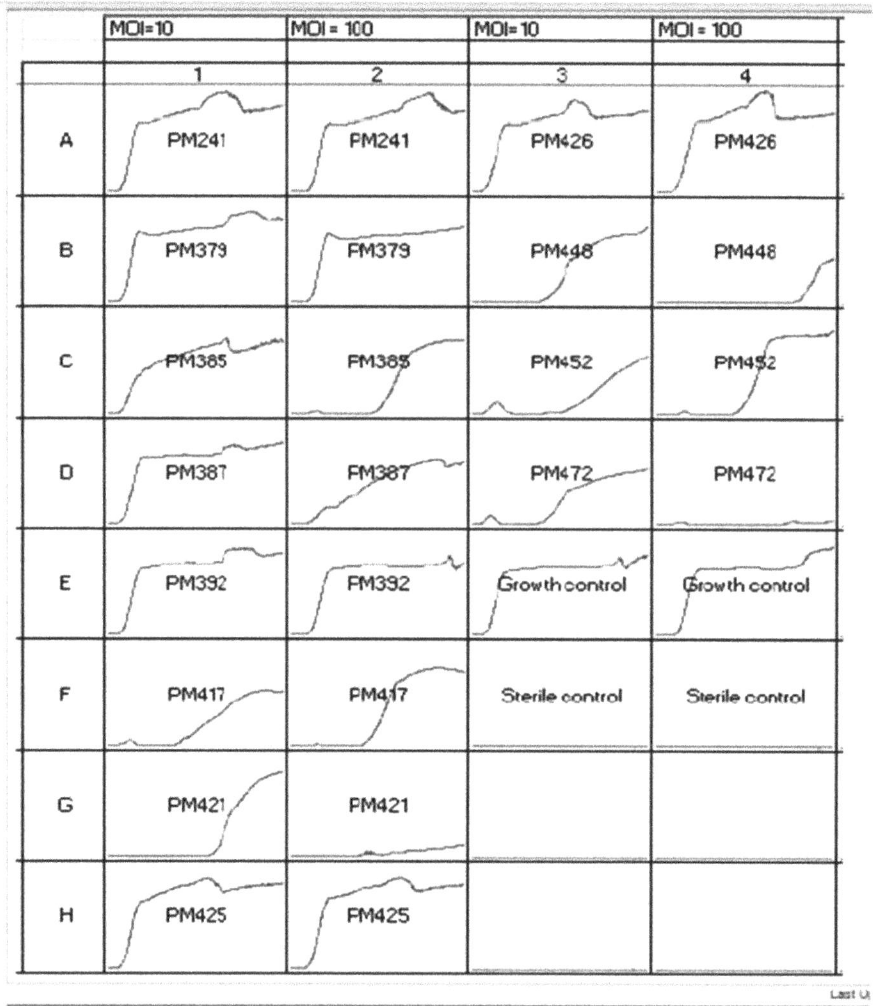

Figure 2. Bacterial growth inhibition curves or "Phagogram" for a compassionate use *Staphylococcus epidermidis* case in a recalcitrant prosthetic joint infection. Different bacteriophages are indicated by PM241-PM472. MOI refers to multiplicity of infection. Growth control is the bacterial isolate with no bacteriophages. Each box has time on the x-axis from 0 to 48 h. This figure shows how growth inhibition testing is conducted to determine potential bacteriophage candidates (PM448, PM472, and PM421). This figure also shows how different MOIs can cause different growth inhibition durations as seen with bacteriophages: PM448, PM472, and PM421.

2.2. *Pharmacology*

The main routes of phage administration that are being investigated in western medicine for the treatment of biofilm infections are local administration directly applied to the infected hardware and intravenous therapy. Eastern European studies have had limited success with topical or oral phage therapies in the treatment of biofilm infections and therefore little interest is present for these methods beyond topical application for burns and wounds [24–26]. Given the novelty of this therapeutic there is a paucity of data with respect to pharmacokinetics of local administration of bacteriophage therapy to biofilms. No data are present to suggest how long locally administrated bacteriophage reside at the infection site, how much is systemically absorbed or the safety of this approach. On the other hand, intravenous bacteriophage therapy has been more widely used and data are present to help guide treatment protocols. Therefore discussion about simple pharmacokinetics is limited to intravenous use.

Distribution: Bacteriophages are expected to be diluted in the whole body volume when given intravenously [27]. In numerous animal studies the titers of bacteriophages after intravenous infusions can be reduced 100–100,000-fold within 30 min of infusion [27]. Animal studies have shown distribution to various other organs including but not limited to heart, lungs, brain, skeletal muscle, bone marrow, and genitourinary tract [27]. However there are no data on intravenous bacteriophage therapy distribution to joints, spinal hardware, Left ventricular assist devices (LVADs) or other spaces that could have poor vascularization.

Metabolism: This is the chemical modification of bacteriophage therapy to reduce its activity. With bacteriophage therapy this occurs mainly through inactivation by the human immune system by neutralizing antibodies [28]. Neutralizing antibody responses have occurred with all forms of bacteriophage administration and this is a theoretical concern for long duration bacteriophage therapies [28,29].

Elimination: Elimination occurs mainly through hepatic clearance. In 1969, using a T4 bacteriophage, Inchley demonstrated that the liver phagocytosed and eliminated more than 99% of the bacteriophages within 30 min after systemic administration [30]. Other studies have supported this extensive hepatic elimination [30–33]. In one compassionate use case, 50 min after intravenous administration no bacteriophage could be detected in patient's serum [34].

Based on these data, intravenous bacteriophage therapies are likely to have significant reduction in titers, secondary to volume of distribution and hepatic elimination. Therefore, achieving MOIs similar to what occurs with in vitro susceptibility testing may be difficult. With the use of bacteriophage therapy applied directly to biofilm infections, MOIs may be similar to what was observed with in vitro susceptibility testing. However, limited pharmacological data have been found to help direct dosing, duration or safety of local bacteriophage administration.

2.3. Safety

Unbeknownst to most, humans are exposed to low titers of bacteriophages on a continual basis [35]. Eastern European medicine has used bacteriophage therapy for close to 100 years with few significant adverse reactions being reported [36]. However, given the extensive hepatic clearance, western medicine is entertaining the use of high titers (greater than 10^9) of intravenous bacteriophage therapy and direct injection of high titers of bacteriophages directly to biofilm infections. Limited safety studies have been conducted using these techniques beyond a phase 1 clinical trial evaluating a three-bacteriophage cocktail with titers of 1×10^9 plaque-forming unit (PFU) twice a day for 14 days to *Staphylococcus aureus* bacteremia [37].

While intravenous bacteriophage therapy has been used in the past with limited adverse events, recent compassionate use cases have shown two adverse events [38,39]. One occurred in the treatment of chronic pseudomonas left ventricular assist device (LVAD) infection in which no success occurred with low titers of intravenous bacteriophage therapy and subsequent bacteriophage therapy with high titers of 1×10^{11} PFU induced fever, shortness of breath and wheezing [38]. These symptoms resolved with supportive medical care but continued with repeat dosing with the same titers. When titers were diluted to 1×10^{10} PFU, the authors document that no adverse events occurred [38]. Endotoxin units were well below the United States Food and Drug Administration approved limit. In the other case, a significant transaminitis occurred after three doses of daily intravenous bacteriophage therapy with titers of 2.7×10^9 PFU in the treatment of a recalcitrant methicillin-resistant *Staphylococcus aureus* prosthetic joint infection. No causative etiology other than bacteriophage therapy could be found [39]. After cessation of bacteriophage therapy liver function returned to normal after 14 days. These two cases suggest that an upper limit may exist with respect to the titers that can be intravenously infused without exposing patients to potential adverse events. However only further safety trials with high titers given intravenously or directly to sites of biofilm infections will be able to assess safety and if there is a ceiling for the amount of titers that can be given.

2.4. Resistance Development

With longer bacteriophage therapies, concern arises for the development of resistance. Resistance usually occurs from bacterial modifications of cell surface receptors or down regulation of receptors used in phage–bacteria attachment [40,41]. Other means of resistance can occur through adaptive systems such as the CRISPR–Cas9 system that cleaves phage DNA thus not allowing for progeny phage to be created [40]. Means to overcome or prevent resistance from occurring include use of cocktails of bacteriophages and bacteriophage substitutions. Bacteriophage cocktails are a group of different bacteriophages that theoretically use different attachment receptors. Therefore, if resistance develops to one receptor, the cocktail should continue to be effective. A recent study showed the frequency of spontaneous induction of resistance to a cocktail of three *Staphylococcus aureus* bacteriophages was no greater than 3×10^{-9} [42]. Bacteriophage substitutions are simply changing therapy to a different bacteriophage that has lytic activity to the bacterium.

Bacteriophage resistance can occur rapidly causing formation of resistant variants that are immune to further bacteriophage infection [41]. This could impede effectiveness of bacteriophage therapy but resistance may also come at a cost to the bacterium especially when antimicrobial agents are present [41]. Moreover, bacteriophage-resistant bacteria often lack important surface features that are responsible for bacterial virulence [41]. Nonetheless resistance is an important factor that should be accounted for especially with prolonged bacteriophage treatments. In a case series of 10 intravenous bacteriophage only cases, resistance occurred in a significant portion of patients and required bacteriophage substitutions [38]. Resistance development is dependent on complex interplays of MOIs, growth inhibition durations and other bacteriophage–bacteria interactions [41]. Therefore resistance might develop rapidly or slower depending on these complex interactions. Determining in vitro resistance development to a clinical isolate is not routinely conducted, but could be easily assessed with susceptibility testing by evaluating the bacterial overgrowth for resistant variants. Resistance development is an important parameter that can have ramifications on efficacy and reproducibility of treatment protocols. Therefore it might be prudent to routinely test for and standardize what an acceptable level of in vitro resistance development is for different infectious processes to reduce further problems of reproducibility and improve efficacy of treatment protocols.

2.5. Synergistic or Antagonistic Activity with Antibiotics

While resistance is an important parameter so is compatibility with systemic antibiotics which may have synergistic or antagonistic activity with bacteriophage therapy. Theoretically, antibiotics that inhibit protein synthesis (rifampin, tetracyclines, linezolid and others) can inhibit phage gene expression and therefore be antagonistic [43]. Antibiotics that inhibit cell wall synthesis inhibitors such as beta-lactams are potentially more synergistic [43]. These findings have been reinforced in numerous in vitro studies [43]. It has also been documented that concentrations of antibiotics also have important ramification of synergistic or antagonistic activity with higher antibiotic concentrations tending to be more antagonistic compared to lower concentrations which tend to be more synergistic [43]. It is interesting that in vivo studies have shown more synergistic activity of antibiotics with bacteriophage therapy then antagonism [15–23]. Spatial and temporal interactions of antibiotics and bacteriophages in vivo likely account for this synergistic activity [43]. It should be reinforced that biofilm bacteria reside where there is poor vascularization and therefore very low concentrations of systemic antibiotics may make phage–antibiotic compatibility less of an issue in vivo [43]. Testing for in vitro for phage–antibiotic compatibility is not commonly conducted. As with resistance development and susceptibility testing, it may be prudent to ensure bacteriophage–antibiotic compatibility with the systemic antibiotics that are planned to be used thus allowing for more reproducible treatment protocols.

2.6. Clinical Biofilms

In vitro bacteriophage biofilm studies are traditionally conducted in static environments. These studies are usually devoid of human plasma proteins, lack in vivo stressors and normally remove planktonic infections before experiments are conducted. However, in vivo, planktonic infections overly clinical biofilm infections and are what causes the majority of the symptoms that patient's experience. Without eradicating these planktonic bacteria, bacteriophage therapy protocols will have to account for the planktonic infection and the biofilm infection. This adds complexity to the use of bacteriophage therapy and potentially further hinders reproducibility given the heterogeneity of these planktonic infections.

Other clinical factors that should be considered include: stability of infected hardware and importance of manual debridement of biofilms. Stability of hardware must be assessed to ensure retaining these materials is possible. This is usually conducted by imaging but manual inspection and manipulation is the most advantageous way to assess the ability to retain these materials. Manual debridement of biofilms has also been shown to be synergistic with respect to bacteriophage activity in biofilms [16,17]. This synergistic activity is likely a result of better bacteriophage penetration into biofilm and exposing biofilm bacteria to bacteriophages [16,17].

2.7. Conclusions

The parameters discussed show that currently bacteriophage therapy is not a therapeutic that can be used similarly to conventional antibiotics. In addition relying mainly on bacteriophage's ability to self-replicate is unlikely to be beneficial beyond isolated case reports given the complexity of these other parameters. Rather thoughtful consideration of many parameters needs to be considered to devise effective, reproducible treatment protocols. Most of these parameters discussed are intertwined but standardization is lacking. Given the heterogeneity of these parameters glaring issues of reproducibility are present at this nascent stage of bacteriophage therapy. To reduce these reproducibility issues standardizing some of these parameters might be needed which include: minimal duration of growth inhibition, resistance testing, bacteriophage–antibiotic compatibility and ensuring in vitro bacteriophage biofilm activity. This may allow for more rigorous testing of reproducible protocols to therefore definitively determine if this therapeutic has efficacy in treating clinical biofilm infections.

3. Current Theoretical Bacteriophage Protocols for Chronic Biofilm Infections

Many recent compassionate use cases have been conducted recently to treat clinical biofilm infections (prosthetic joint infections, LVAD infections, vascular graft infections and others). Two main approaches are being used in western medicine which include: intravenous bacteriophage therapy and the use of surgical interventions to directly inject bacteriophages to site of the biofilm. Table 1 discusses the advantages and disadvantages to each approach in relation to the parameters discussed above. Both approaches involve adjuvant bacteriophage therapy in combination with standard of care systemic antibiotics. Further review of recent case reports with respect to the different approaches is discussed here.

3.1. Case Studies of Intravenous Bacteriophage Therapy in Biofilm Infections

Intravenous bacteriophage therapy has been attempted to treat prosthetic joint infections, ventricular assist devices, vascular graft infections and other hardware infections [38,44–46]. In one case series, the authors describe the use of bacteriophage therapy for two *Pseudomonas* LVAD infections with prolonged intravenous bacteriophage therapies with unsuccessful outcomes [38]. The same author also treated a *Staphylococcus aureus* LVAD infection with intravenous bacteriophage therapy and the was documented as a success, but the patient continued to have culture positive *Staphylococcus aureus* infection at the time of LVAD explant, suggesting the inability of intravenous bacteriophage therapy to eradicate the biofilm infection [38,44]. Another case report treated a *Klebsiella pneumonia* prosthetic joint infection with 8 weeks of intravenous bacteriophage therapy with improvement of symptoms [45]. However the patient remains on chronic indefinite oral suppression antibiotics, limiting the ability to assess if eradication of the clinical biofilm was achieved.

Intravenous bacteriophage therapy is optically attractive in that no surgery is needed. However at the present time no case report has definitively shown the ability to eradicate clinical biofilms with this approach. The theoretical concern with intravenous bacteriophage therapy alone is the entrapment of bacteriophages in the planktonic infection limiting exposure of bacteriophages to the biofilm bacteria. In correlation, bacteriophages are extensively cleared by the liver and in vivo biofilms are usually poorly vascularized. Therefore achieving theoretical MOIs seen with in vitro "susceptibility" testing requires very high titers of infused bacteriophages. These high titers may be limited by potential adverse reactions [38,39]. Further complicating intravenous only therapies is the need for prolonged durations driven by limited bacteriophages reaching their bacterial biofilm targets thereby leading to the development of resistance and neutralizing antibodies. These variables when combined cause numerous confounding variables that may cause significant issues of reproducibility at this nascent stage of bacteriophage therapy.

Table 1. Advantages and disadvantages of intravenous and direct injection of bacteriophage therapy for clinical biofilm infections.

	Direct Bacteriophage Therapy in Correlation with Surgical Interventions	**Intravenous Bacteriophage Therapy**
Advantages	Potentially shorter course with less risk of resistance and neutralizing antibodies occurring Direct injection of high titers to biofilm thereby achieving theoretical MOIs similarly to in vitro testing Removes majority of planktonic infection Ensures hardware salvageable Ensures no other pathogens present Allows for manual scrubbing of biofilm	Circumvent surgery and risks of general anesthesia No wounds created that thus no risk for further infections No confounders with proving efficacy either it works or does not work
Disadvantages	Risks of Anesthesia Risks of poor wound healing Chance for introduction of another pathogen during surgical interventions	Have to treat both planktonic and biofilm infection Limited ability to achieve MOIs that were tested with in vitro testing Limited identification of all pathogens involved to match to bacteriophage therapy Unable to assess prosthesis stability beyond radiographic findings Longer therapy with higher risk of resistance and neutralizing antibodies occurring

3.2. Case Studies of Direct Injection of Bacteriophages to Biofilms with Surgical Intervention

The addition of bacteriophage therapy with debridement and irrigation surgeries is the other approach that has been used in several case studies [38,47–50]. This approach involves injection of high titers of bacteriophage phages directly at the site of the biofilm infection thereby circumventing hepatic clearance. The goal of this approach is to potentially cure these infections without need for removal of the hardware. However the risks of a surgical procedure are present and therefore this approach is optically less desirable.

There have been several compassionate use case reports that have shown successful eradication of biofilm infections which include: chronic orthopedic hardware infections, LVAD infection, vascular graft infection, cardiothoracic surgery infections [38,47–50]. In these case reports different durations of bacteriophage therapy were used. Some cases only required single doses given at the time of surgery while others used drains to continually instill bacteriophage therapy for 7 to 10 days. All cases described no recurrence of bacterial infections while patients were off antimicrobial therapies thereby showing eradication of bacterial biofilms. However with surgical debridement, successful eradication of bacterial biofilm is confounded by the uncertainty of whether it was bacteriophage therapy that was the reason for clearance or if it was the surgical intervention itself. This questioning occurs because success occurs with these surgical debridement procedures without adjuvant bacteriophage therapy albeit at low rates. In addition, limited data are present to help direct safety, appropriate dosing and durations of directly administered bacteriophage therapies but this approach may allow for more standardized reproducible protocols.

4. Conclusions

Many aspects of bacteriophage therapy allow this therapeutic to be an attractive adjuvant therapeutic in the treatment of biofilm infections but much work is needed before definitive efficacy trials are to be conducted. The various parameters discussed here should allow researchers to be more cognizant of the current inherent limitations of bacteriophage therapy. However, given the heterogeneity of these parameters, projected issues of reproducibility are glaring. Therefore, standardizing some of these parameters is warranted to formulate reproducible protocols that will allow for rigorous testing of this therapeutic in the treatment of biofilm infections.

Acknowledgments: Phagomed are acknowledged for providing and authorization of the use of Figure 2.

References

1. Mah, T.F.; O'Toole, G.A. Mechanisms of biofilm resistance to antimicrobial agents. *Trends Microbiol.* **2001**, *9*, 34–39. [CrossRef]
2. Wille, J.; Coenye, T. Biofilm dispersion: The key to biofilm eradication or opening Pandora's box? *Biofilm* **2020**, *2*, 100027. [CrossRef]
3. Stewart, P.S. Antimicrobial Tolerance in Biofilms. *Microbiol. Spectr.* **2015**, *3*. [CrossRef] [PubMed]
4. Van Acker, H.; Van Dijck, P.; Coenye, T. Molecular mechanisms of antimicrobial tolerance and resistance in bacterial and fungal biofilms. *Trends Microbiol.* **2014**, *22*, 326–333. [CrossRef] [PubMed]
5. Kaplan, J.B. Biofilm dispersal: Mechanisms, clinical implications, and potential therapeutic uses. *J. Dent. Res.* **2010**, *89*, 205–218. [CrossRef]
6. Abedon, S.T. Ecology of Anti-Biofilm Agents II: Bacteriophage Exploitation and Biocontrol of Biofilm Bacteria. *Pharmaceuticals* **2015**, *8*, 559–589. [CrossRef]
7. Hanlon, G.W. Bacteriophages: An appraisal of their role in the treatment of bacterial infections. *Int. J. Antimicrob. Agents* **2007**, *30*, 118–128. [CrossRef]
8. Hadas, H.; Einav, M.; Fishov, I.; Zaritsky, A. Bacteriophage T4 development depends on the physiology of its host Escherichia coli. *Microbiology* **1997**, *143*, 179–185. [CrossRef]
9. Doolittle, M.M.; Cooney, J.J.; Caldwell, D.E. Tracing the interaction of bacteriophage with bacterial biofilms using fluorescent and chromogenic probes. *J. Ind. Microbiol.* **1996**, *16*, 331–341. [CrossRef]
10. Lewis, K. Persister cells. *Annu. Rev. Microbiol.* **2010**, *64*, 357–372. [CrossRef]
11. Pearl, S.; Gabay, C.; Kishony, R.; Oppenheim, A.; Balaban, N.Q. Nongenetic individuality in the host-phage interaction. *PLoS Biol.* **2008**, *6*, e120. [CrossRef] [PubMed]
12. Chan, B.K.; Abedon, S.T. Bacteriophages and their enzymes in biofilm control. *Curr. Pharm. Des.* **2015**, *21*, 85–99. [CrossRef] [PubMed]
13. Tait, K.; Skillman, L.C.; Sutherland, I.W. The efficacy of bacteriophage as a method of biofilm eradication. *Biofouling* **2002**, *18*, 305–311. [CrossRef]
14. Yilmaz, C.; Colak, M.; Yilmaz, B.C.; Ersoz, G.; Kutateladze, M.; Gozlugol, M. Bacteriophage therapy in implant-related infections: An experimental study. *J. Bone Jt. Surg. Am.* **2013**, *95*, 117–125. [CrossRef]

15. Chaudhry, W.N.; Concepción-Acevedo, J.; Park, T.; Andleeb, S.; Bull, J.J.; Levin, B.R. Synergy and Order Effects of Antibiotics and Phages in Killing Pseudomonas aeruginosa Biofilms. *PLoS ONE* **2017**, *12*, e0168615. [CrossRef]
16. Mendes, J.J.; Leandro, C.; Corte-Real, S.; Barbosa, R.; Cavaco-Silva, P.; Melo-Cristino, J.; Górski, A.; Garcia, M. Wound healing potential of topical bacteriophage therapy on diabetic cutaneous wounds. *Wound Repair Regen.* **2013**, *21*, 595–603. [CrossRef]
17. Kaur, S.; Harjai, K.; Chhibber, S. Bacteriophage mediated killing of Staphylococcus aureus in vitro on orthopaedic K wires in presence of linezolid prevents implant colonization. *PLoS ONE* **2014**, *9*, e90411. [CrossRef]
18. Morris, J.L.; Letson, H.L.; Elliott, L.; Grant, A.L.; Wilkinson, M.; Hazratwala, K.; McEwen, P. Evaluation of bacteriophage as an adjunct therapy for treatment of peri-prosthetic joint infection caused by Staphylococcus aureus. *PLoS ONE* **2019**, *14*, e0226574. [CrossRef]
19. Cobb, L.H.; Park, J.; Swanson, E.A.; Beard, M.C.; McCabe, E.M.; Rourke, A.S.; Seo, K.S.; Olivier, A.K.; Priddy, L.B. CRISPR-Cas9 modified bacteriophage for treatment of Staphylococcus aureus induced osteomyelitis and soft tissue infection. *PLoS ONE* **2019**, *14*, e0220421. [CrossRef]
20. Ibrahim, O.; Sarhan, S.; Salih, S. Activity of Isolated Staphylococcal Bacteriophage in Treatment of Experimentally Induced Chronic Osteomyelitis in Rabbits. *Adv. Anim. Vet. Sci.* **2016**, *4*, 593–603. [CrossRef]
21. Kishor, C.; Mishra, R.R.; Saraf, S.K.; Kumar, M.; Srivastav, A.K.; Nath, G. Phage therapy of staphylococcal chronic osteomyelitis in experimental animal model. *Indian J. Med. Res.* **2016**, *143*, 87–94. [PubMed]
22. Wroe, J.; Johnson, C.; Garcia, A. Bacteriophage delivering hydrogels reduce biofilm formation in vitro and infection in vivo. *J. Biomed. Mater. Res. A* **2020**, *108*, 39–49. [CrossRef] [PubMed]
23. Międzybrodzki, R.; Borysowski, J.; Weber-Dąbrowska, B.; Fortuna, W.; Letkiewicz, S.; Szufnarowski, K.; Pawełczyk, Z.; Rogóż, P.; Kłak, M.; Wojtasik, E.; et al. Clinical aspects of phage therapy. *Adv. Virus Res.* **2012**, *83*, 73–121.
24. Jault, P.; Leclerc, T.; Jennes, S.; Pirnay, J.P.; Que, Y.-A.; Resch, G.; Rousseau, A.F.; Ravat, F.; Carsin, H.; Floch, R.L.; et al. Efficacy and tolerability of a cocktail of bacteriophages to treat burn wounds infected by Pseudomonas aeruginosa (PhagoBurn): A randomised, controlled, double-blind phase 1/2 trial. *Lancet Infect. Dis.* **2019**, *19*, 35–45. [CrossRef]
25. Rhoads, D.D.; Wolcott, R.D.; Kuskowski, M.A.; Wolcott, B.M.; Ward, L.S.; Sulakvelidze, A. Bacteriophage therapy of venous leg ulcers in humans: Results of a phase I safety trial. *J. Wound Care* **2009**, *18*, 237–243. [CrossRef] [PubMed]
26. Dąbrowska, K. Phage therapy: What factors shape phage pharmacokinetics and bioavailability? Systematic and critical review. *Med. Res. Rev.* **2019**, *39*, 2000–2025. [CrossRef] [PubMed]
27. Jerne, N.K.; Avegno, P. The development of the phage-inactivating properties of serum during the course of specific immunization of an animal: Reversible and irreversible inactivation. *J. Immunol.* **1956**, *76*, 200–208.
28. Łusiak-Szelachowska, M.; Zaczek, M.; Weber-Dąbrowska, B.; Międzybrodzki, R.; Kłak, M.; Fortuna, W.; Letkiewicz, S.; Rogóż, P.; Szufnarowski, K.; Jończyk-Matysiak, E.; et al. Phage neutralization by sera of patients receiving phage therapy. *Viral. Immunol.* **2014**, *27*, 295–304. [CrossRef]
29. Inchley, C.J. The actvity of mouse Kupffer cells following intravenous injection of T4 bacteriophage. *Clin. Exp. Immunol.* **1969**, *5*, 173–187.
30. Jonczyk-Matysiak, E.; Weber-Dabrowska, B.; Owczarek, B.; Międzybrodzki, B.; Łusiak-Szelachowska, M.; Łodej, N.; Górski, A. Phage-phagocyte interactions and their implications for phage application as therapeutics. *Viruses* **2017**, *9*, 150. [CrossRef]
31. Nelstrop, A.E.; Taylor, G.; Collard, P. Studies on phagocytosis. II. in vitro phagocytosis by macrophages. *Immunology* **1968**, *14*, 339–346. [PubMed]
32. Reynaud, A.; Cloastre, L.; Bernard, J.; Laveran, H.; Ackermann, H.-W.; Licois, D.; Joly, B. Characteristics and diffusion in the rabbit of a phage for Escherichia coli 0103. Attempts to use this phage for therapy. *Vet. Microbiol.* **1992**, *30*, 203–212. [CrossRef]
33. LaVergne, S.; Hamilton, T.; Biswas, B.; Kumaraswamy, M.; Schooley, R.T.; Wooten, D. Phage Therapy for a Multidrug-Resistant Acinetobacter baumannii Craniectomy Site Infection. *Open Forum. Infect. Dis.* **2018**, *5*, ofy064. [CrossRef] [PubMed]
34. Górski, A.; Weber-Dabrowska, B. The potential role of endogenous bacteriophages in controlling invading pathogens. *Cell. Mol. Life Sci.* **2005**, *62*, 511–519. [CrossRef] [PubMed]

35. Sulakvelidze, A.; Alavidze, Z.; Morris, J.G., Jr. Bacteriophage therapy. *Antimicrob. Agents Chemother.* **2001**, *45*, 649–659. [CrossRef]
36. Petrovic Fabijan, A.; Lin, R.C.Y.; Ho, J.; Maddocks, S.; Zakour, N.L.B.; Iredell, J.R.; Westmead Bacteriophage Therapy Team. Safety of bacteriophage therapy in severe Staphylococcus aureus infection. *Nat. Microbiol.* **2020**, *5*, 465–472. [CrossRef]
37. Aslam, S.; Lampley, E.; Wooten, D.; Karris, M.; Benson, C.; Strathdee, S.; Schooley, R.T. Lessons Learned from First Ten Consecutive Cases of Intravenous Bacteriophage Therapy to Treat Multidrug Resistant Bacterial Infections at a Single Center in the US. *Open Forum. Infect. Dis.* **2020**, *7*, ofaa389. [CrossRef]
38. Doub, J.B.; Ng, V.Y.; Johnson, A.J.; Slomka, M.; Fackler, J.; Horne, B.; Brownstein, M.J.; Henry, M.; Malagon, F.; Biswas, B. Salvage Bacteriophage Therapy for a Chronic MRSA Prosthetic Joint Infection. *Antibiotics* **2020**, *9*, 241. [CrossRef]
39. Jackson, S.A.; McKenzie, R.E.; Fagerlund, R.D.; Kieper, S.N.; Fineran, P.C.; Brouns, S.J. CRISPR-Cas: Adapting to change. *Science* **2017**, *356*, eaal5056. [CrossRef]
40. Oechslin, F. Resistance Development to Bacteriophages Occurring during Bacteriophage Therapy. *Viruses* **2018**, *10*, 351. [CrossRef]
41. Lehman, S.M.; Mearns, G.; Rankin, D.; Cole, R.A.; Smrekar, F.; Branston, S.D.; Morales, S. Design and Preclinical Development of a Phage Product for the Treatment of Antibiotic-Resistant Staphylococcus aureus Infections. *Viruses* **2019**, *11*, 88. [CrossRef] [PubMed]
42. Abedon, S.T. Phage-Antibiotic Combination Treatments: Antagonistic Impacts of Antibiotics on the Pharmacodynamics of Phage Therapy? *Antibiotics* **2019**, *8*, 182. [CrossRef] [PubMed]
43. Aslam, S.; Pretorius, V.; Lehman, S.M.; Morales, S.; Schooley, R.T. Novel bacteriophage therapy for treatment of left ventricular assist device infection. *J. Heart Lung Transpl.* **2019**, *38*, 475–476. [CrossRef] [PubMed]
44. Cano, E.J.; Caflisch, K.M.; Bollyky, P.L.; Van Belleghem, J.D.; Patel, R.; Fackler, J.; Brownstein, M.J.; Horne, B.; Biswas, B.; Henry, M.; et al. Phage Therapy for Limb-threatening Prosthetic Knee Klebsiella pneumoniae Infection: Case Report and In Vitro Characterization of Anti-biofilm Activity. *Clin. Infect. Dis.* **2020**, ciaa705. [CrossRef] [PubMed]
45. Duplessis, C.; Stockelman, M.; Hamilton, T.; Merril, G.; Brownstein, M.; Bishop-lilly, K.; Schooley, R.; Henry, M.; Horne, B.; Sisson, B.M.; et al. A Case Series of Emergency Investigational New Drug Applications for Bacteriophages Treating Recalcitrant Multi-drug Resistant Bacterial Infections: Confirmed Safety and a Signal of Efficacy. *J. Intensive Crit. Care* **2019**, *5*, 11.
46. Ferry, T.; Leboucher, G.; Fevre, C.; Herry, Y.; Conrad, A.; Josse, J.; Batailler, C.; Chidiac, C.; Medina, M.; Lustig, S.; et al. Salvage Debridement, Antibiotics and Implant Retention ("DAIR") With Local Injection of a Selected Cocktail of Bacteriophages: Is It an Option for an Elderly Patient With Relapsing Staphylococcus aureus Prosthetic-Joint Infection? *Open Forum. Infect. Dis.* **2018**, *5*, ofy269. [CrossRef]
47. Onsea, J.; Soentjens, P.; Djebara, S.; Merabishvili, M.; Depypere, M.; Spriet, I.; De Munter, P.; Debaveye, Y.; Nijs, S.; Vanderschot, P.; et al. Bacteriophage Application for Difficult-to-treat Musculoskeletal Infections: Development of a Standardized Multidisciplinary Treatment Protocol. *Viruses* **2019**, *11*, 891. [CrossRef]
48. Rubalskii, E.; Ruemke, S.; Salmoukas, C.; Boyle, E.C.; Warnecke, G.; Tudorache, I.; Shrestha, M.; Schmitto, J.D.; Martens, M.A.; Rojas, S.V.; et al. Bacteriophage Therapy for Critical Infections Related to Cardiothoracic Surgery. *Antibiotics* **2020**, *9*, 232. [CrossRef]
49. Tkhilaishvili, T.; Winkler, T.; Müller, M.; Perka, C.; Trampuz, A. Bacteriophages as Adjuvant to Antibiotics for the Treatment of Periprosthetic Joint Infection Caused by Multidrug-Resistant Pseudomonas aeruginosa. *Antimicrob. Agents Chemother.* **2019**, *64*, e00924-19. [CrossRef]
50. Mulzer, J.; Trampuz, A.; Potapov, E.V. Treatment of chronic left ventricular assist device infection with local application of bacteriophages. *Eur. J. Cardio-Thorac. Surg.* **2020**, *57*, 1003–1004. [CrossRef]

3

Phage-Bacterial Dynamics with Spatial Structure: Self Organization around Phage Sinks can Promote Increased Cell Densities

James J. Bull [1,2,3,*], Kelly A. Christensen [4,5], Carly Scott [4,6], Benjamin R. Jack [7], Cameron J. Crandall [6] and Stephen M. Krone [4,5,8,*]

1 Department of Integrative Biology, University of Texas, Austin, TX 78712, USA
2 The Institute for Cellular and Molecular Biology, University of Texas, Austin, TX 78712, USA
3 Center for Computational Biology and Bioinformatics, University of Texas, Austin, TX 78712, USA
4 Department of Mathematics, University of Idaho, Moscow, ID 83844, USA; chri4898@vandals.uidaho.edu (K.A.C.); scot9278@vandals.uidaho.edu (C.S.)
5 Center for Modeling Complex Interactions, University of Idaho, Moscow, ID 83844, USA
6 Department of Biological Sciences, University of Idaho, Moscow, ID 83844, USA; cjcrandall91@gmail.com
7 The Institute for Cellular and Molecular Biology, University of Texas, Austin, TX 78712, USA; benjamin.r.jack@gmail.com
8 Institute for Bioinformatics and Evolutionary Studies, University of Idaho, Moscow, ID 83844, USA
* Correspondence: bull@utexas.edu (J.J.B.); krone@uidaho.edu (S.M.K.)

Abstract: Bacteria growing on surfaces appear to be profoundly more resistant to control by lytic bacteriophages than do the same cells grown in liquid. Here, we use simulation models to investigate whether spatial structure per se can account for this increased cell density in the presence of phages. A measure is derived for comparing cell densities between growth in spatially structured environments versus well mixed environments (known as mass action). Maintenance of sensitive cells requires some form of phage death; we invoke death mechanisms that are spatially fixed, as if produced by cells. Spatially structured phage death provides cells with a means of protection that can boost cell densities an order of magnitude above that attained under mass action, although the effect is sometimes in the opposite direction. Phage and bacteria self organize into separate refuges, and spatial structure operates so that the phage progeny from a single burst do not have independent fates (as they do with mass action). Phage incur a high loss when invading protected areas that have high cell densities, resulting in greater protection for the cells. By the same metric, mass action dynamics either show no sustained bacterial elevation or oscillate between states of low and high cell densities and an elevated average. The elevated cell densities observed in models with spatial structure do not approach the empirically observed increased density of cells in structured environments with phages (which can be many orders of magnitude), so the empirical phenomenon likely requires additional mechanisms than those analyzed here.

Keywords: biofilm; phage therapy; resistance; bacteriophage; models; agent based; mass action

---

1. Introduction

Bacteriophages are ubiquitous predators of bacteria, and they have long been entertained as having possible therapeutic utility in medicine. However, therapeutic utility is typically a matter of controlling the bacterial populations, and population control is not easily inferred from the mere fact that individuals of one species can kill individuals of another species. The difference between killing that achieves population control and killing that has little effect on the population rests on quantitative properties of the killing. Fortunately, phages are easily manipulated in the lab and thus easily studied to address dynamics and the control of bacterial populations.

The history of work on phage-bacterial dynamics has been dominated by liquid cultures in which bacteria are suspended as single cells at uniform density. Such cultures are routinely modeled as ordinary differential equations (ODEs) with assumptions of "mass action." Mass action refers to an environment in which all individuals are "well mixed," as would occur in a chemostat or batch culture, and so collisions occur at random. In such a system (see Equation (7)), interaction terms appear as products of bulk densities and essential parameters are easily estimated. The typical outcome following a lytic phage assault on a dense population of sensitive bacteria in liquid is killing of the bacterial population by many orders of magnitude, followed by a rebound of bacteria genetically resistant to the phage [1,2] with possible long-term coevolutionary arms races [3]. This work has led to many insights about bacterial and bacteriophage biology but has also given rise to a perception that bacterial escape from phages is chiefly through evolution of genetic resistance. However, we now know that many bacteria spend much of their lives in structured environments such as biofilms and aggregates, and bacterial biology in structured environments is fundamentally different than in liquid suspensions [4–6]. Spatially structured bacterial populations are difficult to control—they may persist seemingly indefinitely amid ongoing phage attack (they also survive antibiotic attack), and this persistence does not appear to be from genetic resistance [7–13]. Understanding the nature of this coexistence may be critical to phage therapy. Is it spatial structure itself that allows bacterial escape, or is it an indirect consequence of spatial structure on bacterial habits that allows the escape?

The goal of this study is to use models to understand the maintenance of high densities of sensitive bacteria amid phage attack in spatially structured environments. Our ultimate motivation is to develop phage interventions for controlling bacteria, which requires understanding of how bacteria normally escape. Does spatial structure per se allow for easy persistence, or does escape require cells to behave differently in structured environments than in liquid ones? We use computational models to explore the dynamic nature of the phage-bacterial interaction in spatially structured populations, identifying which mechanisms enable bacterial persistence at high densities. The empirical evidence is that sensitive bacteria easily persist, but identifying a process that may reasonably account for the coexistence is challenging.

2. Empirical Anomalies and Possible Causes

Various observations on bacteria grown under spatial structure suggest that genetically sensitive bacteria can be maintained as the dominant population in the presence of phage, at least in the short term [8,10–12,14]. The environmental contexts in these examples are diverse. The phage typically reduce bacterial numbers 1 or more orders of magnitude, but the remaining population is predominantly sensitive and persists at a much higher density than would occur in liquid. The phage sensitivity of residual populations is sometimes measured directly or is inferred from dynamic principles, such as the continuing high output of phage (which could not grow on genetically resistant cells). In some cases, the surviving bacterial strain is a genetic mutant that is fundamentally sensitive to phage but exhibits reduced adsorption (e.g., mucoidy); the bacteria are merely maintained at higher levels than explicable by basic dynamics principles (e.g., [15]).

As one striking example, Darch et al. [14] grew *Pseudomonas aeruginosa* in a synthetic sputum medium; cell numbers were measured non-destructively with confocal microscopy. The cells grew in aggregates. Addition of phage to an established culture resulted in a less than 1-log drop in bacterial numbers (measured in situ). However, when the bacteria were grown in liquid (albeit in different media), addition of phage resulted in a 7-log drop. In a second example, Lu and Colins [10] grew 24 h *E. coli* biofilms in peg-lid microtiter plates (0.2 mL volumes per well). After media replacement, 24 h treatment with phage T7 led to approximately a 2-log reduction in cell density, but close to 10^5 cells remained (their Fig. 3B). However, treatment with a T7 phage engineered to encode an enzyme that degrades a bacterial matrix component led to another nearly 2-log reduction in cell density. Density of the enzyme-free phage was $\approx 5 \times 10^8$/mL in the surrounding liquid. The fact that the enzyme had such a profound effect indicates that sensitive cells were sequestered from the no-enzyme phage while surrounded with a phage density that should have been more than sufficient to eliminate nearly all of them.

Compared to mass action, the most obvious consequence of spatial structure is local variation in the abundance of bacteria and phage. However, this spatial variation arises, reproduction of phage and bacteria enhances that variation, whereas diffusion diminishes it. Structure leads to expanding concentrations of bacteria (colonies) and to high concentrations of phages near bacterial clusters that have been invaded [16–18]. The spatial variation in abundance will interact with any of several factors that could be contributors to the long-term co-maintenance of sensitive bacteria and lytic phages, as follows.

Resource concentration. Phage growth is known to be reduced on cells that are starved [19,20], a phenomenon easily appreciated from the halting of plaque growth on plates after the bacterial lawn matures. In spatial environments, high concentrations of bacteria will depress resources locally, suppressing phage growth in those zones.

Barriers and gradients. Spatial structure allows the local buildup of substances exuded from cells, such as expolysaccharides (EPS), ions, signalling molecules, and outer membrane vesicles [1,8,21]. These agents may trap phages, drive phages away with electrostatic forces, or alter the concentration of factors necessary for phage adsorption.

Phage-adsorbing debris. The remnants of cells lysed by phages may continue to adsorb phage perhaps irreversibly and thereby reduce the number of phage encountering live cells. Spatial structure will facilitate the buildup of debris around clusters of cells.

Co-infection and superinfection. Phage growth with spatial structure will often concentrate phages around cells, which for many phages will lead to high numbers of phages infecting the same cell [18]. This property will reduce the effective number of phage progeny and may allow cells to reach higher densities than in liquid.

Altered gene expression. Cells may vary gene expression specifically in response to surface attachment or signals received from adjacent cells (e.g., [22]). Changes in gene expression are not necessarily effects of spatially structured dynamics per se, but gene expression changes may themselves enable phage-bacterial co-existence. As an example, non-genetic variation in receptor abundance on cells can lead to high levels of the survival of genetically sensitive bacteria challenged with phages [23–26]. If bacterial growth with spatial structure amplifies variation in gene expression, that variation could enable bacterial escape and subsequent growth, more than in liquid.

3. Perspective: Does Spatial Structure Increase Bacterial Density?

The question addressed here is whether phage and cell dynamics that are spatial in nature allow cells to attain a higher density than if everything is well mixed. As our approach uses mathematical and computational models, this question requires understanding the difference between spatial structure and well-mixed conditions. Phage dynamics have traditionally been modeled under the assumptions of mass action, which assumes cells and phages are fully mixed and that interactions occur at rates determined by population averages. Mass action means that cells and phage have no assigned locations; they just exist. This mathematical convenience allows the process to be studied with ordinary differential equations [1,27–29]. With spatial structure, the locations of cells and phages are tracked over time, and interactions are location dependent. Typically, phages move through diffusion and cells remain in fixed locations (adjacent to parent cells). Thus, high densities of cells or phages can build up in parts of the environment while other parts have few or no individuals. Phage killing is local to the areas of high phage density.

Extensive computational analyses of spatially structured phage-bacterial dynamics have been undertaken in a few previous studies [16–18]. This pioneering work described many properties of dynamics unique to spatial structure, such as strong spatial co-localization of bacteria and phage, as well as spatial structure enabling coexistence over a wider range of parameter values than does mass action (due to greater oscillations with mass action).

Our study uses that foundation to ask a specific question: does spatially structured phage dynamics per se maintain a greater cell density than under mass action? The fact that spatial structure more easily allows coexistence [17] might suggest that spatial structure also increases bacterial density, but the effect of spatial structure was reported to stem from reduced global oscillations rather than an increase in (mean) bacterial density. Reduced oscillations could lead to greater coexistence without affecting mean density.

The reason for using models to study these processes is to develop understanding that cannot feasibly be obtained from empirical studies alone. The models allow control of variables so that effects of single variables can be isolated. From there, one may proceed to empirical studies to test specific processes.

4. Setting the Stage for Evaluating the Effect of Spatial Structure: Biological Consequences of Mass Action Are Well Studied

We use a variety of computational approaches to understand phage-bacterial dynamics in spatially structured environments. Whereas the outcomes of simulations are easy to interpret, understanding the causal parameters can be challenging because of the many environmental details that must simultaneously be specified to model dynamics in space. To help understand simulation results, and especially to motivate the types of analyses done with simulations, we offer a brief review of specific mass action results from previous studies using ordinary differential equations.

1. Mass action does not preclude high cell density. Although the typical pattern of phage-bacterial dynamics under mass action is one in which phages decimate the bacterial populations, there are mass action conditions in which high densities of sensitive bacteria can be maintained, typically with a low adsorption rate [28].
2. Maintenance of phages and bacteria requires some form of phage death. The ODE models typically assume a constant rate of phage death or clearance from the system.
3. Numerical solutions to the equations often exhibit undamped and even accelerating oscillations [17,28,29]. The oscillations complicate comparisons of cell density across systems (see below).

5. Formal Spatial Structure

We use computational simulations to consider the formal dynamics of phage and bacteria with spatial structure. Our simulations were based on a two-dimensional 'grid' of sites and included a mix of stochastic (random) and deterministic processes. In these models, every cell, phage or other agent has a location on the grid; at each time step, infection, reproduction and movement may occur (explained in Methods). These models have many components similar to those in mass action models, but with explicit spatial structure and rates that are locally determined. We are primarily interested in whether and how spatial structure affects the cell density maintained in the presence of phages. The grid models include versions that enforce spatial structure as well as mass action versions, although nearly all trials assumed spatial structure. In the mass action versions of the grid models, each individual gets relocated every time step.

Biologically, there are two general types of bacterial avoidance of phages that may be entertained. One is that bacteria are protected from phages, whether by reduced adsorption rate or by surrounding themselves with anti-phage protection. The second is that cells either produce or associate with phage-killing products but are otherwise intrinsically susceptible when phages encounter them. We focus on the latter here, chiefly because it is non-trivial. It is otherwise clear that fully protected bacteria will be able to grow to the limits permitted by the environment—as is well known from ODE models allowing evolution of genetically resistant bacteria. If spatially structured cell growth combined with phage death does not intrinsically promote higher bacterial densities by several orders of magnitude, then protection of individual bacteria becomes plausible as the main driver.

A challenge in switching from mass action to spatial structure lies in accommodating attachment of phage to bacteria. With mass action models, an adsorption rate coefficient (k) subsumes both the chance encounter of a bacteria with phage and the rate at which the phage sticks to the bacterium given an encounter [1]. With spatial structure, we are forced to separate encounter from attachment because the two processes are operating at different scales in different parts of the environment [16].

Although some types of physiological protection of cells may be imposed by the environment (e.g., temperature, metal ions that affect adsorption, pH), of interest here is how the bacteria can potentially influence the local environment to enact protection by blocking encounter with phages. Excretion of extracellular polysaccharides and other substances may directly slow or block phage access altogether, and some of the extracellular matrix may effectively kill phages by binding them irreversibly. Dead cells and outer membrane vesicles may act as decoys that bind phages and cause them to eject their genomes.

6. Results

The maintenance of sensitive cells amid phage attack depends fundamentally on phage density and thus on phage death mechanisms. In a closed environment with cells and phages, such as a flask, the absence of phage death (or other form of permanent loss/sequestration) will ensure that phage ultimately eliminate all sensitive cells. Once cells are abundant, even phages with poor adsorption rates will ultimately increase to such densities that cells are rapidly eliminated. In the absence of cells being completely protected from phage, some form of phage death is required to prevent the ultimate buildup of phage to the point that all cells are killed. While it is obvious that fully protected cells can grow with impunity in the presence of phages, it is less obvious how the interplay between phage growth and death will collaborate to allow coexistence of sensitive cells and phage. The latter is our focus here—how phage death mechanisms influence the density of cells maintained.

6.1. The Nature of Phage Death Used Here: EPS and Cellular Debris

We will model two phage death mechanisms: adsorption to exopolysaccharides (EPS) and adsorption to dead cells (debris). The main difference in implementation of these two mechanisms is that EPS is treated as a spatially static and permanent mechanism of phage death; debris is also assumed to be spatially static, but its creation waxes and wanes as phage kill more or fewer cells, and it is not permanent, instead having an intrinsic decay rate. The association of debris with phage abundance may lead to substantially different outcomes than with a static phage sink. EPS will be the mechanism employed in all but the last set of studies presented here (for reasons explained below).

We accept that the empirical evidence from liquid cultures does not support a major role of debris in causing phage death (e.g., phage titers in lysed cultures are often stable for months—even when the lysate is not filtered or cleared of bacterial debris—J.J. Bull personal observations). The implementation of death by debris is offered in the spirit of any mechanism that rises and falls with phage attack on cells. Furthermore, if debris is short-lived, it may have an impact but the mechanism be difficult to detect empirically. We note that our mechanisms of phage death do not necessarily obey any empirically established process, mostly for lack of effort to detect such processes. Nonetheless, our assumed processes are seemingly more realistic than the usual assumption of a constant, intrinsic phage death rate, and they fall within the broad realm of mechanisms that cells can use to potentially kill off phages (e.g., outer membrane vesicles). It will be shown that our assumption of a fixed level of permanent EPS is equivalent to a constant phage death rate in mass action models.

Spatial structure will alter the dynamics in several ways [16–18], and indeed, it is likely that different models of spatial structure will do so differently. Most fundamentally, a lack of uniform densities will often result, allowing cells to amplify in zones that are temporarily phage-free. As regards phage death, phage reproduction from individual cells will have progeny phage spatially clustered at least temporarily and thus subject to a common fate. In addition, cells may find refuge and amplify behind materials that bind phage and act as phage sinks.

6.2. A Formal Measure of Whether Cell Density Is Elevated

If spatial structure leads to an elevated cell density above that with complete mixing (mass action), it might seem sufficient to merely observe cell density alone. However, any comparison of cell densities between spatial structure and mass action is not straightforward, in part because there is no single cell density expected under mass action—the cell density, even at equilibrium, depends on many parameters, such as phage burst size, adsorption rate, and death rate, to mention a few. Complicating matters further, mass action processes can themselves lead to a high cell density at equilibrium. Thus, cell density alone cannot tell us whether spatial structure elevates cell density. The effect of spatial structure must be measured via some comparison to cell density in the absence of spatial structure, a comparison that otherwise avoids confounding the many differences between the two types of models.

One such approach is to directly compare cell density when spatial structure is present to that when it is absent in the simulation; abolishing spatial structure can be done by increasing the diffusion rates of phage and cells [16,17]. This approach is free of alternative interpretations, but it has the drawback that bacterial and phage numbers often oscillate with mass action [16,17,28]. Given the limited dynamical range of cell densities afforded by the simulations, bacteria may often go extinct in the simulations even when the equilibrium density is well above extinction (see below).

We adopt a related approach, one that takes advantage of a universal property of equilibrium under mass action, at which phage and bacterial densities are unchanging. Our approach identifies a reproduction number constant that will be used to scale bacterial densities, with a similar use in [29]. Every successful phage infection of a cell will, on average, lead to one new successful infection. This dynamical property of populations in reproductive equilibrium is commonly used in ecology [30]. In the context of phage-bacterial dynamics under mass action, it means that the following equality holds:

$$\frac{\text{rate of productive phage infection}}{\text{all sources of phage loss from the free state}} \times \text{phage fecundity per infection} = 1. \tag{1}$$

The ratio on the LHS (left hand side) is merely the fraction of all rates leading to phage loss that result in phage reproduction. Since only one phage offspring from an infected cell will go to establish a new successful infection, the product equals unity on average. We denote the ratio on the LHS of Equation (1) as α. Phage fecundity per infection, known as burst size, is represented here as b. We have analytically confirmed that $\alpha b = 1$ at equilibrium in various mass action models (e.g., those in [27,28,31]) and not found any that violate the equality.

For the specific sources of phage loss in the spatial models, we propose

$$\alpha = \frac{k_C C}{k_C C + k_I I + k_D D + k_E E} \tag{2}$$

where C, I, D, E represent the densities of uninfected cells, infected cells, debris, and EPS, and k with appropriate subscripts denotes the various attachment/infection probabilities. The time-variable quantities in Equation (2) are C, I, and D, but not all models here allow infection of I and D; moreover, α is an increasing function of C and a decreasing function of I and D.

In this implementation, α is calculated with the parameters used and values observed in the simulations of spatial structure, but the value of α is otherwise interpreted as that which would obtain if the population obeyed mass action. In particular, the quantities in Equation (2) are calculated globally, ignoring the spatial structure that played a role in their generation. The extent to which αb exceeds 1 then measures the effect of spatial structure in conspiring to allow a higher density of cells than would accrue without spatial structure. It indicates, in effect, the added degree of protection experienced by cells in a spatial setting. If, for example, the current value is $\alpha b = 5$ in a spatial simulation, this should be interpreted to mean that if the system suddenly transformed to mass action dynamics, the phage progeny from a burst would infect an average of five uninfected cells. (Of course, this excess of infections would be sustained only briefly.) We have qualitatively confirmed this behavior with spatial simulations that had equilibrated by suddenly (in the middle of the simulation run) increasing phage diffusion and allowing cells to move as an approximation to mass action. Finally, in any trial, the maximum possible value of αb is b, but arbitrarily large values of b can be tested for compatibility with cell maintenance.

The observed αb in spatially structured trials is not a measure of cell density directly. However, in the absence of debris attachment ($k_D = 0$) and superinfection of infected cells ($k_I = 0$), it may be used to calculate the equilibrium cell density expected under mass action. From Equation (2), the cell density satisfying $\alpha b = 1$ is

$$\hat{C} = \frac{k_E E}{k_C(b-1)}. \tag{3}$$

$\hat{C}$ provides a constant baseline against which the observed cell density (C_o) may be compared under the above assumptions. The amplification of cell density due to spatial structure (what we will denote as A_g, for the grid model, in anticipation of defining an A for a second model) is thus the ratio of observed cell density to $\hat{C}$:

$$A_g = \frac{C_o}{\hat{C}}. \tag{4}$$

A_g is dimensionless, thus does not depend on cell density units. For convenience, and to emancipate the results from specific values of grid size, cell densities will be measured as the fraction of patches in the grid occupied by cells.

It is evident from inspection of (4) that A_g must have an upper bound ($A_{ub,g}$) whenever cell density has an upper bound. In our model, the upper bound does not arise from grid size, rather it stems from the maximum ratio of cells to EPS:

$$A_{ub,g} = \frac{1}{\hat{C}} = \frac{k_C(b-1)}{k_E E}, \tag{5}$$

where E is measured as the fraction of the grid occupied by EPS and the 1 in $1/\hat{C}$ is for a grid filled with cells.

The foregoing applies only if the causes of phage death are unchanging. When superinfection occurs or debris traps phages,

$$\hat{C} = \frac{k_I I + k_D D + k_E E}{k_C(b-1)}. \tag{6}$$

As I and D are dynamic variables, their values will not generally be the same at the mass action equilibrium as at equilibrium with spatial structure. The calculation of $\hat{C}$ when superinfection and/or debris are admitted, and thus requires some means of determining those values; it may be possible to put bounds on them, however.

6.3. *Simulations*

6.3.1. Increased Cell Densities Especially with Large Burst Sizes

Any effect of spatial structure on cell density, even relative density, is likely to depend on details of phage and cell biology. To look for generalities that transcend specifics, simulations were studied for each of a variety of EPS levels, burst sizes, diffusion rates, and cell growth rates (Figure 1). There are in fact general trends, especially that spatial structure often leads to higher cell densities than mass action, but only under some conditions, especially large phage burst sizes.

In each trial, our measure of relative cell density, A_g, as well as αb and cell density were averaged over the last 3000 steps of runs lasting 10,000 steps, so that the system should have been approaching its equilibrium behavior and any fluctuations would be averaged out. These trials disallowed superinfection of infected cells and attachment to debris: as explained above, this allows calculation of the cell density expected under mass action ($\hat{C}$). An otherwise equivalent set of trials was run allowing superinfection; the αb values were largely unaffected by superinfection, nearly always differing in the first or second decimal place.

Figure 1 shows averages of A_g from 15 trials with different random number seeds and three initial conditions (the averages shown exclude extinctions). These A_g averages sometimes exceeded 1 by more than an order of magnitude, but were also less than 1 for some parameter combinations (as Figure 1 rounds to the nearest integer, values between 0.5 and 1 are not evident). Not all parameter combinations led to sustained coexistence of bacteria and phage, and parameter combinations leading to extinctions for all 15 trials are omitted from the figure. The largest effects on A_g were from changes in EPS and burst size, but changes in the other parameters also had detectable effects. Some of the effects are easily appreciated; for example, it is expected and observed that higher diffusion rates will shift A_g toward 1, as the system gets closer to mass action—if cells and phage in fact coexist.

As expected from previous work [16,17], these systems did not always go to a static equilibrium. The trials recorded distributions of αb and A_g values for the last 3000 time steps; the distributions were narrow for many parameter combinations but were large for some others. There was no suggestion that high αb or A_g was due to large (or small) oscillations, a point that will become reinforced when considering spatially clustered EPS (below). For example, for trials in the upper right corner of Figure 1C (the highest A_g averages observed), 80% of the αb values from the run were usually contained in a range spanning 1.0 around the average. In general, there was wider variance in αb with larger bursts and small EPS values. Within the same figure panel (the same cell reproduction and diffusion rates), there was wider variance the closer the burst size and EPS values approached the extinction zone in the upper left quadrant, although trials with burst sizes of 2 and 6 typically did not show a wide variance.

All trials in Figure 1 used the same attachment probabilities, k_C and k_E. To see if the patterns generalize, additional trials considered different combinations of attachment rates for three burst sizes and two EPS values (Table 1); diffusion and cell reproduction rates were those of Figure 1C, and superinfection was again precluded. There is overlap in A_g values between burst sizes of 2 and 10 and between 10 and 60. Within an EPS level, the smaller A_g value is associated with the smaller burst (with one exception). However, there does not appear to be any single variable strongly determining A_g value across all variables. It is also clear that both large and small A_g values are not limited to the attachment rates used in Figure 1.

To address the possibility that the observed A_g values are bounded artificially by the model, Table 1 includes the upper-bound A_g value for each set of parameters, $A_{ub,g}$. In some cases, the observed A_g is indeed near its upper bound, raising the possibility that the observed value would be higher with a model structure allowing a higher limit. However, not all high A_g values appear to be constrained in this way. This argument will be addressed further when the model is modified to cluster EPS.

The table includes a parallel set of trials and corresponding A_g values for mass action in the grid model; the ratio of A_g for spatial structure over that for mass action is explicitly the ratio of average cell densities maintained under the two conditions, an empirical comparison that bypasses any use of $\hat{C}$. The major difference between mass action and spatial structure is extinction of the former. For the mass action trials that avoided extinction, none of the spatially structured counterparts had A_g averages as high as 2.0.

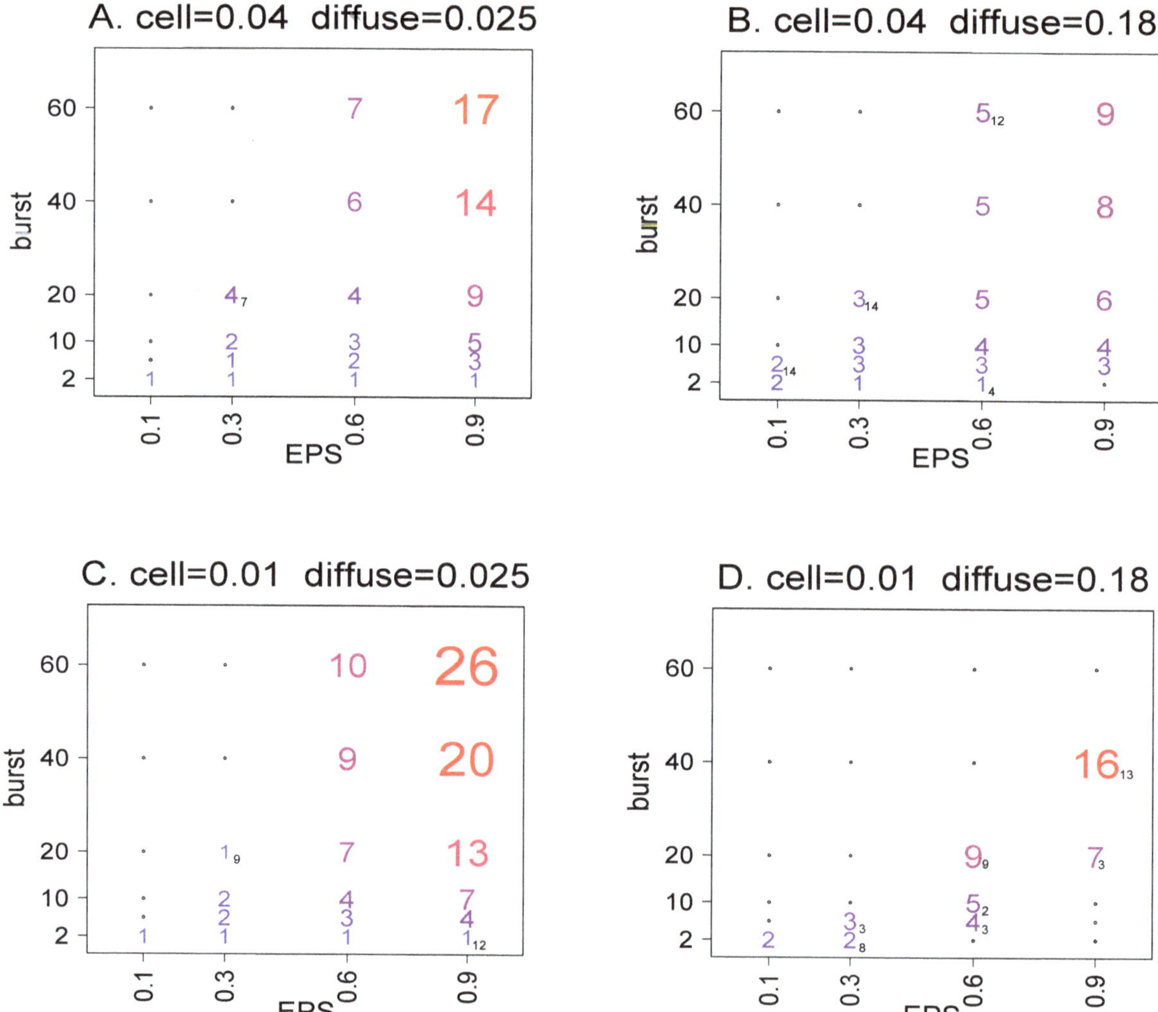

Figure 1. The density of cells maintained in the presence of phage is often increased by spatial structure. Shown in each panel are the A_g values, giving the fold increase in cell density over that with mass action. A_g values are greatly influenced by EPS levels and burst sizes, exceeding 10 only in the upper right quadrant, with large bursts and high EPS densities, and then only for some values of diffusion and cell reproduction rate. Values within each panel give average A_g values from 15 trials each using the same burst and EPS levels, with rate of cell reproduction and phage diffusion rate given at the top of each panel; trials leading to extinction of phage or cells are not included in the averages. EPS was assigned randomly to each patch at the start and remained in the patch for the life of the run; superinfection of infected cells was not allowed ($k_I = 0$), nor was debris attachment ($k_D = 0$). Each trial ran 10,000 time steps, and A was averaged over the last 3000 steps; values are rounded to the nearest integer (values rounded to 1 were often less than 1). A black subscript denotes the number of trials with bacterial and/or phage extinction; a dot indicates that all 15 trials led to extinction. The 'cell=' value given above each panel is the probability that an uninfected cell reproduced at each time step; the 'diffuse=' value is the fraction of phage that left the patch in each time step. In all trials, the adsorption probability to uninfected cells was $k_C = 0.25$, and that to EPS was $k_E = 0.35$.

Table 1. Effect of attachment probabilities on cell density in grid models.

				Spatial		Mass Action		
Burst	**EPS**	k_C	k_E	A_g	*ext*	A_g	*ext*	$A_{ub,g}$
2	0.3	0.05	0.05	1.2	-	1.4	-	3.3
2	0.3	0.05	0.15	0.5	-	1.0	-	1.1
2	0.3	0.05	0.25	0.3	-	-	10	0.7
2	0.3	0.15	0.05	3.1	-	-	10	10.0
2	0.3	0.15	0.15	1.3	-	-	10	3.3
2	0.3	0.15	0.25	0.8	-	1.1	1	2.0
2	0.3	0.25	0.05	5.1	-	-	10	16.7
2	0.3	0.25	0.15	2.2	-	-	10	5.6
2	0.3	0.25	0.25	1.4	-	-	10	3.3
2	0.9	0.05	0.05	—	10	1.0	-	1.1
2	0.9	0.05	0.25	0.2	9	-	10	0.2
2	0.9	0.15	0.05	3.3	8	-	10	3.3
2	0.9	0.15	0.15	1.1	7	1.0	8	1.1
2	0.9	0.15	0.25	0.7	7	-	10	0.7
2	0.9	0.25	0.05	5.5	6	-	10	5.6
2	0.9	0.25	0.15	1.8	7	-	10	1.9
2	0.9	0.25	0.25	1.1	9	-	10	1.1
10	0.3	0.05	0.15	0.8	-	-	10	10.0
10	0.3	0.05	0.25	0.7	-	-	10	6.0
10	0.3	0.15	0.15	1.8	2	-	10	30.0
10	0.3	0.15	0.25	1.3	-	-	10	18.0
10	0.3	0.25	0.15	0.9	4	-	10	50.0
10	0.3	0.25	0.25	2.0	-	-	10	30.0
10	0.9	0.05	0.05	4.4	-	-	10	10.0
10	0.9	0.05	0.15	2.9	-	-	10	3.3
10	0.9	0.05	0.25	1.9	-	1.1	4	2.0
10	0.9	0.15	0.05	9.7	-	-	10	30.0
10	0.9	0.15	0.15	7.7	-	-	10	10.0
10	0.9	0.15	0.25	5.5	-	-	10	6.0
10	0.9	0.25	0.05	14.4	-	-	10	50.0
10	0.9	0.25	0.15	12.2	-	-	10	16.7
10	0.9	0.25	0.25	9.2	-	-	10	10.0
60	0.9	0.05	0.15	8.8	-	-	10	21.9
60	0.9	0.05	0.25	8.2	-	-	10	13.1
60	0.9	0.15	0.15	17.3	-	-	10	65.6
60	0.9	0.15	0.25	18.0	-	-	10	39.3
60	0.9	0.25	0.15	31.4	1	-	10	109.3
60	0.9	0.25	0.25	25.0	-	-	10	65.6

Average amplification of cell density (A_g) due to spatial structure compared to the amplification under mass action across a range of EPS values, burst sizes, and attachment probabilities (k_C, k_E). Columns 5 and 6 are for spatial structure, 7 and 8 for mass action. For each combination, the A_g shown in the row is the mean of 10 runs differing in the random seed and spanning 2 different initial concentrations of phage and bacteria (extinctions were excluded from the averages, and superinfection was not allowed). Both EPS values (0.3, 0.9) were tested at each burst size (2, 10, 60) for each possible combination of k_C and k_E in (0.5, 0.15, 0.25); rows are omitted when all 10 trials resulted in extinction for both mass action and spatial structure (17 cases, including all nine trials with a burst of 60 and EPS value of 0.3); numbers of extinctions are otherwise given when more than 0. A_g modestly exceeds 1.0 due to oscillations in density being asymmetric around 1.0. The mass action assumptions were applied in the grid model, so the model parameters are directly comparable except that cells and phage were randomly assigned to locations each generation.

6.3.2. Understanding the Puzzle of Why Larger Phage Burst Sizes Lead to Higher Cell Densities

The results show clearly that some sets of parameter values lead to large elevations of cell density. The next step is to understand how this elevation happens. In particular, some patterns seem to defy intuition, such as why our relative cell density measures (A_g and αb) increase with b when holding other parameters constant. It is clear that increasing burst size will affect whether cells and phage are both maintained indefinitely, but the fact that αb changes with b indicates that some properties of the infection do not scale proportionally with burst. (αb is more easily addressed in this respect than is A_g.) Changing EPS abundance is also expected to affect coexistence, but the reason for its affect on αb is not clear. Understanding this absence of proportionality is potentially critical to understanding the effect of spatial structure on cell density, and is addressed next.

To understand how spatial structure enables A_g (and thus αb) to exceed 1 and why A_g varies with b, additional statistics were calculated for the parameter combinations used in Figure 1C (Table 2). The statistics included (i) losses of phage to EPS, (ii) the spatial association of cells and phage with EPS (probability that an uninfected cell or free phage was found in a patch with EPS), and (iii) the proportion of infections that happened in patches with EPS. As true of Figure 1, (i) all statistics were averaged over the last 3000 time steps of 10,000 step runs, and (ii) all statistics were averaged over all runs that led to coexistence.

One striking observation is that, holding all other parameters constant, increases in burst size led to directly corresponding increases in phage lost to EPS, while the losses to uninfected cells were only slightly affected. Thus, as burst size increased, the fraction of phage lost to EPS increased disproportionately. Proportionality is expected unless the association of phage or cells with EPS is changing.

Table 2. Spatial grid model outcomes with random placement of EPS, no superinfection or debris.

Burst	EPS	A_g	$A_{ub,g}$	αb	P→E	C:E	P:E	I:E
2	0.1	0.9	7.1	0.9	1.0	0.2	0.01	0.10
2	0.3	1.0	2.4	1.0	1.0	0.5	0.02	0.19
2	0.6	1.1	1.2	1.0	1.0	0.6	0.03	0.25
2	0.9	0.8	0.8	0.9	1.0	0.9	0.04	0.27
6	0.3	1.9	11.9	1.6	5.0	0.5	0.02	0.34
6	0.6	2.9	6.0	2.2	5.0	0.8	0.06	0.51
6	0.9	3.9	4.0	2.6	5.0	0.9	0.09	0.59
10	0.3	1.9	21.4	1.8	9.0	0.4	0.02	0.37
10	0.6	4.3	10.7	3.2	9.0	0.8	0.07	0.58
10	0.9	6.9	7.1	4.3	9.0	0.9	0.12	0.69
20	0.3	0.5	45.2	0.5	18.6	0.4	0.02	0.39
20	0.6	6.8	22.6	5.2	19.0	0.8	0.08	0.65
20	0.9	13.2	15.1	8.2	19.0	0.9	0.17	0.79
40	0.6	9.5	46.4	7.8	39.0	0.7	0.08	0.68
40	0.9	20.4	31.0	13.7	39.0	1.0	0.24	0.87
60	0.6	10.1	70.2	8.8	59.0	0.7	0.08	0.67
60	0.9	26.1	46.8	18.4	59.0	1.0	0.28	0.90

For these numerical trials, parameter values and initial conditions were as in Figure 1C. For each combination of burst size and EPS, the output values shown in the row are the means of 15 runs differing in the random seed and spanning three different initial concentrations of phage and bacteria. All four EPS values (0.1, 0.3, 0.6, 0.9) were tested at each burst size (2, 6, 10, 20, 40, 60); values are not shown when all 15 trials resulted in extinction. The numbers of extinctions for the data shown are given in Figure 1. Burst is phage burst size. EPS is the fraction of grid sites containing EPS, assigned randomly. A_g is the magnitude to which total grid cell density is increased above that expected with mass action. P→E is the average number of phage per burst lost to EPS. C:E is the fraction of uninfected cells found in patches with EPS. P:E is the fraction of free phage found in patches with EPS. I:E is the fraction of infections occurring in patches with EPS.

A second observation is that uninfected cells are somewhat associated with EPS (the association is often only modestly greater than the fraction of patches with EPS), whereas free phage are strongly associated with an absence of EPS. These latter observations suggest that spatial structure favors the retention of cells and phage into separate refuges where they are differentially protected from loss.

There are also apparent trends that, as burst size increases, (i) an increasing proportion of all infections happen on patches with EPS, and (ii) phage are increasingly associated with EPS. As burst size increases, the phage appears to be spreading to less protected areas and incurring greater loss.

6.3.3. Reasons for Higher Cell Densities Become Clearer When EPS Is Clumped: Cells Have More Protection from Spatial Structure

The patterns seen in Tables 1 and 2 are somewhat noisy. Those trials assigned EPS randomly to patches across the grid. Although random assignment may be realistic, it may also complicate understanding. Random assignment gives rise to varied and inconsistent boundaries between EPS-containing and EPS-free regions, possibly complicating inferences about associations of phage and cells with EPS. A clustering of EPS into a single area can overcome those difficulties by ensuring that all trials have the same boundaries around EPS. Trials were conducted so that EPS was laid down contiguously within the grid (adjacent rows were filled until the total EPS allotment was reached). This design resulted in a band of EPS on the grid. One straightforward effect of deterministic clustering is that the size of the boundary between EPS and EPS-free zones is now unaffected by the overall level of EPS. Table 3 provides values from a set of runs corresponding to those in Table 2.

Table 3. Spatial grid model outcomes with deterministically clustered EPS, no superinfection or debris.

Burst	EPS	A_g	$A_{ub,g}$	αb	P→E	C:E	P:E	I:E
2	0.1	0.7	7.1	0.8	1.0	1.0	0.00	0.274
2	0.3	0.7	2.4	0.8	1.0	1.0	0.00	0.273
2	0.6	0.7	1.2	0.8	1.0	1.0	0.00	0.276
2	0.9	0.7	0.8	0.8	1.0	1.0	0.00	0.272
6	0.1	3.3	35.7	2.4	4.9	1.0	0.00	0.594
6	0.3	3.5	11.9	2.5	4.9	1.0	0.00	0.593
6	0.6	3.5	6.0	2.5	4.9	1.0	0.00	0.594
6	0.9	3.5	4.0	2.5	5.0	1.0	0.01	0.600
10	0.1	5.8	64.3	3.9	8.9	1.0	0.00	0.699
10	0.3	6.2	21.4	4.1	8.9	1.0	0.00	0.698
10	0.6	6.3	10.7	4.1	8.9	1.0	0.00	0.697
10	0.9	6.3	7.1	4.1	9.0	1.0	0.01	0.703
20	0.1	11.7	135.7	7.6	19.0	1.0	0.00	0.805
20	0.3	12.9	45.2	8.1	19.0	1.0	0.00	0.805
20	0.6	13.2	22.6	8.2	19.0	1.0	0.00	0.805
20	0.9	13.4	15.1	8.3	19.0	1.0	0.01	0.804
40	0.1	22.4	278.6	14.6	39.2	1.0	0.00	0.889
40	0.3	26.0	92.9	16.0	39.2	1.0	0.00	0.889
40	0.6	26.9	46.4	16.3	39.2	1.0	0.00	0.890
40	0.9	27.2	31.0	16.4	39.0	1.0	0.02	0.887
60	0.1	30.5	421.4	20.5	59.4	1.0	0.00	0.935
60	0.3	38.0	140.5	23.5	59.3	1.0	0.00	0.943
60	0.6	40.1	70.2	24.3	59.3	1.0	0.01	0.942
60	0.9	40.8	46.8	24.5	59.0	1.0	0.04	0.939

For these numerical trials, parameter values were as in Figure 1C, except that EPS was laid down deterministically in a single cluster. For each combination of EPS and burst size, the output values shown in the row are the means of 15 trials differing in the random seed, spanning three different initial abundances of phage and cells. The range of values as a percent of the mean obtained from the 15 trials never exceeded 11%, except for P:E (the range reaching as high as 110% of the mean, which was invariably tiny). No extinctions occurred. Notation is as in Table 2.

Patterns are clearer than with random EPS assignment and support intuition about the effect of spatial structure in enabling high cell densities over those with mass action:

1. A_g (αb) is now moderately constant across different EPS levels within the same burst size. The constancy is stronger at smaller burst sizes. This suggests that the width of the EPS zone itself is unimportant to the properties being measured until bursts get large.

2. The span of A_g (αb) values across the table is higher than with random EPS, not profoundly so, and some A_g (αb) are consistently less than 1, even when $A_{ub,g}$ cannot have imposed the low value. Spatial structure does not invariably increase cell density over mass action.
3. Phage and cells coexist over a wider range of parameter values with clustered EPS than with random EPS. There were no extinctions, in contrast to the many extinctions when EPS was placed randomly.
4. The association of cells with EPS and phage avoidance of EPS is more extreme than with random placement of EPS.
5. There is now a consistent trend that increasing burst size increases the fraction of infections occurring in patches with EPS.
6. Within a burst size, the value A_g is far more stable than is the $A_{ub,g}$, suggesting that the observed A_g is not often constrained by the upper bound.

An intuitive interpretation of these results is that free phage and uninfected cells tend to occupy different patches (phages live in EPS-free patches, cells live in patches with EPS: Figure 2). At low burst sizes, phage are lost to EPS at a high enough rate relative to burst that they virtually only persist in patches without EPS, and they amplify when cells migrate into those patches. This pattern can be argued from the fraction of infections that occur in EPS-free patches. As burst size increases, phages increasingly diffuse into zones with EPS, where they encounter otherwise protected cells. However, these successful infections also result in high rates of phage lost to EPS.

Burst sizes measured from infected cells grown in rich media are often much larger than those evaluated here [1]. However, it should first be appreciated that our simulations of spatial structure are two-dimensional, and a smaller burst size will operate in two dimensions than in three. Since our 2D model characterizes the horizontal spread of phage, it is appropriate to think of only a fraction of the full 3D burst contributing to horizontal spread. Since the volume of a thin slice (say of thickness equal to a tenth of the radius) that intersects the center of a sphere of radius r is less than 10% of the volume of the sphere, a full 3D burst B should correspond to an analogous 2D burst of size $b < B/10$. For example, a burst of 60 in two dimensions corresponds to a burst of over 600 in three dimensions.

Nonetheless, trials with burst sizes of 100 and 300 were evaluated for the same EPS levels and adsorption rates as in Table 3. Analyses of these large bursts were reserved for the clumped EPS model because of the repeatability of outcomes provided by this model. The largest A_g values were observed for the EPS levels of 0.9: 48 for a burst of 100 and 66 for a burst of 300. Thus, increasing burst sizes several-fold led to only modest increases in A_g values. As in Table 3, nearly all phage per burst were lost to EPS. All trials with EPS of 0.1 and a burst of 300 went extinct, revealing that phage can indeed overwhelm cells if the EPS is clustered in small enough patches (no extinctions were observed for the smaller bursts in Table 3). Furthermore, strong oscillations were typical of all trials, again suggesting that, with the larger burst sizes, phages are invading deeper into the EPS-protected refuges. These dynamical effects of large burst sizes on extinction and dynamics would likely disappear with sufficiently large grid sizes (much larger than 10,000 patches) because the zones of EPS protection would be larger and thus require phages to traverse greater distances before reaching the centers of the EPS zones. From the perspective of how spatial structure contributes to an elevated density of cells, larger bursts increase the elevation, but much less than proportionally.

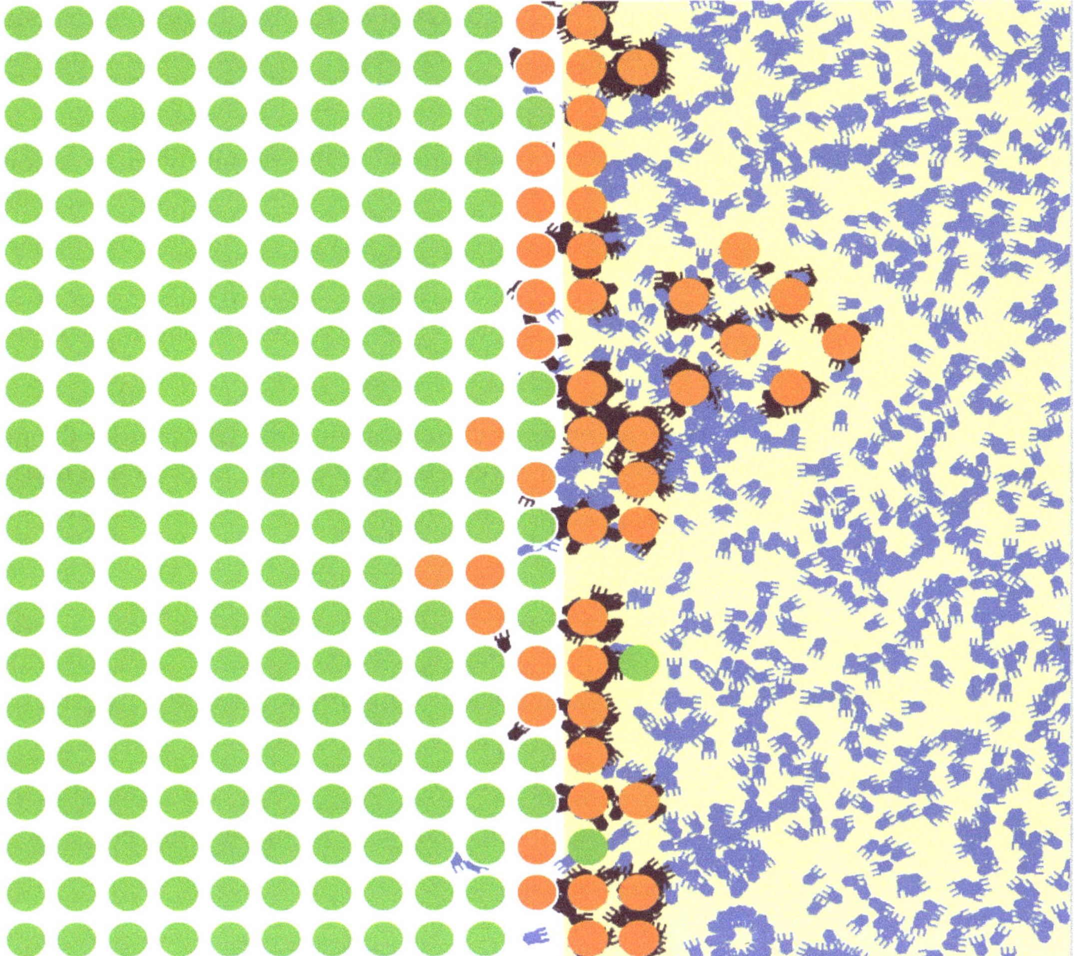

Figure 2. Illustration of self-organization of phages and cells with clumped EPS. White background indicates EPS, yellow is absence of EPS. A green (orange) circle is an uninfected (infected) cell. A blue or black legged icon is a phage (blue is free, black is attached to a cell). Phages are mostly confined to the EPS-free zone and the first row of EPS. Figure was generated from a NetLogo trial with a grid size of 21×21, a burst of 20, diffusion step size of 0.45 and attachment probabilities as in Figure 1C. There were 32 phage (partially obscured by cells) in the first three rows of EPS; αb for the entire grid was 7.26.

6.3.4. Average Densities under Differential Equation Mass Action Are Also Sometimes Elevated but Not as Much and for a Different Reason

The analysis so far has compared simulated cell densities under spatial structure to densities expected for mass action equilibrium, except for a few trials in Table 1. It is well known that models of mass action dynamics do not obey equilibrium for wide parameter ranges, instead exhibiting either stable oscillations or accelerating oscillations [29]. It is thus possible that average cell densities under mass action will themselves systematically differ from the expected equilibrium. That is, A-values for mass action may not equal 1, as has been implied above.

Two efforts were undertaken to calculate A-values for mass action: a simulated version of mass action based on adding 'mixing' to the spatial grid model, and a version based on an ODE model. The first mass action model merely modified the simulation code of spatial structure so that phage and cells were each assigned grid positions randomly every time step. However, the comparison of A-values for spatial structure and mass action is most informative when the A-values for spatial structure are well above 1, as those are the only cases in which there appears to be a meaningful effect of spatial structure on cell density. As was shown in Table 1, cell-phage coexistence under mass action was obtained only with parameter values for which the spatial structure A_g values were

1–2. (Increasing the grid size 9-fold did not lead to coexistence for any informative combinations either.) The A-values under mass action were sometimes higher, but the main result is that mass action extinction was always the outcome for parameter combinations leading to even moderate A_g under spatial structure.

The second approach used ordinary differential equation (ODE) models of mass action:

$$\begin{aligned} \dot{C} &= rC(1 - C/K) - \kappa CP, \\ \dot{P} &= b\kappa C_L P_L - \kappa CP - \delta P, \end{aligned} \tag{7}$$

with the "dot" indicating time derivative, parameters in Table 4, and a subscript L indicating the value L time units in the past. The $(1 - C/K)$ term slows bacterial growth as cell density nears K, the carrying capacity.

In contrast to the comparison of mass action and spatially structured trials under the grid model, it is not practical to directly compare cell densities between the grid model and an ODE model because of the much higher cell densities enabled by the ODE model. This realization motivates the use of a parallel A statistic for the ODE model. To wit, equilibrium cell density under this ODE model is

$$\bar{C} = \frac{\delta}{\kappa(b-1)}$$

and hence it is this quantity that observed cell densities are compared to when defining an ODE-based A value:

$$A_{ode} = \frac{C}{\bar{C}}$$

also dimensionless (the subscript *ode* indicating the ODE model). Its upper limit is

$$A_{ub,ode} = K/\bar{C}. \tag{8}$$

Table 4. Model variables and parameters.

Notation	Description	Units
Variables		
C	density of uninfected bacteria	/mL
P	density of phage	/mL
Parameters		
κ	adsorption rate of phage to cells	mL/min
δ	loss rate of phage to EPS	/min
b	burst size of phage	
L	lysis time	min
K	carrying capacity of environment	/mL

Using ODEs presents the additional challenge establishing a correspondence between attachment probabilities in the grid model to attachment rates in the ODE model. To develop such a correspondence, we used the fact that, over a single unit of time (1 min in ODE corresponds to 1 time step in grid-based model), a phage avoids EPS in the grid-based model with probability $1 - k_E E$ and in the ODE model with probability $e^{-\delta}$. Thus, $\delta = -\ln(1 - k_E E)$ is an approximate equivalence. For $k_E = 0.35$ and $E \in 0.1, 0.3, 0.6, 0.9$, this gives a range for δ of (0.04, 0.38), but the range goes down to 0.005 for the lowest k_E and E values used in Table 1. A similar basis was used to obtain equivalence between k_C and κ; in contrast to the equivalence for EPS, however, cell density is not fixed, so it is necessary to choose a density for the equivalence. Here, that density was the maximum for the system (K for the ODE versus 1 in the grid model). For those cell densities and the k_C values used in Table 1, κ was in the range (5×10^{-11}, 3×10^{-10}). For an ODE model scaled per-minute, these are reasonable values [28], although on the low end for some phages [26]. An exact correspondence between mass action and spatial models is not required, of course, because we are interested in whether any realistic mass action process can give high A-values; the conversions derived above merely suggest that the ODE model equivalence lies in established regions of parameter space for phages grown in liquid culture.

ODE numerical trials were run for 50,000 time steps using appropriate parameters (Table 5). Many parameter combinations led to expanding oscillations and premature termination of the run (effective extinction). Coexistence of cells and phage was obtained for many runs as well, typically with stable oscillations. For those, average A_{ode} values ranged from slightly above 1 to 10. The average exceeds 1.0 because of the asymmetry in the range of values: A_{ode} periodically goes up to the limit ($A_{ub,ode}$) but can go no lower than 0 (reflecting an asymmetry in the range of bacterial densities).

The highest A_{ode} averages were associated with the highest oscillations in cell densities (up to 18 orders of magnitude for the trial with an average A_{ode} of 10). No attempt was made to evaluate parameter space comprehensively, as our goal was merely to discover whether sustained oscillations resulted in a deviation of A_{ode} from 1.0. In the absence of oscillations, A_{ode} was 1.0, as expected (one example shown).

Summary of ODE model versus spatial grid model. For the differential equation model, an average A_{ode} above 1 is due entirely to sustained oscillations, whereas for the spatial grid model, an elevated A_g is not from oscillations but is intrinsic to the dynamics. Thus, the mechanism of high A-values are completely different for spatial structure and mass action; in the former, they are intrinsic to the environment and are approximately constant. In the latter, they arise because of oscillations in cell density and the asymmetry of limits on A.

Table 5. A_{ode} values for the ODE mass action model.

A_{ode}	$A_{ub,ode}$	**Burst**	δ	κ	L	r
3.9–4.1	9.0	10	0.1	1×10^{-10}	20	0.03
1.7	4.5	10	0.1	5×10^{-11}	20	0.03
5.8	18.0	10	0.05	1×10^{-10}	20	0.03
1.1	3.0	10	0.3	1×10^{-10}	20	0.03
4.2–4.4	9.0	10	0.1	1×10^{-10}	25	0.03
1.0	1.9	20	0.3	3×10^{-11}	20	0.03
1.2	3.3	20	0.4	7×10^{-11}	20	0.03
5.0	9.5	20	0.2	1×10^{-10}	20	0.03
5.6–5.8	9.8	60	0.3	5×10^{-11}	25	0.04
3.8	7.4	60	0.4	5×10^{-11}	20	0.03
10.1–10.2	39.3	60	0.045	3×10^{-11}	21	0.03

A_{ode} values for a small sample of numerical trials of Equation (7) in which bacteria-phage coexistence was observed for the full 50,000 time units. Parameter combinations leading to extinctions are not shown and often resulted with small changes in a single parameter from a parameter set in which coexistence was otherwise observed. A_{ode} was calculated as the arithmetic mean of cell density divided by $\delta/(\kappa(b-1))$; averages were calculated every 10,000 time units spanning time 10,000 to 50,000, and when the four values differed, the range is given. Parameters used in the trial are defined in Table 4. Carrying capacity K was 10^9 for all trials.

6.3.5. Debris: Adding Greater Reality Does Not Change the Trends

The preceding results from the grid model exclude all mechanisms of phage death except irreversible attachment to EPS, and EPS locations and levels were fixed. Other cell-based mechanisms of phage death are plausible and likely temporary. To consider whether our results continue to hold when other phage death mechanisms are present, we expanded the spatial grid model in include cellular debris—remnants of lysed cells that cause phage to bind irreversibly or inject their genomes non-productively. In mass action (liquid culture), this effect appears to be negligible empirically, as phage concentrations are often stable over months ([1], and personal observations). It is unknown whether debris may constitute a greater element of phage death in biofilms and other structured habitats, but we entertain it as an example of a possibly general phenomenon of local phage death resulting from the lysis of cells. Furthermore, the killing effect of debris may be short-lived, thus difficult to detect empirically, but such effects can be studied in the models.

Following [16,31,32], debris was introduced as infected cells that persisted after death (after lysing). In our trials, they were assigned a fixed lifespan, during which they could act as a phage sink in the same capacity as an infected (but unlysed) cell; α is correspondingly recalculated to include this new loss term, and, because of its inclusion, we can no longer use (3) to calculate an expected cell density under mass action. Our presentation is thus of αb instead of A, but αb is a suitable proxy. Additionally, superinfection of infected cells was allowed in these trials. The main effect of this debris model is that the dead cell is present after burst and thus is an additional source of death in the patch when phage densities are highest. Even limiting debris longevity to a mere two time steps had a huge effect on shifting the source of phage loss from EPS to debris but had only a modest effect on αb (as well as on coexistence) (Table 6, columns were added to indicate phage lost to debris and infected cells). Coexistence of phage and cells was typically not observed when debris was present and EPS was absent (not shown), but this outcome is necessarily sensitive to debris longevity (our trials assumed a moderately short life for debris).

Table 6. Random EPS with debris lasting two steps, superinfection allowed.

EPS	Burst	αb	P→C	P→I	P→E	P→D	C:E	P:E	I:E
0.1	6	2.2	1.08	0.71	1.58	2.58	0.17	0.01	0.097
0.3	6	2.4	1.07	0.60	1.83	2.50	0.49	0.02	0.218
0.6	6	2.8	1.11	0.74	1.69	2.46	0.68	0.04	0.257
0.9	6	2.7	1.14	0.83	1.61	2.46	0.90	0.05	0.255
0.1	10	0.3	1.13	1.22	3.51	4.28	0.14	0.00	0.100
0.3	10	3.1	1.13	0.92	3.85	4.10	0.48	0.02	0.272
0.6	10	3.9	1.17	1.04	3.80	3.99	0.76	0.05	0.356
0.9	10	4.4	1.25	1.35	3.44	3.96	0.90	0.07	0.343
0.3	20	3.9	1.24	1.62	9.06	8.09	0.43	0.02	0.297
0.6	20	6.4	1.26	1.42	9.60	7.72	0.77	0.07	0.451
0.9	20	8.7	1.40	1.86	9.16	7.59	0.91	0.11	0.461
0.3	40	4.2	1.47	2.97	19.71	16.12	0.36	0.02	0.272
0.6	40	10.4	1.38	1.88	21.62	15.13	0.76	0.08	0.501
0.9	40	16.4	1.56	2.16	21.62	14.67	0.93	0.17	0.558
0.6	60	13.5	1.47	2.30	33.67	22.55	0.75	0.08	0.510
0.9	60	22.4:	1.63	2.23	34.45	21.69	0.95	0.20	0.616

αb values and other properties of dynamics when debris is included and superinfection of infected cells is allowed. Dead cells persisted for two time steps after cell lysis and acted as a phage sink during this time (adsorption to debris was the same as to live cells, 0.25). Parameter values were otherwise as in Figure 1C. For each combination of EPS and burst size, the output values shown in the row are the means of 15 trials differing in the random seed and using three different initial densities of cells and phage. All four EPS values were tested at each burst size; values are not shown when all 15 trials resulted in extinction. For those rows shown, 10 extinctions occurred for (EPS = 0.9, burst =6), 13 extinctions for (0.1, 10), and two extinctions each for (0.9, 10) and (0.3, 40). Ranges of the 15 values as a per cent of the mean were mostly less than 20% and never exceeded 42%, except that the range of αb values was almost as large as the mean for (0.3, 40); some of those trials experienced large variation in αb values with occasional low numbers of cells. Notation as in Table 2, with $P \rightarrow I$ indicating the approximate number of phage per burst lost to infected cells and $P \rightarrow D$ indicating the loss to debris. In contrast to Tables 1–3, A_g is not provided because the baseline calculation of equilibrium cell density for mass action includes terms that depend on dynamics.

7. Discussion

Phage and their hosts exist in a predator–prey relationship, the dynamics of which have been modeled for over half a century. These models have assumed population structures of well-mixed environments (mass action), both for mathematical convenience and because laboratory studies of phage have used conditions that represent mass action—flasks in shakers and chemostats. However, it is increasingly evident that bacteria grown in biofilms and other spatial contexts are able to persist at much higher densities than apparent from the models, and it is not clear why. This study used a computational approach to investigate the simple question of whether and how spatially structured cell and phage growth might allow higher equilibrium cell densities than with the well mixed conditions of mass action. This question is motivated by empirical observations suggesting that genetically sensitive cells are often profoundly more protected from phage when grown with structure (e.g., biofilms or aggregates) than when grown in liquid. By uncovering the mechanisms behind these high densities, it may be possible to improve the prospects for phage therapy.

Our main findings are:

1. Spatial structure sometimes, but not always, led to cell densities above those maintained at equilibrium under mass action. However, average cell densities under mass action were also often greater than expected at equilibrium. Any effect of spatial structure in elevating cell densities thus appears to be less than an order of magnitude.
2. The mechanisms of 'elevated' cell densities are different between spatial structure and mass action. The effect of spatial structure appears to stem from phage and cells dynamically sorting to occupy different patches in the environment, with cells in patches that otherwise kill phage, and phage occupying patches that did not kill them but were largely free of cells. The elevation under mass action arises from sustained oscillations, due to a large dynamic range for $A > 1$ but A being bounded to lie above 0.
3. Under spatial structure, increasing burst size was usually observed to increase the relative cell density—to increase the effect of spatial structure in raising cell density—holding other parameters constant. However, a high abundance of environmental protection (EPS) contributed to relative cell density; phage diffusion rates, cell reproduction rates and attachment rates also had influences.
4. The burst size effect was shown to result from a curious effect of the spatial segregation between phages and cells. At higher burst sizes, phages increasingly invaded refuges occupied by cells and suffered proportionally greater losses. Thus, the per capita phage loss to EPS was higher with higher burst sizes, thus accounting for their poorer efficacy in suppressing cell density.

7.1. Back to Nature: Do Our Spatial Models Explain What We Observe?

Our efforts were primarily to look for mechanisms that might promote high cell densities as observed in nature. Having found possible mechanisms, the question then turns whether those mechanisms do indeed operate in nature. The latter question is empirical and is a far greater challenge than merely identifying possible mechanisms. Understanding of the empirical side of phage-bacterial dynamics with spatial structure is rudimentary, and our discussion of it is correspondingly speculative. It is premature to suggest that the mechanisms promoting high cell density in our models are empirically important, but they at least suggest directions of inquiry. Indeed, a recent study accounts for bacterial colony survival amid phage attack merely by considering the rate of colony growth versus the rate of phage penetration; when the colony reaches a certain size before phage encounter, it grows faster than the rate at which phage can penetrate—due in no small part to the large number of phages infecting the same cell in the close confines of the bacterial colony [33]. In their model, therefore, cells persist in spatial structure because phages are slow to invade the structure and because many different phage infect the same cell—an effect we intentionally excluded in most of our trials.

The largest effect of spatial structure on cell density observed in our trials is well short of the apparent effects of spatial structure observed in some empirical systems. Furthermore, mass action models were also observed to maintain average cell densities above the expected equilibrium, albeit that this elevated average arises from oscillations. In some natural systems, cells are maintained at densities several orders of magnitude above those in liquid systems. It could be that the cell density increase under spatial structure observed in a numerical trial is artificially bounded by the construct of the model, hence that a more realistic model would exhibit a far higher equilibrium cell density. While a larger grid size or allowing multiple cells per site could increase the dynamic range of A, we speculate that a fully 3D system would better capture the large cell densities seen in biofilms that are subjected to phage attack. Imagining our clustered EPS zone as a 2D slice of a biofilm, a 3D version would have a two-dimensional (surface) interface between the protected and unprotected regions. This surface would be more permeable to phage incursions, but the potential gain in cell density in the EPS zone when going from a 2D to a 3D model could vastly increase the dynamic range of A.

An alternative interpretation is that empirically high cell densities arise with spatial structure mostly from mechanisms other than those considered here. At one extreme, cells grown with structure may be resistant to infection. This resistance need not even be genetic [23–26]. Resistance could stem from changes in gene expression that arise when cells are attached to surfaces. Such gene expression changes could lower phage receptor densities or could lead to the secretion of protective layers.

Alternatively, cell protection with spatial structure could be an automatic consequence of limited diffusion and not even involve changes in gene expression. Thus, if cells normally secrete diffusible substances that can form gradients or protective boundaries, spatial structure would allow those gradients to form and protect cells from all sides, whereas liquid culture would not. In contrast, our models allowed protection purely from phage death: cells could escape phage merely because phage were killed before they could attack cells. That phage death was spatially structured, allowing cells to associate with refuges within that structure. Spatial structure offers many possible mechanisms of cellular escape from phages, and our models point a direction toward more biologically comprehensive processes. Empirical progress in understanding bacterial escape will obviously be useful in directing further modeling efforts.

7.2. Our Models in Context

Whereas it is straightforward to measure an average cell density with spatial structure any time cells and phage are maintained, it is difficult to use the same approach to determine the cell density that would obtain under the same conditions if phage and cells were fully mixed: the dynamic ranges of cell and phage densities are limited in the simulations, and the oscillations that typically accompany mass action dynamics lead to extinctions in finite populations, even when the average densities are well above the extinction threshold. We thus developed a metric for calculating the equilibrium cell density expected under mass action that could be compared to the cell densities observed in many of the simulations.

For cells to persist amid phages, the cells must either be fully protected from infection (i.e., some form of resistance, genetic or otherwise), or phages must die often enough to keep from overwhelming the cells. We explored the latter process here. Many of our observations as regards dynamics with spatial structure are similar to those of [17], but we took the analysis one step farther by making a comparison of the effect of spatial structure versus mass action on cell density. Another difference is that we did not impose an intrinsic phage death rate, instead allowing phages to die either from sticking to spatially static substances that could in principle be produced by cells (exopolysaccharide, or EPS), or from infection of 'debris,' represented here as short-lived parts of dead cells that persist after lysis (inspired by [31,32]). EPS, which is fixed spatially in our model, and thereby allows cells and phages to differentially organize around them, is similar to the fixed refuge model in [17], the main difference being that we have a specific mechanism for inhibiting phage growth. In our model, superinfection results in phage loss; results in our Figure 1 and Tables 1–3 specifically precluded superinfection, but parallel trials that allowed superinfection yielded similar outcomes. In [16], superinfection is beneficial to phage since it is assumed to inhibit lysis with a resultant increase in burst size; in [17], there is no superinfection.

Our chief interest in this study was to evaluate the effect of spatial structure on long-term or equilibrium cell density, comparing it to the density expected under mass action. For the purpose of evaluating the effect of spatial structure on phage-bacterial coexistence, Heilman et al. [17] provided a direct comparison of coexistence under the the two conditions. However, oscillations in cell and phage densities under mass action often led to extinction in the grid-based simulations of mass action we attempted, except in cases for which spatial structure appeared to have a small or no elevating effect on cell density. To evaluate the effect of mass action on cell density for cases of interest, we used an ordinary differential equation model, with parameters chosen to correspond to those of the spatial structure model.

To evaluate the effect of spatial structure on cell density, compared to mass action, we used the well-known principle that, in populations at reproductive equilibrium, each individual merely replaces itself, on average—each offspring has one successful offspring during its lifetime (in asexual populations). For a phage with burst size b, this means that for each infection of a cell that survives to burst, only one of those b progeny will itself establish a surviving infection. We defined α as the ratio of successful infections divided by all sources of free phage loss, hence this equilibrium condition is $\alpha b = 1$. Under some conditions easily implemented in numerical trials, this equilibrium condition can be used to calculate an equilibrium cell density for mass action. The dimensionless statistic A was then used as the ratio of observed cell density over the equilibrium cell density under mass action—the 'amplification' effect of spatial structure. This statistic could be derived for the grid model (with or without spatial structure) and for the ODE model of mass action, allowing easy comparisons of the effect of different structures.

Across different parameter combinations in the model of spatial structure, grid-based A_g values ranged from slightly less than 1 to nearly 30. Thus, spatial structure sometimes conspired to reduce cell density below that maintained with mass action, but also commonly led to an elevation of cell density—depending on parameter values. However, a similar elevation of average density was also observed under mass action whenever the dynamics exhibited sustained oscillations.

A large effect on A was from burst size (b). It was not immediately clear why increasing burst size should increase the effect of spatial structure on cell density, so various metrics of phage dynamics were analyzed, and a simple explanation was found. The environmental structure allows cells to reside in protected areas (those with EPS) and phages to exist in death-free areas (those without EPS). This is a type of self organization due to the different causes of death for cells (phage kill them) and phage (EPS kills them). When this organization is established, infections result from cells growing into unprotected areas and/or phage diffusing into zones in which they are rapidly killed but where cells reside. The balance between these two processes shifts as burst size is increased—a larger burst means that phages diffuse further into protected-cell zones, but at a cost that more phage progeny are killed. It is also clear that large burst sizes result in the EPS-free zone being essentially devoid of bacteria; this is reflected in a large fraction of infections being limited to the EPS zone. In contrast, with low burst sizes, cells are growing into unprotected zones, where they are killed by phages and where phages do not die (as in Figure 2). In the case of no superinfection or debris attachment, it is also clear that the denominator in A decreases as a function of b.

7.3. Caveats

One potentially important omission from our models is local variation in cell growth rate (as might be mediated by variation in resource concentration). Bacterial growth is known to be important to phage growth (e.g., [1]), with starved cells reducing burst sizes and increasing times to lysis [34]; a change in susceptibility of cell populations at high density requires non-standard models and leads to alternative stable states of the bacterial system even with mass action [35]. Biofilms are thought to be highly structured for resources and consequent cell growth rates [9,36]. To what extent starvation of cells or delayed spread of phages contributes to high cell densities is not addressed by our model but is certainly a worthy avenue of further analysis. Also excluded are temperate phages, whereby infection can lead to a viable cell carrying the phage genome (a lysogen); dynamics of temperate phages with spatial structure presents a fundamentally different set of challenges [37].

The theory advanced here motivates the empirical search for phage death mechanisms, especially those that operate with spatial structure. We yet know little of how rapidly phage are inactivated by exopolysaccharides, outer membrane vesicles, or other materials produced in situ. Such measurements will be difficult when phages are actively growing on live cells in structured environments, but it should be possible to inactivate cells while leaving the structure intact, then measuring the effect on phages.

8. Methods: Simulation Model Basics

Three computer programs were used to model spatial dynamics: a program written in C, a program written in Python, and a program written in NetLogo. Due to its superior runtime and versatility, the C program was used for all results presented; the Python program was written to verify the C program results. The Netlogo program was used early in the study to visualize spatial dynamics and develop intuition about the processes. All three models are broadly similar to those in [16,17].

The C code was also adapted to model mass-action dynamics in a grid model. This version of mass action allows an "apples-to-apples" comparison of mass action and spatial dynamics on the same computational platform—including finite population size and identical parameters. With finite population size, the grid based mass action model is stochastic and thus differs somewhat from an ODE-based mass action model. (The randomness actually disappears in the limit as population size goes to infinity.) Aside from the randomness and heightened probability of extinction due to finite population size in simulations of grid-based mass action, they produce similar behavior to numerical solutions of ODE-based mass action.

C program for spatial grid model. The spatial C program was typically run with a 100×100 grid of patches with no boundary effects (migration on a torus). Figure 1 and Tables 1–3 were generated using this program. All phage, infected cells, dead cells, and EPS were assigned to a patch, and all interactions of phage within a patch occurred with other entities in that patch. A patch could harbor at most one cell (infected or uninfected), but in runs allowing debris (dead cells), a dead cell could occur in a patch with an infected or uninfected cell. Independent phage infection probabilities were assigned to the entities of EPS, cells, infected cells, and dead cells, such that a phage could remain uninfected or infect only one of the other entities. Once infected, cells had a finite lifespan (20 steps).

Within a time step, phage migration from a patch was limited to its eight neighbors, with probabilities according to a truncated symmetric, bivariate normal distribution centered on the patch and with a single variance parameter, as follows. Writing

$$f(x,y) = \frac{1}{2\pi\sigma^2} e^{-\frac{(x^2+y^2)}{2\sigma^2}}, \tag{9}$$

if $F(z) = P(Z \leq z)$ denotes the cumulative distribution of the standard (1-dimensional) normal, we have the following probabilities for phage diffusion to the eight patches (of side length 1) in the basic neighborhood:

center patch: A^2 (no diffusion),
each "orthogonal" neighboring patch: AB,
each diagonal patch: B^2,
where $A = 2F(0.5/\sigma) - 1$ and $B = F(1.5/\sigma) - F(0.5/\sigma)$.
These values were normalized by dividing each by $C = A^2 + 4AB + 4B^2$ to give the fractions of phage diffusing and remaining in the central patch.

In our trials, most of the probability was to remain on the central patch (no diffusion), so a phage was unlikely to move to a neighboring patch in a single time step. Phage diffusion was calculated deterministically (assigning appropriate fractions of the phage in a patch to that patch and the eight neighboring patches), but the overall net effect of migration on the patch was converted to an integral value by assigning any decimal fraction to 0 or 1 with a random draw in proportion to its magnitude.

Cell reproduction was permitted in every time step, each cell's reproductive fate chosen randomly according to a fixed probability, and independently of other cells' fates. Cells could reproduce only if one or more of their eight neighboring patches were unoccupied by a live cell (infected or uninfected), and preference was given that a daughter cell move into an orthogonal (off-diagonal) patch. All runs began with cells distributed randomly to 30% of patches and phage distributed randomly to 30% of patches (a patch getting phage received a burst size of phage).

C program for mass action grid model. For mass action, the C program was altered in three ways: (i) after burst and before new infections were allowed, all individuals in the entire population of phage were randomly assigned to patches in the grid; (ii) localized phage diffusion was turned off; and (iii) after cell reproduction, the entire population of infected and uninfected cells was reassigned to new patches, with at most one cell (infected or not) per patch. All other aspects of the mass-action C code are identical to those in the spatial C code, allowing us to assess the effects of spatial structure using the same computational platform. There was no simulation of mass-action dynamics in the case of spatially clumped EPS since only the amount of EPS makes a difference in this case.

Python program for spatial grid model. The second spatial simulation, written in Python, assumed a 20×20 grid of patches without boundary effects. This simulation served as a prototype for the C simulation, and operates similarly with some exceptions. During each time step in the simulation, following a randomized order, each patch executed cell lysis (if applicable), cell reproduction, infection, and phage diffusion. Then, the simulation repeated the same steps in the next randomly-selected patch until all patches were updated for that time step. Contrast this process with the C simulation, where a single event (e.g., lysis) executed across all patches before the next type of event (e.g., reproduction) executed. In the Python simulation, phage and cells only diffused to orthogonal patches. Allowing for diagonal diffusion did not qualitatively impact the simulation results, as long as both phage and cells followed similar diffusion rules. Early simulations in which cells were allowed to diffuse diagonally (but phage were not) decreased the proportion of infections (I:E) that occurred in EPS under deterministic EPS clustering, and also made I:E sensitive to EPS abundance. Such disparity in diffusion capabilities of phage and cells was determined to be unrealistic, so in the C version of the program, both cells and phage were allowed to diffuse both orthogonally and diagonally. In summary, the differences between the Python and C simulations are minor, and both simulations produced comparable output.

NetLogo program for spatial grid model. The third spatial simulation, written in the agent-based platform NetLogo, assumed a 51×51 grid of patches without boundary effects. This discrete-time simulation updates all patches simultaneously according to probabilities that are based on the current configuration. It is similar to the C simulation except for the following: (a) individual phage diffuse randomly and independently by taking steps in random directions with a prescribed step size; (b) nutrient-dependent cell growth and lysis, where an initial allocation of nutrient was provided and then replenished periodically by pulsing in fresh nutrient across the grid (though the simulations used here had nutrient pulsing every time step to match the nutrient-independent dynamics of the other two simulations); (c) the offspring of a reproducing cell is placed at one of the eight neighboring patches as long as there is space available. Reproduction is suppressed whenever all these local patches are at their carrying capacity; and (d) an approximation to mean-field dynamics is simulated by using large phage step size and random placement of cell offspring (but no subsequent cellular diffusion). Trends observed with the NetLogo program were similar to those with the other two programs.

The choices of a 20×20 grid size for the Python simulation, a 51×51 grid size for the NetLogo simulation, and a 100×100 grid size for the C simulation were made because of computational constraints but are arbitrary. An increase in grid size moderately increased αb in some conditions and decreased it in others. However, the magnitude of these changes was small, and the larger grid size simulations showed smaller variances in αb than in smaller grid size simulations. For example, in one set of simulations with the C program (EPS = 0.9, burst = 60, random placement of EPS), αb was 18.19, 17.98, 17.96 at grid sizes of 30×30, 100×100, and 300×300, respectively. Thus, the choice of grid size does not affect the overall trends in αb described here.

Numerical ODE trials were carried out with Mathematica 11.1.0 (Wolfram Research Inc., Champaign, IL, USA) using NDSolve.

9. Conclusions

Phages are predators of bacteria. Their predator-prey dynamics have been studied for decades in the ideal conditions of liquid culture, where a reasonable agreement has been obtained between models and observations. More recent studies of phages and bacteria grown on surfaces and other 'structured' environments suggest that bacterial densities are often much higher than expected from liquid culture results.

Our study focused on the simple question of how spatial structure alone might allow densities of sensitive cells to be maintained at higher levels than in liquid. Our approach relied on computational models in which bacteria could escape phage only by residing adjacent to environmental phage traps, such as exopolysaccharide or cellular debris that irreversibly binds phage. We found that these types of environments could enable an elevation of cell density in which phage and cells self-organized into different regions of the environment: cells persisted in protected areas, phages persisted in areas that lacked phage-killing agents. However, the magnitude to which cell densities were elevated was always less than 2 orders of magnitude, often less than one order—and less than reported in empirical contexts. Other mechanisms are thus needed to account for bacterial survival amid phage attack in structured environments.

Acknowledgments: We thank Benji Oswald for assistance with the IBEST computer cluster. We are pleased to acknowledge the following grant support for this work: to B.R.J. and J.J.B.: National Institutes of Health Grants R01 GM 088344 and GM 122079; to K.C. and C.S.: National Science Foundation UBM (DMS-1029485); to S.MK.: Center for Modeling Complex Interactions at the University of Idaho (NIH grant P20GM104420), and the IBEST Computational Resources Core (NIH grant UL1 TR000423).

Author Contributions: J.J.B. and S.M.K. conceived of the problem, the general approach and were responsible for all analytical work. All authors contributed to one or more simulation codes and carried out trials. The manuscript was written by J.J.B. and S.M.K.

Abbreviations

The following abbreviations are used in this manuscript:

ODE ordinary differential equations
EPS exopolysaccharide

References

1. Adams, M.H. *Bacteriophages*; Interscience Publishers: New York, NY, USA, 1959.
2. Bohannan, B.J.M.; Lenski, R.E. Linking genetic change to community evolution: Insights from studies of bacteria and bacteriophage. *Ecol. Lett.* **2000**, *3*, 362–377.
3. Weitz, J.S.; Hartman, H.; Levin, S.A. Coevolutionary arms races between bacteria and bacteriophage. *Proc. Natl. Acad. Sci. USA* **2005**, *102*, 9535–9540.
4. Donlan, R.M.; Costerton, J.W. Biofilms: Survival mechanisms of clinically relevant microorganisms. *Clin. Microbiol. Rev.* **2002**, *15*, 167–193.
5. Briandet, R.; Lacroix-Gueu, P.; Renault, M.; Lecart, S.; Meylheuc, T.; Bidnenko, E.; Steenkeste, K.; Bellon-Fontaine, M.N.; Fontaine-Aupart, M.P. Fluorescence correlation spectroscopy to study diffusion and reaction of bacteriophages inside biofilms. *Appl. Environ. Microbiol.* **2008**, *74*, 2135–2143.
6. Alhede, M.; Kragh, K.N.; Qvortrup, K.; Allesen-Holm, M.; van Gennip, M.; Christensen, L.D.; Jensen, P.O.; Nielsen, A.K.; Parsek, M.; Wozniak, D.; et al. Phenotypes of Non-Attached Pseudomonas aeruginosa Aggregates Resemble Surface Attached Biofilm. *PLoS ONE* **2011**, *6*, e27943.
7. Hanlon, G.W.; Denyer, S.P.; Olliff, C.J.; Ibrahim, L.J. Reduction in exopolysaccharide viscosity as an aid to bacteriophage penetration through Pseudomonas aeruginosa biofilms. *Appl. Environ. Microbiol.* **2001**, *67*, 2746–2753.

8. Sutherland, I.W.; Hughes, K.A.; Skillman, L.C.; Tait, K. The interaction of phage and biofilms. *FEMS Microbiol. Lett.* **2004**, *232*, 1–6.
9. Xavier, J.B.; Foster, K.R. Cooperation and conflict in microbial biofilms. *Proc. Natl. Acad. Sci. USA* **2007**, *104*, 876–881.
10. Lu, T.K.; Collins, J.J. Dispersing biofilms with engineered enzymatic bacteriophage. *Proc. Natl. Acad. Sci. USA* **2007**, *104*, 11197–11202.
11. Cornelissen, A.; Ceyssens, P.J.; T'Syen, J.; Van Praet, H.; Noben, J.P.; Shaburova, O.V.; Krylov, V.N.; Volckaert, G.; Lavigne, R. The T7-related Pseudomonas putida phage phi-15 displays virion-associated biofilm degradation properties. *PLoS ONE* **2011**, *6*, e18597.
12. Hosseinidoust, Z.; Tufenkji, N.; van de Ven, T.G.M. Formation of biofilms under phage predation: Considerations concerning a biofilm increase. *Biofouling* **2013**, *29*, 457–468.
13. Soothill, J. Use of bacteriophages in the treatment of *Pseudomonas aeruginosa* infections. *Expert Rev. Anti-Infect. Ther.* **2013**, *11*, 909–915.
14. Darch, S.E.; Kragh, K.N.; Abbott, E.A.; Bjarnsholt, T.; Bull, J.J.; Whiteley, M. Phage Inhibit Pathogen Dissemination by Targeting Bacterial Migrants in a Chronic Infection Model. *mBio* **2017**, *8*, doi:10.1128/mBio.00240-17.
15. Schmerer, M.; Molineux, I.J.; Bull, J.J. Synergy as a rationale for phage therapy using phage cocktails. *PeerJ* **2014**, *2*, e590.
16. Heilmann, S.; Sneppen, K.; Krishna, S. Sustainability of virulence in a phage-bacterial ecosystem. *J. Virol.* **2010**, *84*, 3016–3022.
17. Heilmann, S.; Sneppen, K.; Krishna, S. Coexistence of phage and bacteria on the boundary of self-organized refuges. *Proc. Natl. Acad. Sci. USA* **2012**, *109*, 12828–12833.
18. Taylor, B.P.; Penington, C.J.; Weitz, J.S. Emergence of increased frequency and severity of multiple infections by viruses due to spatial clustering of hosts. *Phys. Biol.* **2016**, *13*, 066014.
19. Robb, S.M.; Woods, D.R.; Robb, F.T. Phage growth characteristics on stationary phase Achromobacter cells. *J. Gen. Virol.* **1978**, *41*, 265–272.
20. Los, M.; Golec, P.; Łoś, J.M.; Weglewska-Jurkiewicz, A.; Czyz, A.; Wegrzyn, A.; Wegrzyn, G.; Neubauer, P. Effective inhibition of lytic development of bacteriophages lambda, P1 and T4 by starvation of their host, Escherichia coli. *BMC Biotechnol.* **2007**, *7*, doi:10.1186/1472-6750-7-13.
21. Manning, A.J.; Kuehn, M.J. Contribution of bacterial outer membrane vesicles to innate bacterial defense. *BMC Microbiol.* **2011**, *11*, 258.
22. Erez, Z.; Steinberger-Levy, I.; Shamir, M.; Doron, S.; Stokar-Avihail, A.; Peleg, Y.; Melamed, S.; Leavitt, A.; Savidor, A.; Albeck, S.; et al. Communication between viruses guides lysis-lysogeny decisions. *Nature* **2017**, *541*, 488–493.
23. Lenski, R.E. Dynamics of interactions between bacteria and virulent bacteriophage. *Adv. Microb.Ecol.* **1988**, *10*, 1–44.
24. Chapman-McQuiston, E.; Wu, X.L. Stochastic receptor expression allows sensitive bacteria to evade phage attack. Part I: Experiments. *Biophys. J.* **2008**, *94*, 4525–4536.
25. Chapman-McQuiston, E.; Wu, X.L. Stochastic receptor expression allows sensitive bacteria to evade phage attack. Part II: Theoretical analyses. *Biophys. J.* **2008**, *94*, 4537–4548.
26. Bull, J.J.; Vegge, C.S.; Schmerer, M.; Chaudhry, W.N.; Levin, B.R. Phenotypic resistance and the dynamics of bacterial escape from phage control. *PLoS ONE* **2014**, *9*, e94690.
27. Campbell, A. Conditions for the existence of bacteriophage. *Evolution* **1961**, *15*, 143–165.
28. Levin, B.R.; Stewart, F.M.; Chao, L. Resource—Limited growth, competition, and predation: A model and experimental studies with bacteria and bacteriophage. *Am. Nat.* **1977**, *977*, 3–24.
29. Weitz, J.S. *Quantitative Viral Ecology: Dynamics of Viruses and Their Microbial Hosts*; Princeton University Press: Oxford, UK, 2015.
30. Charnov, E.L. *Life History Invariants: Some Explorations of Symmetry in Evolutionary Ecology*; Oxford University Press: Oxford, UK, 1993.
31. Aviram, I.; Rabinovitch, A. Dynamical types of bacteria and bacteriophages interaction: Shielding by debris. *J. Theor. Biol.* **2008**, *251*, 121–136.
32. Rabinovitch, A.; Aviram, I.; Zaritsky, A. Bacterial debris-an ecological mechanism for coexistence of bacteria and their viruses. *J. Theor. Biol.* **2003**, *224*, 377–383.

33. Eriksen, R.S.; Svenningsen, S.L.; Sneppen, K.; Mitarai, N. A growing microcolony can survive and support persistent propagation of virulent phages. *Proc. Natl. Acad. Sci. USA* **2018**, *115*, 337–342.
34. Bryan, D.; El-Shibiny, A.; Hobbs, Z.; Porter, J.; Kutter, E.M. Bacteriophage T4 Infection of Stationary Phase *E. coli*: Life after Log from a Phage Perspective. *Front. Microbiol.* **2016**, *7*, 1391.
35. Weitz, J.S.; Dushoff, J. Alternative stable states in host-phage dynamics. *Theor. Ecol.* **2008**, *1*, doi:10.1007/s12080-007-0001-1.
36. Nadell, C.D.; Drescher, K.; Foster, K.R. Spatial structure, cooperation and competition in biofilms. *Nat. Rev. Microbiol.* **2016**, *14*, 589–600.
37. Mitarai, N.; Brown, S.; Sneppen, K. Population dynamics of phage and bacteria in spatially structured habitats using phage λ and *Escherichia coli*. *J. Bacteriol.* **2016**, *198*, 1783–1793.

4

Characterization of a Lytic Bacteriophage as an Antimicrobial Agent for Biocontrol of Shiga Toxin-Producing *Escherichia coli* O145 Strains

Yen-Te Liao [1], Alexandra Salvador [1], Leslie A. Harden [1], Fang Liu [1,3], Valerie M. Lavenburg [1], Robert W. Li [2] and Vivian C. H. Wu [1,*]

1 Produce Safety and Microbiology Research Unit, Department of Agriculture (USDA), Agricultural Research Service (ARS), Western Regional Research Center (WRRC), Albany, CA 94710, USA; yen-te.liao@ars.usda.gov (Y.-T.L.); alexandra.salvador@ars.usda.gov (A.S.); leslie.harden@ars.usda.gov (L.A.H.); fang.liu@ars.usda.gov (F.L.); Valerie.lavenburg@ars.usda.gov (V.M.L.)

2 Animal Genomics and Improvement Laboratory, Department of Agriculture (USDA), Agricultural Research Service (ARS), Beltsville, MD 20705, USA; Robert.Li@ars.usda.gov

3 College of Food Science and Engineering, Ocean University of China, Qingdao 266100, China

* Correspondence: vivian.wu@ars.usda.gov

Abstract: Shiga toxin-producing *Escherichia coli* (STEC) O145 is one of the most prevalent non-O157 serogroups associated with foodborne outbreaks. Lytic phages are a potential alternative to antibiotics in combatting bacterial pathogens. In this study, we characterized a *Siphoviridae* phage lytic against STEC O145 strains as a novel antimicrobial agent. *Escherichia* phage vB_EcoS-Ro145clw (Ro145clw) was isolated and purified prior to physiological and genomic characterization. Then, in vitro antimicrobial activity against an outbreak strain, *E. coli* O145:H28, was evaluated. Ro145clw is a double-stranded DNA phage with a genome 42,031 bp in length. Of the 67 genes identified in the genome, 21 were annotated with functional proteins, none of which were *stx* genes. Ro145clw had a latent period of 21 min and a burst size of 192 phages per infected cell. The phage could sustain a wide range of pH (pH 3 to pH 10) and temperatures (−80 °C to −73 °C). Ro145clw was able to reduce *E. coli* O145:H28 in lysogeny broth by approximately 5 log at 37 °C in four hours. These findings indicate that the Ro145clw phage is a promising antimicrobial agent that can be used to control *E. coli* O145 in adverse pH and temperature conditions.

Keywords: STEC-specific bacteriophage; whole genome sequencing; STEC O145 strains; antimicrobial agent

---

1. Introduction

Shiga toxin-producing *Escherichia coli* (STEC) is a notorious foodborne pathogen that can cause severe illness, such as hemolytic uremic syndrome (HUS), which has a high mortality rate among young children and the elderly [1]. The first known STEC outbreak occurred in 1982 and was associated with the consumption of undercooked hamburger patties contaminated with *E. coli* O157:H7 strains [2]. Since then, the number of STEC-related infections, including the serogroups of O157 and non-O157 with O26, O45, O103, O111, O121, and O145 in particular, has increased every year, with an estimated 176,000 cases, 2400 hospitalizations, and 20 deaths annually in the U.S. [3]. In recent years, foodborne illnesses associated with consuming contaminated produce have increased [4]. STEC is one of the most frequently-occurring bacterial pathogens, responsible for about 18% of produce-associated outbreaks in the United States [5]. Next to STEC O157, STEC O145 is the most widespread pathogen among the top six non-O157 STEC serogroups associated with human infections in the U.S. [6,7]. In 2010,

STEC-O145-contaminated romaine lettuce led to a serious foodborne outbreak in multiple states [8]. Infections caused by STEC O145 strains have been reported around the world [9,10].

To trace the contamination source, Carter et al. compared various STEC O145 strains isolated from different environmental sources that had previously been implicated in produce-associated outbreaks including animal feces (cattle and pigs), sediment, surface water around produce-growing regions, and other environmental sources [11]. The authors found that although these strains belonged to the same serogroup (O145), they had significant phenotypic variation that could be associated with natural selection as a result of exposure to different environmental stresses. The changing phenotypic characteristics of these pathogens and/or the development of antimicrobial resistance could challenge existing antimicrobial interventions. A previous study revealed that several weak acids that were effective against *E. coli* O157:H7 were insufficient to control non-O157 STEC strains [12]. Therefore, alternative approaches are needed to prevent the spread of these pathogens.

Bacteriophages (or phages) are some of the most highly diverse and abundant entities in the biosphere, being approximately 10 times more prevalent than bacteria [13]. Phages may have different associations with their bacterial hosts primarily due to two different infection cycles: lytic and lysogenic [14]. Due to concerns surrounding antibiotic resistance as well as advantages of host specificity of lytic phages against the bacterial hosts, interest in isolating and characterizing various lytic phages is growing to use phages as an alternative to antibiotics in controlling bacterial pathogens [15]. Another study evaluated the effectiveness of seven phages isolated from different sources on the reduction of *E. coli* O157:H7 in a post-harvest setting [16]. The authors found that the most promising phage, with strong lytic effects, was isolated from municipal wastewater; it resulted in approximately 2.5 and 3.5 log colony forming unit (CFU)/g reduction in *E. coli* O157:H7 on cut green pepper and spinach leaves after phage treatment, respectively. Amarillas et al. isolated and characterized a phage from horse feces that was capable of infecting multidrug-resistant *E. coli* O157:H7 strains and some *Salmonella* strains [17]. Another study isolated two T5-like phages from food samples; these phages were able to infect different species of pathogens including STEC O152 and O103, *Shigella sonnei*, *Salmonella*, multi-drug resistant *E. coli*, and generic *E. coli* strains [18]. Tolen et al. evaluated the effectiveness of current available prototype bacteriophage intervention on the reduction of STEC O157 and non-O157 strains inoculated on cattle hide [19]. However, none of these commercial phage products targets STEC O145 strains.

The studies discussed above primarily focused on the antimicrobial activities of phages targeting either *E. coli* O157:H7 or other antibiotic-resistant *E. coli* strains; similar information regarding phages that are lytic against non-O157 STEC is relatively scarce. Therefore, the objective of this study was to characterize a bacteriophage isolated from non-fecal compost and to examine its potential as a novel biocontrol agent for STEC O145 strains.

2. Results

2.1. Genomic Analyses of Ro145clw

In this study, *Escherichia* phage vB_EcoS-Ro145clw (also known as Ro145clw) was isolated from non-fecal compost samples using *E. coli* O145 (RM10808) as the primary host strain. After purification, the extracted phage DNA was sequenced; the assembled phage genome had 4350× coverage. Phage Ro145clw has a 42,031 bp double-stranded DNA and an average G + C content of 50.6%. The BLASTn results showed that both *Escherichia* phage K1G (GenBank accession #GU196277) and *Escherichia* phage P AB-2017 (GenBank accession #KY295898), belonging to the family *Siphoviridae,* had the highest nucleotide similarity to phage Ro145clw. Further JSpeciesWS analysis revealed that Ro145clw shared an 84.05% and 83.58% average nucleotide identity based on BLAST (ANIb) with K1G and P AB-2017 phages, respectively. These results indicated that the Ro145clw genome belongs to the *Siphoviridae* family.

Genome annotation predicted 67 putative open reading frames (ORFs), of which 21 encoded functional proteins that were associated with phage DNA replication, packaging, structural proteins, and host cell lysis (Supplementary, Table S1). The six annotated ORFs in the Ro145clw genome associated with DNA replication included putative thermostable DNA polymerase I, putative helicase, transcriptional repressor DicA, putative helicase-primase, putative PD-(D/E)XK nuclease superfamily protein, and putative calcineurin-like phosphoesterase superfamily domain protein. At least nine predicted ORFs in Ro145clw were annotated as phage structural proteins in Ro145clw, including tail protein, tail assembly chaperone protein, tail fiber, head protein, major capsid protein, decoration protein, and tape measure protein. Three consecutive ORFs in Ro145clw (ORF_51, ORF_52, and ORF_53) coded for putative holin-like class II, holin-like class I, and endolysin, respectively, were associated with forming a holin-dependent host cell lysis system [20]. Both ORF_51 and ORF_52 shared 92% and 95% average nucleotide identity, respectively, with their counterparts in phage G AB-2017, whereas ORF_53 shared 86% average nucleotide identity to the gene encoding lysozyme in *Escherichia* phage P AB-2017 [21]. Two spanin proteins encoded by ORF_66 and ORF_67 were located downstream of the cell lysis system in the Ro145clw genome and were associated with the final step of cell lysis by breaking the structure of the outer membrane of the host cell to release the phage progenies [22]. No virulence genes (such as *stx*, antibiotic-resistance genes, or tRNAs) were found in Ro145clw. PhageTerm analysis predicted that phage Ro145clw had a headful DNA packaging mechanism with a preferred packaging (*pac*) site [23].

Comparative analysis showed that phages Ro145clw and K1G shared similar ORF content (Figure 1); however, one ORF-encoding tailspike protein that was present in K1G was absent in Ro145clw. One putative tail fiber protein encoded by ORF_21 and four hypothetical proteins encoded by ORF_10, ORF_11, ORF_45, and ORF_46 in the Ro145clw genome were absent in the K1G phage genome (Figure 1). Phylogenetic analysis of terminase showed that Ro145clw was closely related to the phage K1ind2 (Figure 2A), indicating a similar headful packaging strategy. The analysis of both genes encoding tail and endolysin indicated that Ro145clw had a close evolutionary relationship with phage VB EcoS-Golestan (Figure 2B,E). The genes encoding tape measure protein and holin-like class I in Ro145clw showed maximum similarity with the counterparts in phage L AB-2017 (Figure 2C) and phage ST2 (Figure 2D), respectively.

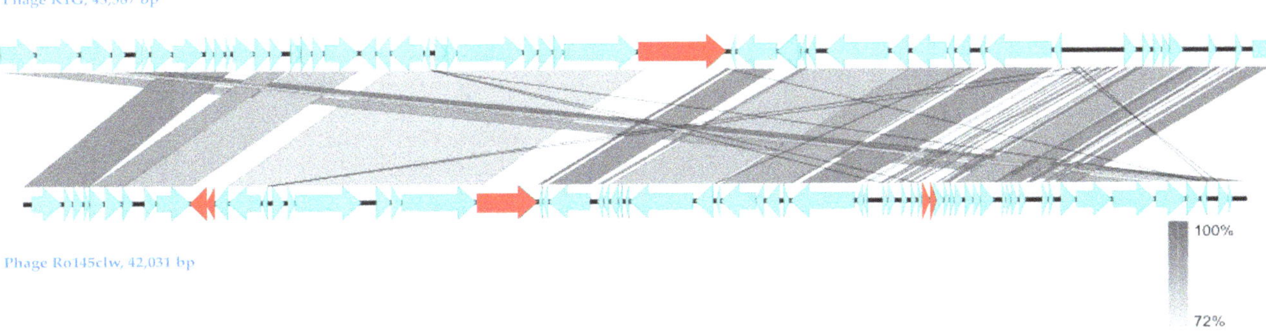

Figure 1. Genome comparison of Ro145clw and its reference phage K1G, using BLASTn and visualization with EasyFig. Genome maps of phages K1G and Ro145clw are presented as turquoise blue arrows, which indicate the order of annotated open reading frames (ORFs) from left to right along the phage genomes. Regions of sequence similarity are connected by a gray-scale shaded area, and the unshared ORFs are highlighted in red. Capital letters indicate the ORFs associated with (A) putative tail assembly chaperone, (B) tape measure, (C) putative structural, (D) tail, and (E) major capsid protein observed on the SDS-PAGE gel (refer to Figure 6).

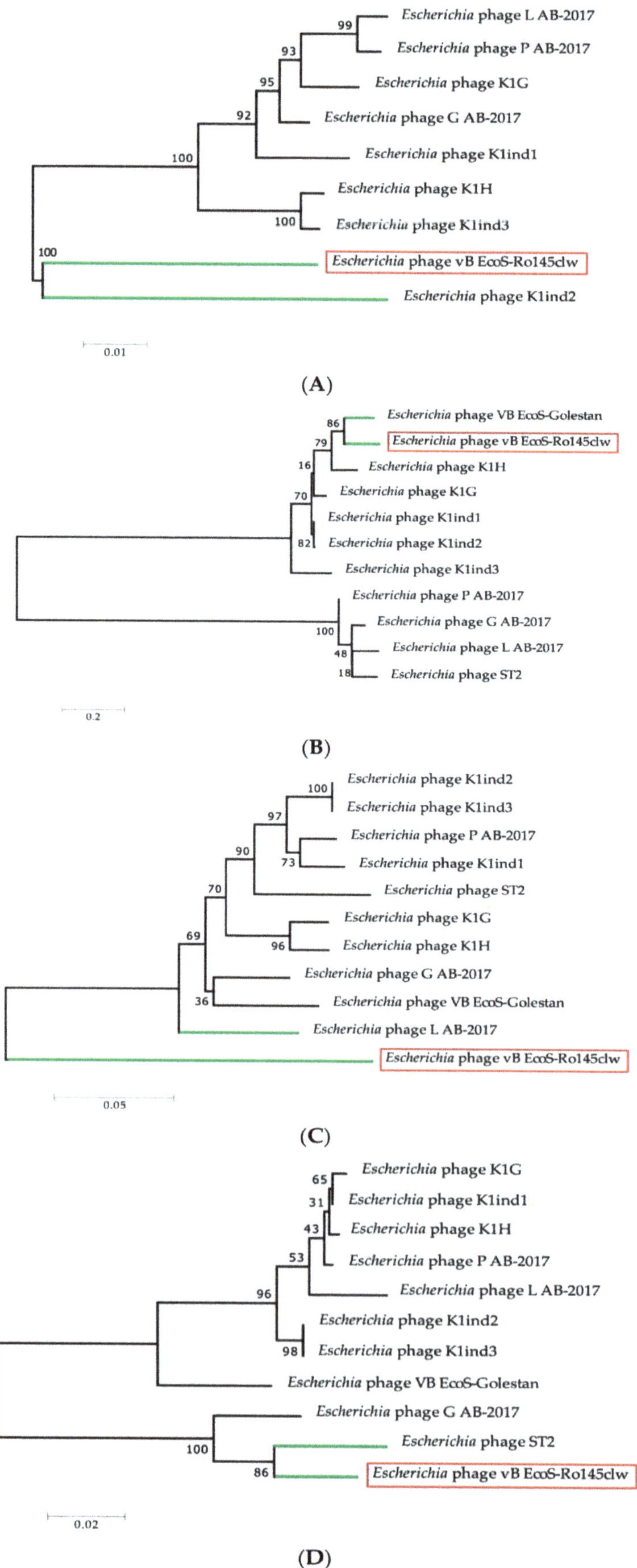

Figure 2. *Cont.*

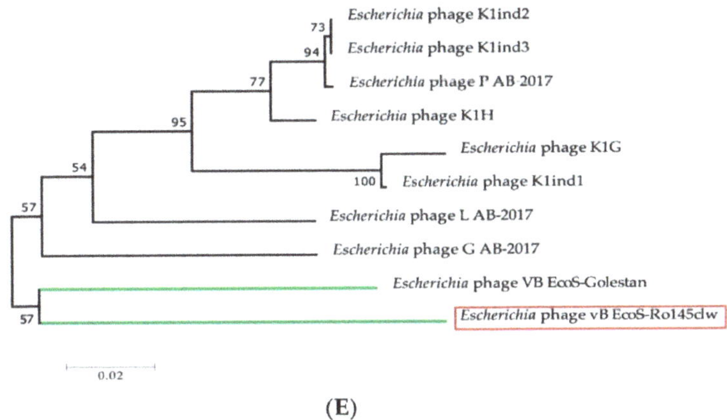

(E)

Figure 2. Neighbor-joining phylogenetic tree of phage vB-EcoS-Ro145clw (highlighted with a red box) and the closely-related K1glikevirus reference genomes based on the Clustal Omega alignment of the sequences of (**A**) terminase, (**B**) tail protein, (**C**) tape measure, (**D**) holin-like class I, and (**E**) endolysin. Numbers next to the branches are bootstrap values (500 replicates). The scale represents the homology percentage. Green lines are used to indicate the closest evolutionary relationship between the reference phages and phage vB-EcoS-Ro145clw.

2.2. Morphology and Host Range of Ro145clw

Phage Ro145clw displayed a morphology containing an icosahedral head approximately 58–62 nm in diameter and a long non-contractile tail 122.7 ± 2.5 nm in length, which is typical of phages belonging to the *Siphoviridae* family (Figure 3). Ro145clw contained a base plate structure that resembled a rosette with three to four leaves, with an estimated diameter of 27.3 ± 2.5 nm.

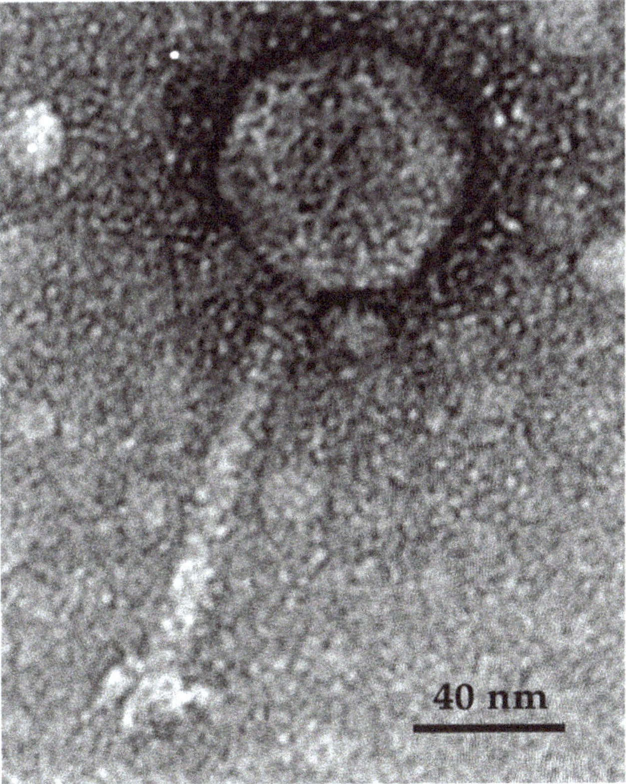

Figure 3. Transmission electron microscopy image of phage Ro145clw with a long and non-contractile tail, showing *Siphoviridae* morphology.

The results of the spot test assay indicated that phage Ro145clw is able to produce a lysis zone on the selected STEC O145 strains, with complete lysis against all the environmental STEC O145 strains, but incomplete lysis against the outbreak strains including RM13514, RM13516, RM12581, and RM12761 (Table 1). Efficiency of plating (EOP) was used to determine the productive infection of the test strains in comparison with the primary strain used for phage isolation. The results showed that the *E. coli* O145:NM strain had a high phage-producing efficiency similar to that of the primary host strain, and four *E. coli* O145 strains (RM8732, RM11691, RM9872, and RM12367) had high phage-producing efficiency (EOP > 0.5) after phage Ro145clw infection (Table 1). One *E. coli* O145:H-strain had medium phage-producing efficiency, and four *E. coli* O145:H28 strains resulted in inefficient phage production (EOP < 0.001).

Table 1. Host range and efficiency of plating (EOP) of phage Ro145clw against different serogroups of Shiga toxin-producing *Escherichia coli* (STEC) and *Salmonella* strains.

Strains	Strain Ref. No.	EOP $^{\alpha}$
STEC O26	*E. coli* O26:H18 (RM17857), *E. coli* O26:H- (RM18118) *E. coli* O26:H- (RM18132), *E. coli* O26:H- (RM17133)	R *
STEC O103	*E. coli* O103:H2 (RM12551), *E. coli* O103:H2 (RM13322) *E. coli* O103:H- (RM8356), *E. coli* O103:H- (RM10744)	R
STEC O121	*E. coli* O121:H19 (RM10046), *E. coli* O121:H19 (RM10068) *E. coli* O121:H- (RM8082), *E. coli* O121:H- (RM12997)	R
STEC O111	*E. coli* O111:H2 (RM13483), *E. coli* O111:H- (RM13789) *E. coli* O111:H- (RM11765), *E. coli* O111:H8 (RM14488)	R
STEC O145	*E. coli* O145:H+ (RM8732)	0.73
	E. coli O145:H+ (RM11691)	0.64
	E. coli O145:H+ (RM12367)	0.67
	E. coli O145:H- (RM10808)	H ^
	E. coli O145:H28 (RM9872)	0.59
	E. coli O145:H28 (RM13514)	<0.001
	E. coli O145:H28 (RM13516)	<0.001
	E. coli O145:H28 (RM12761)	<0.001
	E. coli O145:H28 (RM12581)	<0.001
	E. coli O145:NM (SJ23)	1.05
	E. coli O145:H- (94-0491)	0.29
STEC O45	*E. coli* O45:H- (RM10729), *E. coli* O45:H- (RM13726) *E. coli* O45:H- (RM13745), *E. coli* O45:H- (RM13752)	R
STEC O157	*E. coli* O157:H7 (RM18959), *E. coli* O157:H7 (RM18961) *E. coli* O157:H7 (RM18972), *E. coli* O157:H7 (RM18974) *E. coli* O157:H7 (ATCC 43888)	R
Salmonella	*Salmonella* Montevideo 51, *Salmonella* Newport H1073 *Salmonella* Heidelberg 45955, *Salmonella* Enteritidis PT30 *Salmonella* Typhimurium 14028	R

$^{\alpha}$ EOP was conducted on spot test-positive strains and is presented with a value that was calculated by the ratio of phage titer on test bacterium relative to the phage titer on the primary bacterium used for isolation. High production efficiency is EOP ≥ 0.5, medium production efficiency is 0.5 > EOP ≥ 0.1, low production efficiency is 0.1 > EOP > 0.001, and inefficiency of phage production is EOP ≤ 0.001. * R denotes no lysis in the spot test assay. ^ H was the primary bacterial strain used for isolation.

2.3. One-Step Growth Curve

The growth factors of phage Ro145clw, including the eclipse period, latent period, and burst size, were evaluated. The results demonstrated that Ro145clw phage had an approximately 14-min-long eclipse period and a 21-min-long latent period (Figure 4). An average burst size of 192 phages per infected cell was observed at approximately 35 min of incubation at 37 °C (Figure 4).

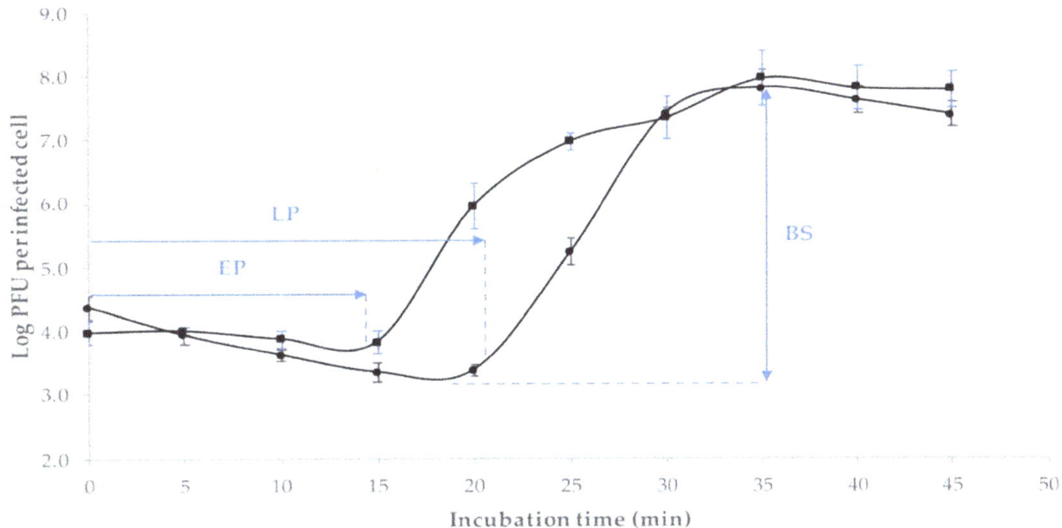

Figure 4. One-step growth curve of the phage Ro145clw using *E. coli* O145 strain (RM10808). The growth parameters of the phage indicate an eclipse period (EP) of 14 min, a latent period (LP) of 21 min, and an average burst size (BS) of 192 phages per infected cell. Closed circles indicate non-chloroform-treated samples; closed squares indicate chloroform-treated samples. The error bars present the standard error of the mean for each time point of the one-step growth curve.

2.4. Phage pH and Temperature Stability

Regardless of the different initial phage concentrations for treatment, Ro145clw was stable at 65 °C and 73 °C during the one-hour investigation, with only 0.1 and 0.3 log plaque-forming unit (PFU)/mL reductions in phage titers, respectively (Figure 5A). The phage stock with an initial concentration of 1×10^{10} PFU/mL in 25% glycerol remained at a similar titer when stored at –80 °C for five months (Supplementary, Table S2). Regarding pH stability, the results showed that phage Ro145clw maintained similar titers ($p > 0.05$) in a range of final pH from 3.1 to 10.5 after incubation at 37 °C for 24 h (Figure 5B). However, the phage titer was significantly reduced at pH 3.1 by 2.2 log PFU/mL compared to other pH treatments ($p < 0.05$). The results indicated that phage Ro145clw was able to be sustained in a wide pH range.

2.5. Analysis of Phage Structural Proteins

The separation of phage proteins by sodium dodecyl sulfate-polyacrylamide gel (SDS-PAGE) revealed five bands related to phage structural proteins, with molecular weights ranging from approximately 37 to 100 kDa (Figure 6). The identified structural proteins included putative tail assembly chaperone, tape measure protein, phage structural protein, tail protein, and major capsid protein, with coverage of amino acid sequences ranging from 11 to 62% by mass spectrometry (Table 2). Five out of eight structural proteins predicted from the genomic data were identified by mass spectrometry. None of the proteins associated with DNA replication or host lysis were detected in the SDS-PAGE gel.

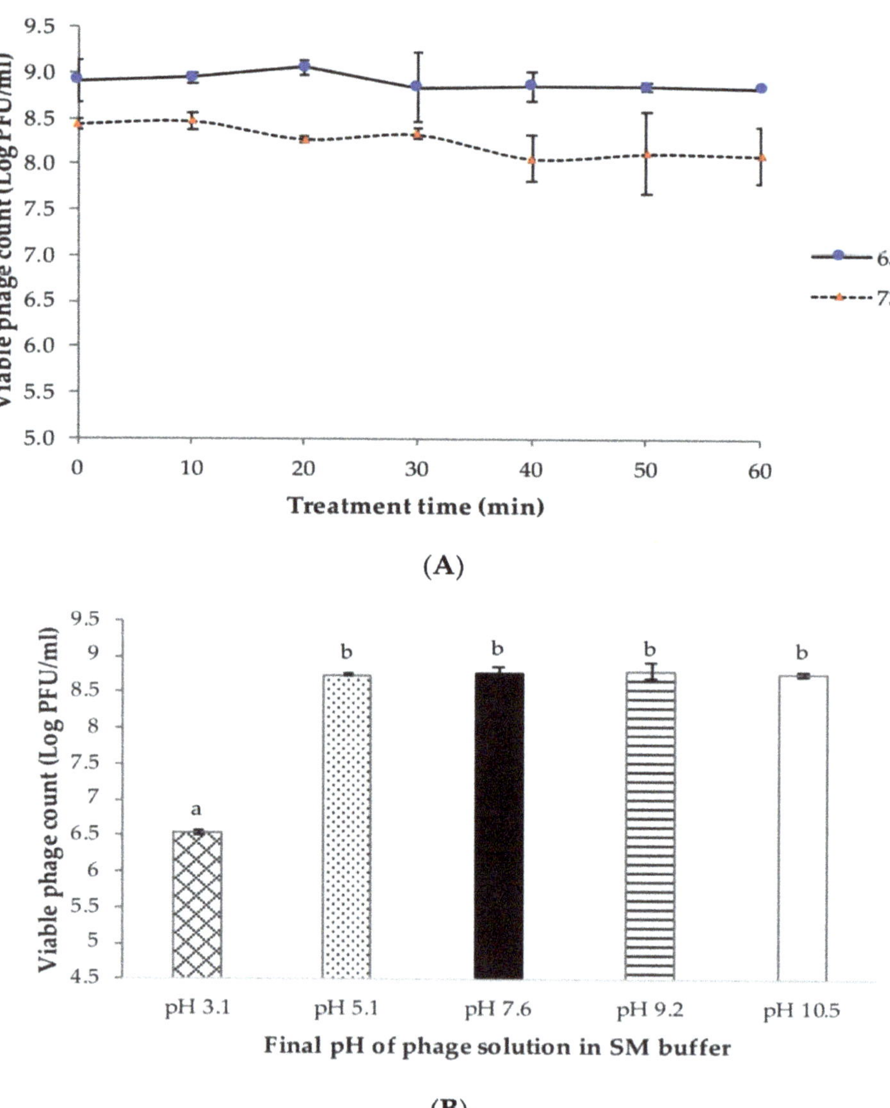

Figure 5. Stability of phage Ro145clw at (**A**) different temperatures (65 °C and 73 °C) for one hour and (**B**) various final pH (pH 3.1, pH 5.1, pH 7.6, pH 9.2, and pH 10.5) for 24 h. No statistical differences were observed between each time point of the thermal stability ($p > 0.05$). For the pH stability test, means of phage titers from different pH treatments that lack common letters (a and b) differ ($p < 0.05$). SM buffers with the initial pH of 2.2, 4.5, 7.5, 10, and 12 were used for the pH test. The error bars show the standard error of the mean (SEM).

Table 2. Structural proteins of phage Ro145clw, identified by matrix assisted laser desorption ionization-time of flight (MALDI-TOF) mass spectrometry.

Gel Band	ORF	Putative Function	Sequence Coverage (%)	No. of Peptides	Predicted Mass (kDa)
A	20	Putative tail assembly chaperone	11	11	95.5
B	17	Tape measure protein	29	16	80.8
C	62	Putative structural protein	22	8	54.7
D	9	Tail protein	25	5	40.9
E	1	Major capsid protein	62	12	37.8

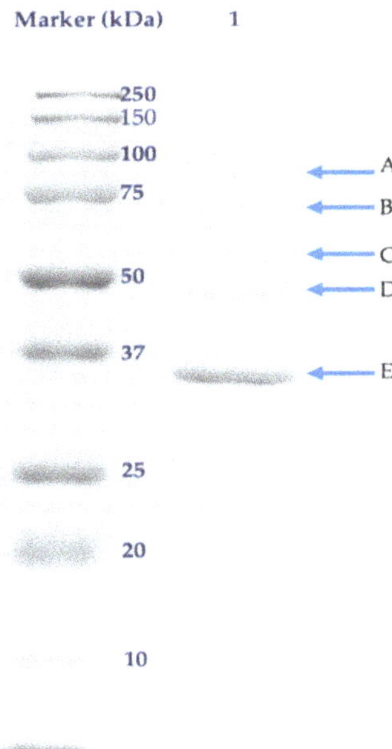

Figure 6. The structural proteins of phage Ro145clw (lane 1) on a 12% SDS-PAGE gel, visualized by Coomassie brilliant blue R-250. A = Putative tail assembly chaperone; B = Tape measure protein; C = Putative structural protein; D = Tail protein; E = Major capsid protein.

2.6. *Antimicrobial Activity against E. coli O145:H28 in Lysogeny Broth (LB)*

The effect of the multiplicity of infection (MOI) of phage Ro145clw on the growth of the *E. coli* O145:H28 strain was monitored in 96-well plates using a spectrophotometer prior to the in vitro bacterial reduction study in LB. Regardless of MOI, the bacteria of all treatment groups started to grow in a similar pattern to the control group before four hours of incubation at 37 °C (Supplementary, Figure S1). However, in contrast to the control, bacterial growth was suppressed (not a prompt decrease) by the treatment of phage Ro145clw; regardless of the MOIs, this was first observed at approximately five hours' incubation, and continued with minimum growth throughout the experiment period (Supplementary, Figure S1). Due to similar bacterial suppression between the treatments of MOI 10 and MOI 100, a MOI of 100 was selected for the in vitro antimicrobial study in LB.

The in vitro antimicrobial effects of Ro145clw against the *E. coli* O145:H28 strain at different temperatures are illustrated in Figure 7. At 37 °C, the culture of *E. coli* O145:H28 without phage treatment (control) increased 0.8 log after two hours of inoculation and reached 9 log CFU/mL after 24 h of incubation. In the treatment group using phage Ro145clw, *E. coli* O145:H28 levels showed significant decreases of 2.87, 5.07, and 3.20 log ($p < 0.05$) in comparison to the control at two, four, and six hours, respectively (Figure 7A). Although the phage-treated culture commenced growing after 4 h of incubation, viable *E. coli* O145:H28 cells were still reduced by 1.25 log ($p < 0.05$) less than the control group after 24 h (Figure 7A). The treated *E. coli* O145:H28 was reduced by 3.51 and 1.05 log after six hours and 24 h of incubation at 25 °C, respectively (Supplementary, Table S3). At 8 °C, the phage treatment resulted in reductions in *E. coli* O145:H28 by 0.82, 1.15, 1.17, and 1.74 log compared to the control group at two, four, six, and 24 h, respectively (Figure 7B). The phage was able to reduce the *E. coli* O145:NM strain with high EOP by approximately 2.7 log more than the reduction of the low EOP strain, *E. coli* O145:H28, after six hours incubation at 25 °C (Supplementary, Table S3). Additionally, the bacteriophage-insensitive mutant (BIM) frequency was $8.70 \pm 1.22 \times 10^{-2}$ for *E. coli* O145:H28 strain and $3.52 \pm 2.27 \times 10^{-5}$ for *E. coli* O145: NM strain. As expected, phage Ro145clw was more common against environmental STEC O145 strain than the outbreak strain.

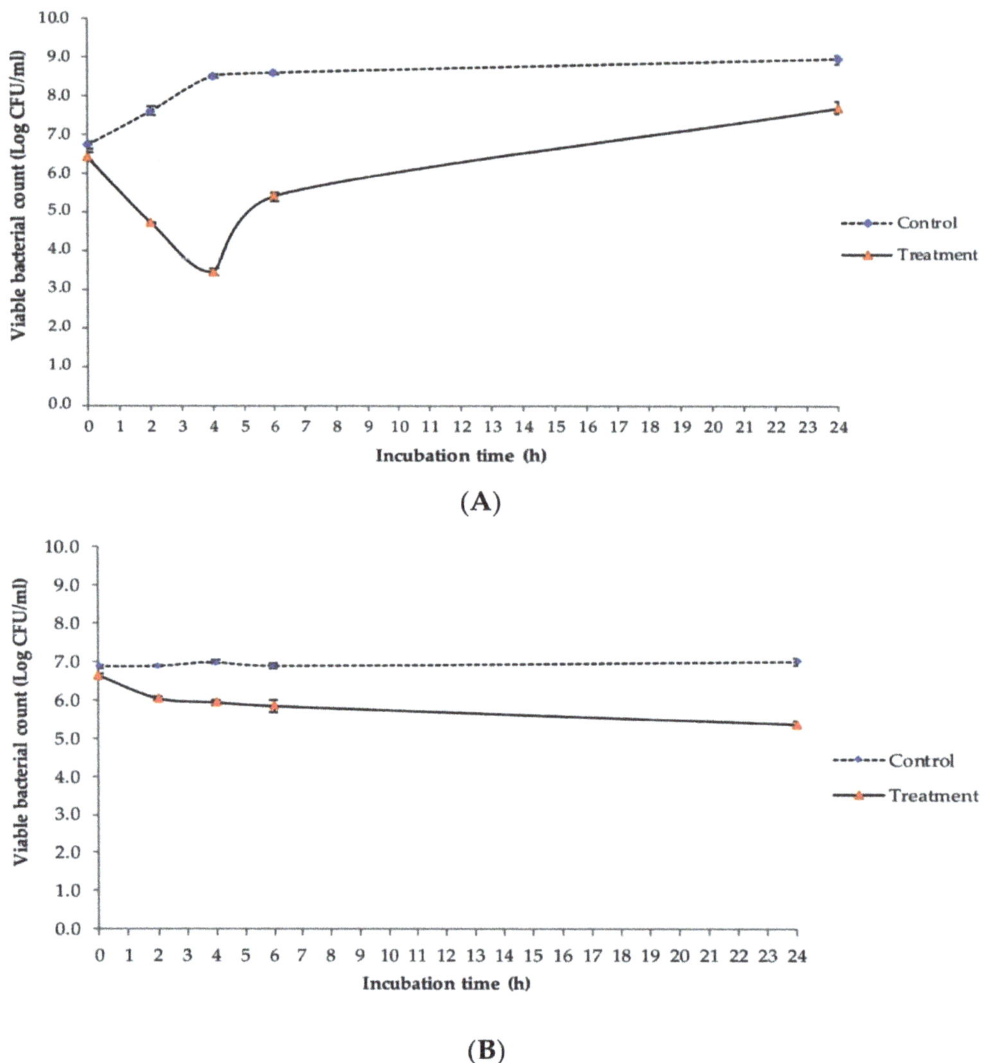

Figure 7. Antimicrobial effects of phage Ro145clw (multiplicity of infection (MOI) of 100) on *E. coli* O145:H28 (RM13514) in LB at (**A**) 37 °C and (**B**) 8 °C for 24 h. The control group contained bacterial culture without phages (dashed line) and the treatment group contained bacterial culture treated with phage Ro145clw (solid line). The error bars present the SEM for each time point of the treatment.

3. Discussion

Increasing numbers of foodborne outbreaks have been associated with food contaminated by non-O157 STEC. Although phages have been studied for their potential to control bacterial pathogens, the number of commercially-available phages and published studies on phages that are lytic against non-O157 STEC are relatively few in comparison with those on STEC O157. In the current study, a new phage, vB_EcoS-Ro145clw (or Ro145clw), which produces lytic activity against STEC O145 strains, was isolated from a non-fecal environment, unlike the majority of STEC-specific phages that have been isolated from animal-associated environments such as feedlots or fecal samples [24,25]. Though the prevalence of STEC-specific phages is highly related to the presence of their STEC hosts, which are commonly found in ruminant feces, our previous study demonstrated that various STEC-specific phages could also be isolated from produce-growing areas in Salinas Valley, CA, U.S. with STEC O145-specific phages being the most prevalent [26].

For biocontrol applications to be developed, knowledge of the genome sequence of lytic phages is critical for ensuring that no lysogenic factors, virulence-related genes, or antibiotic-resistance genes are encoded [27]. The phage Ro145clw contains a 42,031-bp double-stranded DNA genome with an average G + C content of 50.6%, but no tRNA. There are no unwanted genes such as lysogenic genes, *stx*, *eae*, or antibiotic resistance genes present in the Ro145clw genome, which makes the phage suitable for biocontrol uses. Comparative analysis showed that the phage Ro145clw is closely related to a group of phages belonging to the genus *K1gvirus*, with 84.05% BLAST-based ANI over 64% of the aligned K1G phage sequences. No *K1gvirus* phages encode tRNA, and they all have average genome sizes ranging from 42 to 46 kb, with G + C contents over 50%. This evidence suggests that phage Ro145clw might belong to the genus *K1gviru*, according to the Bacterial and Archaeal Viruses Subcommittee description [28]. Phylogenetic analysis indicates that different core genes in the Ro145clw genome have a close evolutionary relationship with different *K1gviru* phages, most likely due to horizontal genetic transfer during the evolutionary process [29,30].

Transmission electron microscopy (TEM) showed that the phage Ro145clw morphology belongs to the family *Siphoviridae*; this result is consistent with the taxonomic classification based on the BLASTn search of the genome. The phage contains a unique rosette-like base plate structure, which is not commonly seen in siphophages, but has been previously described in Rtp [31] and KLPN1 [32] phages. However, the actual function of the structure has not been well elaborated. The host range of Ro145clw is narrow and STEC-O145-specific. The results of this study indicate that environmental STEC O145 strains are more susceptible to phage Ro145clw infection than outbreak strains. The phage has a latent period of 21 min and a burst size of 192 phages per infected cell, which is considered to be a large burst size in comparison with other coliphages such as phiC119 (210 phages per infected cell) and vB_EcoS-B2 (224 phages per infected cell) that are lytic against different *E. coli* strains [17,33]. A previous study demonstrated that a phage with a large burst size is favorable as a biocontrol agent because the phage population could substantially multiply within a short period of time to control the target bacterial cells [34]. A complete cycle of Ro145clw infection against the STEC O145 strain used for isolation took approximately 45 min, which was approximately 20 min and 30 min shorter than those of phage phiC119 [17] and phage PE37 [35], respectively, against *E. coli* O157:H7 strains.

These findings suggest that phage Ro145clw has a relatively short infection cycle against its host strain. Wang et al. isolated a phage, phage AYO145A, that was lytic against STEC O145 strains from bovine feces in Canada [24]. The phage belongs to the family *Myoviridae* and has a narrow host range. Although whole genome sequencing was used to unveil the genomic characters of AYO145A [36], information regarding further physiological characterization, such as the one-step growth curve and the antimicrobial activity of the phage, is lacking. Another study evaluated a number of phages that were lytic against different serogroups of non-O157 STEC that had been isolated from cattle feces in the United States [25]. Their results showed that four myophages that were lytic against STEC O145 had different burst sizes, ranging from 23 to 195 phages per infected cell, and were also able to infect STEC O111 strains. However, a genomic characterization of these phages was not conducted and thus the presence of unwanted genes such as *stx* could not be determined. To the best of our knowledge, our current study is the first to provide both physiological and genomic information regarding a phage specific to STEC O145 strains.

Phage stability is critical and closely associated with the effectiveness of controlling pathogens during application. Previous studies indicate that each phage responds differently to exposure to external stress [25,37]. The results of this study indicate that phage Ro145clw is resistant to a pH change from 5.1 to 10.5, but a reduction of approximately 2.2 log was observed at pH 3.1. Ro145clw is able to withstand pasteurization temperatures (63 and 73 °C), and the thermal stability feature of the phage is likely to be associated with the gene encoding tape measure protein [38]. Son et al. found that a STEC O157-specific phage (isolated from bovine intestine) was susceptible to pH changes, with 1 log PFU/mL reductions at either pH 6 or 8 [35]. Litt et al. found that most phages were able to survive in a pH range from 5 to 9, but dropped off significantly when the pH went higher or lower than this range [25]. The findings of this study indicate the potential utility of phage Ro145clw in a wider range of conditions.

The genomic and biological characterization of phage Ro145clw indicates that the phage has a biocontrol potential for STEC O145 strains. The antimicrobial activities of the phage against an outbreak strain (*E. coli* O145:H28) were evaluated in LB in this study. The results showed that the strain was reduced by 5.07 log after 4 h of incubation at 37 °C and commenced growing for the remaining incubation time. Though the difference was not significant, phage Ro145clw was more active in reducing *E. coli* O145:H28 at 25 °C than at 37 °C during the first quarter of incubation period. However, at 8 °C, the antimicrobial activity of phage Ro145clw decreased. Son et al. reported a similar trend, showing that the phage reduced higher levels of *E. coli* O157:H7 at 25 °C than at 8 °C in LB [35]. The authors also found that phage-treated *E. coli* O157:H7 culture started to grow after 6 h of incubation at room temperature. This trend has been observed in other studies, as the time required for the treated bacterial culture to grow varies from strain to strain [39,40]. However, the mechanisms associated with the phage-treated bacteria's regrowth require further investigation. The antimicrobial activities of phage Ro145clw resulted in a greater reduction in environmental STEC O145 strains than the outbreak STEC O145 strain (RM13514) at room temperature (25 °C). These findings suggest that phage Ro145clw is a suitable biocontrol agent for STEC O145 in pre-harvest environments, such as those present in produce farms.

4. Materials and Methods

4.1. Bacterial Strains Preparation

Three non-pathogenic *E. coli* strains and 14 STEC strains were selected as host strains for the isolation of STEC-specific phages in this study. The *E. coli* strains included ATCC13706, ATCC43888, and DH5α, and the STEC strains included two strains per serogroup of O26, O45, O103, O111, O121, O145, and O157 STEC. These were obtained from the culture collection of the Produce Safety and Microbiology (PSM) Research Unit at the US Department of Agriculture (USDA), Agricultural Research Service (ARS), Western Regional Research Center, Albany, CA, USA. Seven additional STEC O145 strains, including four outbreak strains and five *Salmonella* strains (also obtained from the PSM culture collection), were used to test the antimicrobial activity of the phage (Supplementary, Table S4). All STEC strains were previously isolated from different environmental samples, such as water and animal feces, and were further confirmed with the presence of *eae* and *stx* genes. Fresh cultures of the strains were prepared by inoculating a sterile 5 mL tryptic soy broth (TSB; Difco, Becton Dickinson, Sparks, MD USA) with a loopful of the individual strain, and were incubated overnight at 37 °C prior to use.

4.2. Bacteriophage Isolation

Non-fecal compost samples, derived from composted food scraps and yard trimmings, were collected from a composting operation. For phage isolation, the samples were enriched with a 14-strain STEC cocktail and a 3-strain non-pathogenic *E. coli* cocktail in TSB, supplemented with 10% calcium chloride solution at 37 °C overnight. After centrifugation at 8000× *g*, the supernatant was obtained and used to confirm the presence of STEC-specific phages using a spot test assay against each individual strain of the 14 STEC strains (Supplementary, Table S4). The fresh overnight culture of each STEC strain (0.1 mL) was mixed with 12 mL molten tryptic soy agar (TSA, Difco, Becton Dickinson, Sparks, MD, USA) and poured into a sterile Petri plate. After the strain-mixed agar solidified, 10 μL of the supernatant (obtained from the enrichment) were spotted on the TSA plate and incubated at 37 °C for 24 h. As a result, the supernatant was positive against the STEC O145 strain (RM10808) and further subjected to the phage purification process using a single-layer plaque assay as previously described, with minor modifications [26]. The single-layer plaque assay was conducted immediately after picking a plaque from the previous plaque assay plate for at least three runs, until the plaques were a similar size on the plate. After purification, the phage was propagated with the fresh overnight culture of the STEC O145 host (RM10808) in 40 mL TSB, supplemented with 10 mM of $CaCl_2$ at 37 °C for 24 h. The propagated phage was centrifuged at 8000× *g* for 10 min and filtered through a 0.22-μm filter membrane to remove bacterial debris. The purified phages were subsequently concentrated using a 100 kDa cut-off Amicon Ultra-15 Centrifugal Filter Unit (Merck Millipore, Billerica, MA, USA) prior to downstream analyses such as transmission electron microscopy (TEM) and DNA extraction.

4.3. Whole-Genome Sequencing and Genomic Analysis

Phage DNA was extracted using a phage DNA extraction kit from Norgen Biotek (Thorold, ON, Canada). The DNA library was prepared using a TruSeq Nano DNA Library Prep Kit (Illumina, San Deigo, CA, USA), and the final amplified libraries were quantified by a bioanalyzer (Agilent, Santa Clara, CA, USA) before sequencing. Approximately 6 million 2 × 250 bp pair-end sequence reads were generated using a MisSq Reagent Kit v3 (600-cycle) on the MiSeq platform (Illumina, San Deigo, CA, USA). The quality of raw sequence reads was first checked using FASTQC. The poor sequence reads (below Q30) were then trimmed using Trimmomatic (Galaxy Version 0.36.5, with the setting of average quality required for 30 (= Q30) to trim poor quality reads). A de novo assembly of the resulting quality reads was conducted using Unicycler Galaxy v0.4.6.0 (SPAdes) with default parameters. The final contig was annotated by Prokka (v.1.12.0) with default parameters, followed by manual characterization with PHASTER Webserver [41] and BLASTn against the viral nucleotide sequences obtained from National Center for Biotechnology Information (NCBI) with Geneious (v11.0.4).

The annotated functions of the putative ORFs were confirmed using BLASTp. The prediction of tRNA in the phage genome was accomplished using tRNAscan-SE Search Server [42]. The phage termini and the possible packaging mechanism were predicted according to the in silico determination method proposed in PhageTerm [43]. The new phage sequence was subjected to a BLASTn search to obtain reference phage genomes with high nucleotide similarity from the NCBI database. These reference phage genomes were subjected to analysis with JSpeciesWS [44] to facilitate the taxonomic classification of the newly-isolated phage based on the degree of nucleotide sequence similarity [28]. The comparison of genome maps between phage Ro145clw and its reference genomes was visualized with the EasyFig visualization tool [45]. The presence of antibiotic-resistance genes in the phage genome was identified using the ResFinder (version 3.0) database [46]. Core gene analysis was conducted with CoreGenes3.5 Webserver, and genes with scores higher than 75 were considered core genes [47]. Comparative analysis of the core genes was conducted using the ClustalW algorithm for sequence alignment [48]. The phylogenetic tree was performed with MEGA 7 with the maximum composite likelihood method [49]. The reference phage genomes used in this study of *Escherichia* phage K1G (GenBank accession #GU196277), *Escherichia* phages ST2 (GenBank accession #MF153391), *Escherichia* phage G AB-2017 (GenBank accession #KY295895), and *Escherichia* phage P AB-2017 (GenBank accession #KY295898) were obtained from the NCBI database.

4.4. Biological Characteristics

4.4.1. One-Step Growth Curve

The experiment of a one-step growth curve was performed following the procedures described in Amarillas et al., with subtle modification [17]. The STEC O145 strain was inoculated in TSB and incubated at 37 °C overnight, then sub-cultured in 20 mL TSB at 37 °C until optical density at 600 nm (OD_{600}) was 0.5. Subsequently, phage Ro145clw was added to a bacterial suspension at a MOI of 0.01, and the phage-bacteria mixture was kept at room temperature for 2 min for phage adsorption onto the bacterial cells. After the 2-min adsorption period, the mixture was centrifuged at 10,000× *g* for one minute at 4 °C. The supernatant was removed, and the phage titers were obtained to calculate the residual titers of the phages. The bacterial pellet containing infected strains was gently re-suspended in 20 mL TSB and incubated at 37 °C for 1 h, with sampling at 5-min intervals. At each sampling point, an aliquot of 1 mL of sample was obtained and centrifuged at 10,000× *g* for 30 s at 4 °C, followed by filtration through a 0.22-μm pore-size membrane filter, then a single-layer plaque assay, as described above in duplication. Simultaneously, an additional aliquot of 1 mL phage-infected culture was collected at each time point and treated with $CHCl_3$. After homogenization for 2 min and centrifugation at 10,000× *g* for 2 min, the supernatant was obtained and subjected to serial dilutions prior to the single-layer plaque assay to determine the eclipse period. This entire experiment was conducted in three replications to estimate the burst size and latent period. The latent period was determined as the time that elapsed between the end of adsorption and the first release of phage progeny. The eclipse period was determined as the time period that elapsed between the end of adsorption and the appearance of phage particles within the bacterial cell. Burst size was calculated as the ratio of total number of phage particles produced to the initial number of infected bacterial cells during the latent period [50].

4.4.2. Transmission Electronic Microscopy

The concentrated phage was used to examine the phage morphology with a transmission electron microscope (FEI Tecnai G2). An aliquot of 6 μL was placed on copper mesh PLECO grids (Ted Pella Inc., Redding, CA, USA) and left to set for 1 min at room temperature. Whatman filter paper was used to remove excessive phage lysate, followed by negative staining with an added 8 μL of 0.75% uranyl acetate (Sigma-Aldrich, Darmstadt, Germany) for 30 s staining at room temperature.

4.4.3. Phage Stability

To examine pH susceptibility, 100 μL of the phage lysate was added to 900 μL of SM buffer with the final pH levels of 3.1, 5.1, 7.6, 9.2, and 10.5. Samples were incubated at 37 °C for 24 h. Viable phage particles were enumerated using the plaque assay. For the temperature test, phage lysate was added to SM buffer at a volume ratio of 1:9, and 1 mL of the phage solution was dispensed in sterile tubes prior to thermal treatments (65 and 73 °C). The phage titers were determined by the single-layer plaque assay every 10 min for 60 min. These temperatures were selected to evaluate the stability of Ro145clw in high-temperature processes such as pasteurization. The course of thermal treatment time (60 min) was selected to evaluate the short-term thermal stability of phage Ro145clw. For the stability of frozen storage, an aliquot of 500 μL phage lysate was mixed with glycerol at a final concentration of 25% and stored at −80 °C.

4.5. Structural Protein Analysis

The purified and concentrated phage lysate was subjected to sodium dodecyl sulfate polyacrylamide gel electrophoresis (SDS-PAGE) using a 1D Biorad 12% TGX gel with Precision Plus MW standard marker (2 μL; Biorad, Hercules, CA, USA). Electrophoresis was performed at 100 V for 90 min. The gel was stained using an Imperial™ Protein Stain (ThermoFisher, Waltham, MA, USA) containing a formulation of Coomassie brilliant blue R-250. In-gel digestions were conducted with Trypsin (Promega, Madison, WI, USA) using a Digest Pro digestion robot (Intavis, Köln, Germany). The robot was programmed to perform the in-gel digestion following methods that have been previously published [51,52]. Digested samples were subjected to nanoflow reversed-phase chromatography with an Eksigent NanoLC (Sciex, Framingham, MA, USA) using Picochip 105 mm columns packed with REPROSIL-Pur C18-AQ, 3 μM, 120A packing (New Objectives, Woburn, MA, USA). A 10 μL portion of each digested sample was injected with 2% acetonitrile in water with 0.1% formic acid, with a flow rate of 400 nL/min for 1 h. Elution solvents A and B were 2% acetonitrile in water and acetonitrile, respectively (each containing 0.1% formic acid). Sample elution began with 3% B, ramping up to 10% B at 10 min, then to 25% B at 40 min, then to 40% B at 58 min, returning to 3% B at 60 min. Mass spectral analyses were performed with an Orbitrap Elite (Thermo Fisher Scientific, Waltham, MA, USA), operated in positive ion mode using a top three data-dependent data acquisition method. Survey scans were collected at 60 K resolution in the Orbitrap detector. The top three most intense ions above the threshold of 30 K counts were subjected to collision-induced fragmentation (CID) with normalized collision energy set to 30. The resulting fragment ions were detected in the instrument's linear trap. Dynamic exclusion of precursor ions was set to 6 s. Mascot software (Matrix Science,

Boston, MA, USA) was used to match the tandem mass spectrometry (MS–MS) data to amino acid sequences derived from the nucleotide sequences that were obtained from the phage isolates.

4.6. Antimicrobial Activities

4.6.1. Host Range and Efficiency of Plating

After phage purification, the phage was subjected to the host range test against three non-pathogenic *E. coli*, 28 STEC and five *Salmonella* strains using the spot test assay as described above. For the spot test-positive strains, efficiency of plating (EOP) was used to determine productive infection by using phage particles produced against each susceptible strain in comparison to the phage particles produced against the primary host strain [53]. Fresh overnight cultures of the test strains and of the primary host strain were prepared in TSB at 37 °C for 18 h. After serial dilution, the phage lysates with four dilution factors (10^{-3} to 10^{-7}) were subjected to the single-layer plaque assay separately against all test strains and the primary host strain. The plates were then incubated at 37 °C overnight. The experiment was conducted in three replications. EOP was calculated based on the average of plaque-forming units (PFU) against each test bacterium divided by the average of PFU against the primary bacterium used for isolation. Generally, if the EOP was 0.5 or more, it was classified as having a high phage-producing efficiency. An EOP above 0.1 but below 0.5 indicated a medium-producing efficiency; an EOP between 0.001 and 0.1 indicated a low-producing efficiency; any value under 0.001 represented inefficient phage production.

4.6.2. Bacterial Challenge Assay

The bacterial challenge assay was conducted using a spectrophotometer to monitor bacterial growth treated with different concentrations of phage lysate as previously described, with minor modifications [54]. Prior to the experiment, a fresh overnight culture of *E. coli* O145:H28 was prepared in 5 mL of TSB and incubated at 37 °C for 18 h. Subsequently, the culture was pelleted down at 4000× *g* centrifugation and washed twice with the same volume of fresh TSB. After resuspension in TSB, the bacterial culture was diluted down to 1×10^5 CFU/mL and further dispensed into a 96-well plate, with 200 μL per well; then, phage Ro145clw was added at MOIs of 1, 10, and 100. The plate was monitored in a plate reader with the temperature set at 37 °C. The OD_{600} reading was recorded every 30 min for 18 h.

4.6.3. Determination of Bacteriophage-Insensitive Mutant (BIM) Frequency

The emergence frequency of bacteriophage-insensitive mutant (BIM) was conducted by mixing appropriate volume of overnight cultures of STEC strains [*E. coli* O145:H28 (RM13514) and *E. coli* O145:NM (SJ23)] with phage Ro145clw at MOI of 100. The mixture was added with $CaCl_2$ (10 mM) and $MgSO_4$ (10mM) and then incubated at 37 °C for 10 min. After serial dilutions, the diluted bacterium-phage mixture was plated on MacConkey agar with a top thin layer of TSA (5 mL) and incubated at 37 °C overnight. BIM frequency was determined by dividing the number of surviving bacterial cells by the initial bacterial concentration. The experiments were conducted in 3 replications.

4.6.4. Antimicrobial Activity Test in LB

A fresh overnight culture of *E. coli* O145:H28 was prepared in 10 mL TSB at 37 °C for 18 h. An aliquot of 0.2 mL overnight culture was added to 18.8 mL LB (Invitrogen, Carlsbad, CA, USA) to obtain the final concentration at 1×10^7 CFU/mL. One tube of the bacterial suspension was treated with phage lysates at 1×10^9 PFU/mL (MOI 100). A control group was also prepared by adding the same volume of SM buffer to 20 mL of bacterial suspension. Both the control and treatment were incubated at 8 and 37 °C. At 0, 2, 4, 6, and 24 h of incubation, samples were serially diluted using sterile 0.1% peptone water, and an aliquot of 0.1 mL diluted sample was spread-plated on MacConkey agar plates (BD, Franklin Lakes, NJ, USA). The plates were incubated at 37 °C overnight, and colonies of bacteria were counted. The antimicrobial effects of the phage against *E. coli* O145:H28 (representing a low EOP) and *E. coli* O145: NM (high EOP) were compared using the same method as described at 25 °C.

4.6.5. Statistical Analysis

Experiments were performed with at least three individual repetitions. Bacterial colony counts and phage titers were calculated as CFU/mL or PFU/mL and logarithmically transformed for statistical analysis. Least squares mean (LSM) was performed to compare the means of phage titers using JMP® (Version 12.0.1, SAS Institute Inc., Cary, NC, USA). One-way analysis of variance (ANOVA) with the statistical significance at 5% level was used to evaluate the effects of different pH on the recovery of phage titers. The Student's *t*-test was used to evaluate the viable bacterial count between the control group and treatment group with the phage at each time point.

4.7. Nucleotide Sequence Accession Number

The genome sequence of *Escherichia* phage vB_EcoS-Ro145clw was deposited in GenBank under accession number MG852086. The raw sequence reads were submitted to the NCBI sequence read archive (SRA) with accession number PRJNA525899.

5. Conclusions

In this study, phage Ro145clw, with strong lytic infection against environmental STEC O145 strains, was shown to have a relatively short latent period (21 min) and a large burst size (192 phages per infected cell). The genomic data indicated the absence of unwanted genes including virulence genes, antibiotic-resistance genes, and lysogenic genes in the Ro145clw genome. Phage Ro145clw is resistant to adverse pH and temperature conditions; these features might be associated with the environment from which the phage was isolated. The antimicrobial effects of the phage against environmental STEC O145 strains were more prominent than against outbreak strains. These findings substantiate the potential biocontrol alternative of the phage Ro145clw to prevent the spread of STEC O145 in the pre-harvest environment. The genomic information for phage Ro145clw provides valuable insights into the diversity of the specific lytic phages against STEC strains. Future studies in using phage cocktails may be undertaken to improve the biocontrol effectiveness against outbreak STEC strains.

Supplementary Materials:
Figure S1: Bacterial challenge assay of the phage Ro145clw against outbreak strain *E. coli* O145:H28; Table S1: List of annotated ORFs with the size, location, and predicted functions in the genome of Ro145clw; Table S2: Storage evaluation of phage Ro145clw in 25% glycerol at −80 °C for five months; Table S3: Comparison of the antimicrobial activities of phage Ro145clw (MOI of 100) against different EOP bacterial strains (initial concentration = 7 log CFU/mL) in LB at 25 °C; Table S4: Bacterial strains including *E. coli* and *Salmonella* were used in the present study for either phage isolation or the host range test of the isolated phage.

Author Contributions: Conceptualization, V.C.H.W.; Methodology, Y.-T.L.; Software, R.W.L. and Y.-T.L.; Formal Analysis, R.W.L. and Y.-T.L.; Resources, V.C.H.W.; Data Curation, R.W.L., Y.-T.L., L.A.H., V.M.L. and F.L.; Writing-Original Draft Preparation, Y.-T.L.; Investigation, Y.-T.L., A.S., L.A.H., F.L. and V.M.L.; Writing-Review & Editing, V.C.H.W. and Y.-T.L.; Supervision, V.C.H.W.; Project Administration, V.C.H.W.; Funding Acquisition, V.C.H.W.

Acknowledgments: The authors would like to thank Anne Bates for her assistance in generating part of the host range test and EOP data.

References

1. Tarr, P.I.; Gordon, C.A.; Chandler, W.L. Shiga-toxin-producing *Escherichia coli* and haemolytic uraemic syndrome. *Lancet* **2005**, *365*, 1073–1086. [CrossRef]

2. Riley, L.W.; Remis, R.S.; Helgerson, S.D.; McGee, H.B.; Wells, J.G.; Davis, B.R.; Hebert, R.J.; Olcott, E.S.; Johnson, L.M.; Hargrett, N.T.; et al. Hemorrhagic colitis associated with a rare *Escherichia coli* serotype. *N. Engl. J. Med.* **1983**, *308*, 681–685. [CrossRef] [PubMed]
3. Scallan, E.; Hoekstra, R.M.; Angulo, F.J.; Tauxe, R.V.; Widdowson, M.-A.; Roy, S.L.; Jones, J.L.; Griffin, P.M. Foodborne illness acquired in the United States–Major pathogens. *Emerg. Infect. Dis.* **2011**, *17*, 7–15. [CrossRef] [PubMed]
4. Karmali, M.A. Emerging Public Health Challenges of Shiga Toxin-Producing *Escherichia coli* Related to Changes in the Pathogen, the Population, and the Environment. *Clin. Infect. Dis.* **2017**, *64*, 371–376. [CrossRef] [PubMed]
5. Herman, K.M.; Hall, A.J.; Gould, L.H. Outbreaks attributed to fresh leafy vegetables, United States, 1973–2012. *Epidemiol. Infect.* **2015**, *143*, 3011–3021. [CrossRef] [PubMed]
6. Brooks, J.T.; Sowers, E.G.; Wells, J.G.; Greene, K.D.; Griffin, P.M.; Hoekstra, R.M.; Strockbine, N.A. Non-O157 Shiga toxin-producing *Escherichia coli* infections in the United States, 1983–2002. *J. Infect. Dis.* **2005**, *192*, 1422–1429. [CrossRef] [PubMed]
7. Luna-Gierke, R.E.; Griffin, P.M.; Gould, L.H.; Herman, K.; Bopp, C.A.; Strockbine, N.; Mody, R.K. Outbreaks of non-O157 Shiga toxin-producing *Escherichia coli* infection: USA. *Epidemiol. Infect.* **2014**, *142*, 2270–2280. [CrossRef] [PubMed]
8. Taylor, E.V.; Nguyen, T.A.; Machesky, K.D.; Koch, E.; Sotir, M.J.; Bohm, S.R.; Folster, J.P.; Bokanyi, R.; Kupper, A.; Bidol, S.A.; et al. Multistate outbreak of *Escherichia coli* O145 infections associated with romaine lettuce consumption, 2010. *J. Food Prot.* **2013**, *76*, 939–944. [CrossRef] [PubMed]
9. Rivero, M.A.; Passucci, J.A.; Rodriguez, E.M.; Parma, A.E. Role and clinical course of verotoxigenic *Escherichia coli* infections in childhood acute diarrhoea in Argentina. *J. Med. Microbiol.* **2010**, *59*, 345–352. [CrossRef]
10. De Schrijver, K.; Buvens, G.; Posse, B.; Van den Branden, D.; Oosterlynck, O.; De Zutter, L.; Eilers, K.; Pierard, D.; Dierick, K.; Van Damme-Lombaerts, R.; et al. Outbreak of verocytotoxin-producing *E. coli* O145 and O26 infections associated with the consumption of ice cream produced at a farm, Belgium, 2007. *Euro Surveill.* **2008**, *13*, 8041. [CrossRef]
11. Carter, M.Q.; Quinones, B.; He, X.; Zhong, W.; Louie, J.W.; Lee, B.G.; Yambao, J.C.; Mandrell, R.E.; Cooley, M.B. An Environmental Shiga Toxin-Producing *Escherichia coli* O145 Clonal Population Exhibits High-Level Phenotypic Variation That Includes Virulence Traits. *Appl. Environ. Microbiol.* **2015**, *82*, 1090–1101. [CrossRef] [PubMed]
12. Liao, Y.T.; Brooks, J.C.; Martin, J.N.; Echeverry, A.; Loneragan, G.H.; Brashears, M.M. Antimicrobial interventions for O157:H7 and non-O157 Shiga toxin-producing *Escherichia coli* on beef subprimal and mechanically tenderized steaks. *J. Food Prot.* **2015**, *78*, 511–517. [CrossRef] [PubMed]
13. Hatfull, G.F. Bacteriophage genomics. *Curr. Opin. Microbiol.* **2008**, *11*, 447–453. [CrossRef] [PubMed]
14. Clokie, M.R.J.; Millard, A.D.; Letarov, A.V.; Heaphy, S. Phages in nature. *Bacteriophage* **2011**, *1*, 31–45. [CrossRef] [PubMed]
15. Hagens, S.; Loessner, M.J. Bacteriophage for biocontrol of foodborne pathogens: Calculations and considerations. *Curr. Pharm. Biotechnol.* **2010**, *11*, 58–68. [CrossRef] [PubMed]
16. Snyder, A.B.; Perry, J.J.; Yousef, A.E. Developing and optimizing bacteriophage treatment to control enterohemorrhagic *Escherichia coli* on fresh produce. *Int. J. Food Microbiol.* **2016**, *236*, 90–97. [CrossRef] [PubMed]
17. Amarillas, L.; Chaidez, C.; Gonzalez-Robles, A.; Lugo-Melchor, Y.; Leon-Felix, J. Characterization of novel bacteriophage phiC119 capable of lysing multidrug-resistant Shiga toxin-producing *Escherichia coli* O157:H7. *PeerJ* **2016**, 13. [CrossRef]
18. Svab, D.; Falgenhauer, L.; Rohde, M.; Szabo, J.; Chakraborty, T.; Toth, I. Identification and Characterization of T5-Like Bacteriophages Representing Two Novel Subgroups from Food Products. *Front. Microbiol.* **2018**, *9*, 202. [CrossRef] [PubMed]
19. Tolen, T.N.; Xie, Y.; Hairgrove, T.B.; Gill, J.J.; Taylor, T.M. Evaluation of Commercial Prototype Bacteriophage Intervention Designed for Reducing O157 and Non-O157 Shiga-Toxigenic *Escherichia coli* (STEC) on Beef Cattle Hide. *Foods* **2018**, *7*, 114. [CrossRef] [PubMed]
20. Catalao, M.J.; Gil, F.; Moniz-Pereira, J.; Sao-Jose, C.; Pimentel, M. Diversity in bacterial lysis systems: Bacteriophages show the way. *FEMS Microbiol. Rev.* **2013**, *37*, 554–571. [CrossRef] [PubMed]

21. Baig, A.; Colom, J.; Barrow, P.; Schouler, C.; Moodley, A.; Lavigne, R.; Atterbury, R. Biology and Genomics of an Historic Therapeutic *Escherichia coli* Bacteriophage Collection. *Front. Microbiol.* **2017**, *8*, 1652. [CrossRef] [PubMed]
22. Summer, E.J.; Berry, J.; Tran, T.A.T.; Niu, L.; Struck, D.K.; Young, R. Rz/Rz1 lysis gene equivalents in phages of Gram-negative hosts. *J. Mol. Biol.* **2007**, *373*, 1098–1112. [CrossRef] [PubMed]
23. Oliveira, L.; Tavares, P.; Alonso, J.C. Headful DNA packaging: Bacteriophage SPP1 as a model system. *Virus Res.* **2013**, *173*, 247–259. [CrossRef] [PubMed]
24. Wang, J.; Niu, Y.D.; Chen, J.; Anany, H.; Ackermann, H.W.; Johnson, R.P.; Ateba, C.N.; Stanford, K.; McAllister, T.A. Feces of feedlot cattle contain a diversity of bacteriophages that lyse non-O157 Shiga toxin-producing *Escherichia coli*. *Can. J. Microbiol.* **2015**, *61*, 467–475. [CrossRef] [PubMed]
25. Litt, P.K.; Saha, J.; Jaroni, D. Characterization of Bacteriophages Targeting Non-O157 Shiga Toxigenic *Escherichia coli*. *J. Food Prot.* **2018**, *81*, 785–794. [CrossRef] [PubMed]
26. Liao, Y.-T.; Quintela, I.A.; Nguyen, K.; Salvador, A.; Cooley, M.B.; Wu, V.C.H. Investigation of prevalence of free Shiga toxin-producing *Escherichia coli* (STEC)-specific bacteriophages and its correlation with STEC bacterial hosts in a produce-growing area in Salinas, California. *PLoS ONE* **2018**, *13*, e0190534. [CrossRef]
27. Endersen, L.; Guinane, C.M.; Johnston, C.; Neve, H.; Coffey, A.; Ross, R.P.; McAuliffe, O.; O'Mahony, J. Genome analysis of *Cronobacter* phage vB_CsaP_Ss1 reveals an endolysin with potential for biocontrol of Gram-negative bacterial pathogens. *J. Gen. Virol.* **2015**, *96*, 463–477. [CrossRef]
28. Adriaenssens, E.M.; Brister, J.R. How to Name and Classify Your Phage: An Informal Guide. *Viruses* **2017**, *9*, 70. [CrossRef]
29. Hatfull, G.F.; Hendrix, R.W. Bacteriophages and their genomes. *Curr. Opin. Virol.* **2011**, *1*, 298–303. [CrossRef]
30. Peng, Q.; Yuan, Y. Characterization of a newly isolated phage infecting pathogenic *Escherichia coli* and analysis of its mosaic structural genes. *Sci. Rep.* **2018**, *8*, 8086. [CrossRef]
31. Wietzorrek, A.; Schwarz, H.; Herrmann, C.; Braun, V. The genome of the novel phage Rtp, with a rosette-like tail tip, is homologous to the genome of phage T1. *J. Bacteriol.* **2006**, *188*, 1419–1436. [CrossRef] [PubMed]
32. Hoyles, L.; Murphy, J.; Neve, H.; Heller, K.J.; Turton, J.F.; Mahony, J.; Sanderson, J.D.; Hudspith, B.; Gibson, G.R.; McCartney, A.L.; et al. *Klebsiella pneumoniae* subsp. *pneumoniae*-bacteriophage combination from the caecal effluent of a healthy woman. *PeerJ* **2015**, *3*, e1061. [CrossRef] [PubMed]
33. Xu, Y.; Yu, X.; Gu, Y.; Huang, X.; Liu, G.; Liu, X. Characterization and Genomic Study of Phage vB_EcoS-B2 Infecting Multidrug-Resistant *Escherichia coli*. *Front. Microbiol.* **2018**, *9*, 793. [CrossRef] [PubMed]
34. Nilsson, A.S. Phage therapy–Constraints and possibilities. *Upsala J. Med. Sci.* **2014**, *119*, 192–198. [CrossRef] [PubMed]
35. Son, H.M.; Duc, H.M.; Masuda, Y.; Honjoh, K.I.; Miyamoto, T. Application of bacteriophages in simultaneously controlling *Escherichia coli* O157:H7 and extended-spectrum beta-lactamase producing *Escherichia coli*. *Appl. Microbiol. Biotechnol.* **2018**, *102*, 10259–10271. [CrossRef] [PubMed]
36. Wang, J.; Niu, Y.D.; Chen, J.; McAllister, T.A.; Stanford, K. Complete Genome Sequence of *Escherichia coli* O145:NM Bacteriophage vB_EcoM_AYO145A, a New Member of O1-Like Phages. *Genome Announc.* **2015**, *3*, e00539-15. [CrossRef]
37. Merabishvili, M.; Vervaet, C.; Pirnay, J.-P.; De Vos, D.; Verbeken, G.; Mast, J.; Chanishvili, N.; Vaneechoutte, M. Stability of *Staphylococcus aureus* phage ISP after freeze-drying (lyophilization). *PLoS ONE* **2013**, *8*, e68797. [CrossRef]
38. Geagea, H.; Labrie, S.J.; Subirade, M.; Moineau, S. The Tape Measure Protein Is Involved in the Heat Stability of *Lactococcus lactis* Phages. *Appl. Environ. Microbiol.* **2018**, *84*, e02082-17. [CrossRef]
39. Hudson, J.A.; Billington, C.; Cornelius, A.J.; Wilson, T.; On, S.L.W.; Premaratne, A.; King, N.J. Use of a bacteriophage to inactivate *Escherichia coli* O157:H7 on beef. *Food Microbiol.* **2013**, *36*, 14–21. [CrossRef]
40. Tomat, D.; Migliore, L.; Aquili, V.; Quiberoni, A.; Balagué, C. Phage biocontrol of enteropathogenic and shiga toxin-producing *Escherichia coli* in meat products. *Front. Cell. Infect. Microbiol.* **2013**, *3*, 20. [CrossRef]
41. Arndt, D.; Grant, J.R.; Marcu, A.; Sajed, T.; Pon, A.; Liang, Y.; Wishart, D.S. PHASTER: A better, faster version of the PHAST phage search tool. *Nucleic Acids Res.* **2016**, *44*, W16–W21. [CrossRef] [PubMed]
42. Lowe, T.M.; Chan, P.P. tRNAscan-SE On-line: Integrating search and context for analysis of transfer RNA genes. *Nucleic Acids Res.* **2016**, *44*, W54–W57. [CrossRef] [PubMed]

43. Garneau, J.R.; Depardieu, F.; Fortier, L.C.; Bikard, D.; Monot, M. PhageTerm: A tool for fast and accurate determination of phage termini and packaging mechanism using next-generation sequencing data. *Sci. Rep.* **2017**, *7*, 8292. [CrossRef] [PubMed]
44. Richter, M.; Rossello-Mora, R.; Oliver Glockner, F.; Peplies, J. JSpeciesWS: A web server for prokaryotic species circumscription based on pairwise genome comparison. *Bioinformatics* **2016**, *32*, 929–931. [CrossRef] [PubMed]
45. Sullivan, M.J.; Petty, N.K.; Beatson, S.A. Easyfig: A genome comparison visualizer. *Bioinformatics* **2011**, *27*, 1009–1010. [CrossRef] [PubMed]
46. Zankari, E.; Cosentino, S.; Vestergaard, M.; Rasmussen, S.; Lund, O.; Aarestrup, F.M.; Larsen, M.V. Identification of acquired antimicrobial resistance genes. *J. Antimicrob. Chemother.* **2012**, *67*, 2640–2644. [CrossRef] [PubMed]
47. Mahadevan, P.; King, J.F.; Seto, D. CGUG: In silico proteome and genome parsing tool for the determination of "core" and unique genes in the analysis of genomes up to ca. 1.9 Mb. *BMC Res. Methods* **2009**, *2*, 168. [CrossRef] [PubMed]
48. McWilliam, H.; Li, W.; Uludag, M.; Squizzato, S.; Park, Y.M.; Buso, N.; Cowley, A.P.; Lopez, R. Analysis Tool Web Services from the EMBL-EBI. *Nucleic Acids Res.* **2013**, *41*, W597–W600. [CrossRef] [PubMed]
49. Tamura, K.; Stecher, G.; Peterson, D.; Filipski, A.; Kumar, S. MEGA6: Molecular Evolutionary Genetics Analysis version 6.0. *Mol. Biol. Evol.* **2013**, *30*, 2725–2729. [CrossRef]
50. Adams, M.H. *Bacteriophage*; Interscience Publishers, Inc.: New York, NY, USA, 1959.
51. Shevchenko, A.; Tomas, H.; Havlis, J.; Olsen, J.V.; Mann, M. In-gel digestion for mass spectrometric characterization of proteins and proteomes. *Nat. Protoc.* **2006**, *1*, 2856–2860. [CrossRef]
52. Shevchenko, A.; Wilm, M.; Vorm, O.; Mann, M. Mass spectrometric sequencing of proteins silver-stained polyacrylamide gels. *Anal. Chem.* **1996**, *68*, 850–858. [CrossRef] [PubMed]
53. Mirzaei, M.K.; Nilsson, A.S. Correction: Isolation of phages for phage therapy: A comparison of spot tests and efficiency of plating analyses for determination of host range and efficacy. *PLoS ONE* **2015**, *10*, e0118557. [CrossRef] [PubMed]
54. Fong, K.; LaBossiere, B.; Switt, A.I.M.; Delaquis, P.; Goodridge, L.; Levesque, R.C.; Danyluk, M.D.; Wang, S. Characterization of Four Novel Bacteriophages Isolated from British Columbia for Control of Non-typhoidal *Salmonella in Vitro* and on Sprouting Alfalfa Seeds. *Front. Microbiol.* **2017**, *8*, 2193. [CrossRef] [PubMed]

5

Protective Effects of Bacteriophages against *Aeromonas hydrophila* Causing Motile Aeromonas Septicemia (MAS) in Striped Catfish

Tuan Son Le [1,2], Thi Hien Nguyen [3], Hong Phuong Vo [3], Van Cuong Doan [3], Hong Loc Nguyen [3], Minh Trung Tran [3], Trong Tuan Tran [3], Paul C. Southgate [4] and D. İpek Kurtböke [1,*]

1 GeneCology Research Centre, Faculty of Science, Health, Education and Engineering, University of the Sunshine Coast, 90 Sippy Downs Drive, Sippy Downs, QLD 4556, Australia; tuan.son.le@research.usc.edu.au
2 Research Institute for Marine Fisheries, 224 Le Lai, Ngo Quyen, Hai Phong 180000, Vietnam
3 Research Institute for Aquaculture No. 2, 116 Nguyen Dinh Chieu, District 1, Ho Chi Minh 700000, Vietnam; nguyenhien05@gmail.com (T.H.N.); vohongphuong@gmail.com (H.P.V.); vancuongdisaqua@gmail.com (V.C.D.); hongloc@gmail.com (H.L.N.); trung16893@yahoo.com.vn (M.T.T.); tuantran_695@yahoo.com.vn (T.T.T.)
4 Australian Centre for Pacific Islands Research and Faculty of Science, Health, Education and Engineering, University of the Sunshine Coast, Maroochydore, QLD 4556, Australia; psouthgate@usc.edu.au
* Correspondence: ikurtbok@usc.edu.au

Abstract: To determine the effectivity of bacteriophages in controlling the mass mortality of striped catfish (*Pangasianodon hypophthalmus*) due to infections caused by *Aeromonas* spp. in Vietnamese fish farms, bacteriophages against pathogenic *Aeromonas hydrophila* were isolated. *A. hydrophila*-phage 2 and *A. hydrophila*-phage 5 were successfully isolated from water samples from the Saigon River of Ho Chi Minh City, Vietnam. These phages, belonging to the *Myoviridae* family, were found to have broad activity spectra, even against the tested multiple-antibiotic-resistant *Aeromonas* isolates. The latent periods and burst size of phage 2 were 10 min and 213 PFU per infected host cell, respectively. The bacteriophages proved to be effective in inhibiting the growth of the *Aeromonas* spp. under laboratory conditions. Phage treatments applied to the pathogenic strains during infestation of catfish resulted in a significant improvement in the survival rates of the tested fishes, with up to 100% survival with MOI 100, compared to 18.3% survival observed in control experiments. These findings illustrate the potential for using phages as an effective bio-treatment method to control Motile Aeromonas Septicemia (MAS) in fish farms. This study provides further evidence towards the use of bacteriophages to effectively control disease in aquaculture operations.

Keywords: *Aeromonas hydrophila*; Motile Aeromonas Septicemia; MAS; multiple-antibiotic-resistance; bacteriophage; biological control; striped catfish (*Pangasianodon hypophthalmus*)

---

1. Introduction

Striped catfish (*Pangasianodon hypophthalmus*) is one of the most important farmed fish species, especially in Vietnam, Thailand, Cambodia, Laos and, more recently, the Philippines and Indonesia [1]. Vietnam supplied 90% of catfish production with a value of US$1.1 to 1.7 billion in 2015. Motile Aeromonas Septicemia (MAS), also called haemorrhage disease or red spot disease, causes great losses for farmers (up to 80% mortality) and presents in fish with clinical signs of haemorrhages on the head, mouth, and at the base of fins, a red, swollen vent, and the presence of pink to yellow ascitic fluid [2]. *Aeromonas hydrophila*, *Aeromonas caviae*, and *Aeromonas sobria* species were often isolated from diseased catfish, and new species such as *Aeromonas dhakensis* and *Aeromonas veronii* were also reported by using molecular methods based on the sequencing of the *rpo*D gene [3].

Multiple antibiotic resistance (MAR) of *A. hydrophila* strains has been reported in different countries. Vivekanandhan et al. [4] tested 319 strains of *A. hydrophila* isolated from fish and prawns in South India and indicated that all of them were resistant to methicillin, rifampicin, bacitracin, and novobiocin (99%). Moreover, 21 *Aeromonas* spp. isolated from carp showed resistance to ampicillin and penicillin [5]. Recently, Thi et al. [6] tested antibiotic resistance of 30 strains of *A. hydrophila* isolated from diseased striped catfish in the Mekong Delta from January 2013 to March 2014. The study found that *A. hydrophila* isolates were highly resistant to tetracycline and florfenicol and were completely resistant to trimethoprim, sulfamethoxazole, ampicillin, amoxicillin, and cefalexine.

ALPHA JECT ® Panga 2 vaccine, protecting against *Edwardsiella ictaluri* and *A. hydrophila*, has been approved for market in Vietnam since the early 2017 (https://www.pharmaq.no/updates/pharmaq-fish-va/). However, the cost-effectiveness of vaccine use in catfish production is another obstacle in intensive catfish production. Moreover, the development of a commercial vaccine against *A. hydrophila* has been slow because *A. hydrophia* is biochemically and serologically heterogeneous [7]. Therefore, there is a need for effective, environmentally safe control measures for managing MAS in catfish.

One approach has been the use of bacteriophages (phages) to control pathogenic bacteria in aquaculture operations. Recently, studies related to the use of phages specific to *A. hydrophila* in aquaculture have gained attention. Hsu et al. [8] isolated two *A. hydrophila* phages and three *Edwardsiella tarda* phages to treat disease in eels (*Anguilla japonica*) in vitro. The phages reduced bacterial density by about 1000 times after 2 h when the MOI was 11.5 at 25 °C in the fluid environment. El-Araby et al. [9] demonstrated the effectiveness of bacteriophage ZH1 and ZH2 treatment against *A. hydrophila* in Tilapia, improving the survival rates by up to 82%.

However, so far, treatments using bacteriophages against pathogens causing MAS in catfish have not been studied extensively. The objective of this study was, therefore, to isolate bacteriophages infective in pathogenic *A. hydrophila* with a long-term objective to eradicate this disease-causing pathogen in aquaculture operations.

2. Results

2.1. Prophage Induction

No reduction in the optical density of bacterial suspension treated with Mitomycin C (Table S1, Supplementary Materials) and no clear zones from the spot technique were observed. Therefore, it was concluded that there was no prophage in *A. hydrophila* N17.

2.2. Antibiotic Susceptibility

All isolates were completely (100%) resistant to oxytetracycline, ampicillin, gentamycin and amoxicillin/clavulanic acid, enrofloxacin, and bactrim. Nearly all isolates (83.3%) were resistant to kanamycin and 33.3% were resistant to tetracycline, doxycycline, and ciprofloxacin (Table 1).

Table 1. Antibiogram profile of the *Aeromonas hydrophila* strains tested.

Antibiotics	Number of Resistant Isolates (n = 6)
Tetracycline	2
Oxytetracycline	6
Gentamycin	6
Kanamycin	5
Bactrim (SMX/TMP)	6
Doxycycline	2
Enrofloxacin	6
Amoxicillin/clavulanic acid	6
Ampicillin	6
Ciprofloxacin	2

2.3. Isolation and Characterization of Bacteriophages

The A. hydrophila-phage 2 (or Φ2) and A. hydrophila-phage 5 (or Φ5) were successfully isolated against the propagation hosts used (Figure 1 and Table 2).

Φ2 had an isometric head of 129 nm in diameter with a tail sheath 173 nm long and 15 nm wide. Φ5 was composed of: (i) an isometric head of 120 nm in diameter, (ii) a tail sheath of 198 nm in length and 15 nm in width. All of the phages had contractile tails (Figure 1 and Table 2).

Table 2. Characteristics of bacteriophages against *A. hydrophila* strains.

Φ	Concentration PFU/mL	Head (nm)		Neck (nm)		Tail Sheath (nm)		Genus
		L	W	L	W	L	W	
2	10^9		129	10	15	173	15	*Spounalikevirus*
5	10^{10}		120	15	15	198	15	*Spounalikevirus*

W: width; L: length.

Both phages produced clear plaques with diameters of 0.1 mm (Figure 1).

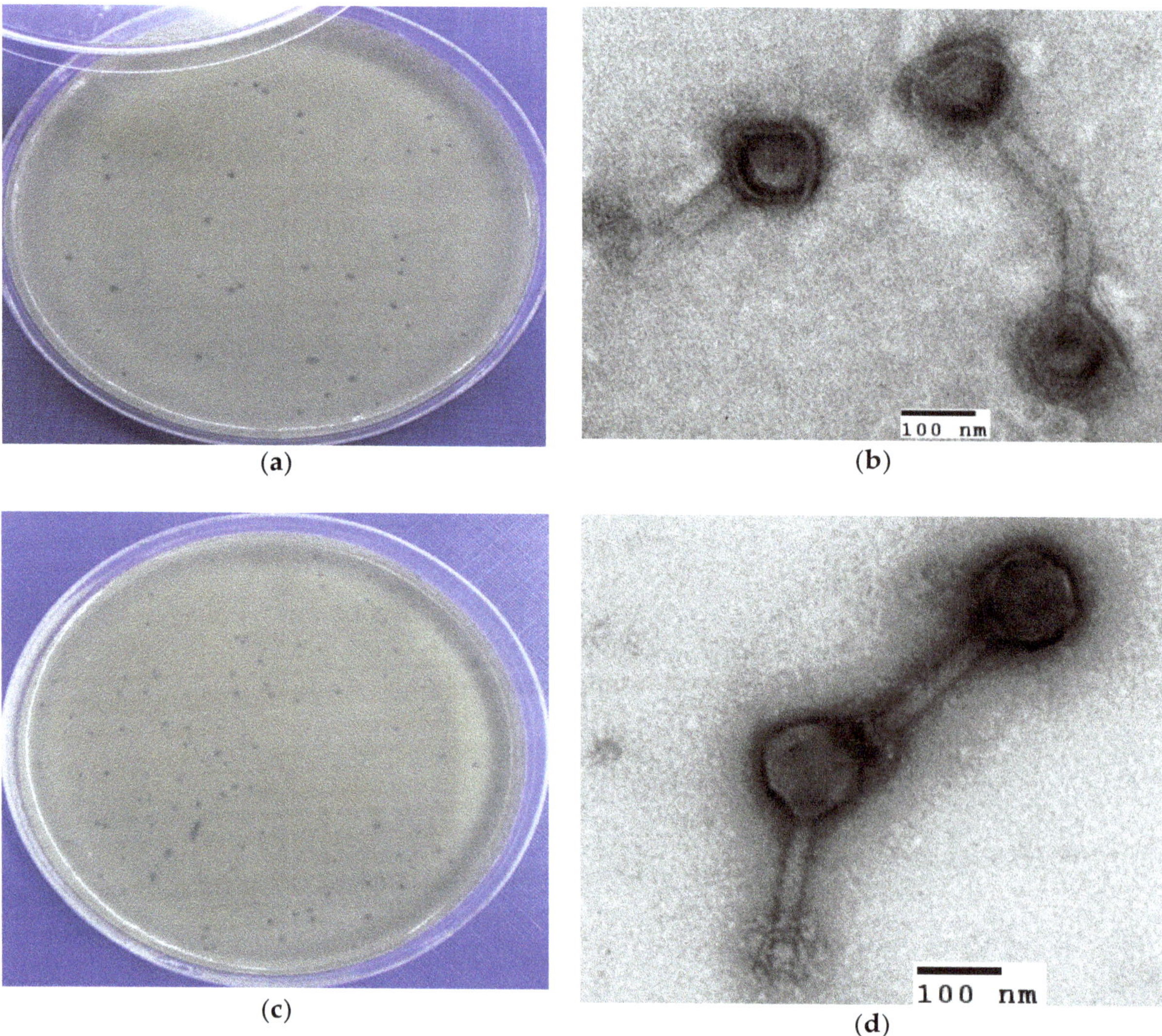

Figure 1. Plaque formation and microphotograph of *A. hydrophila* phages. (**a**,**b**) Φ2 and (**c**,**d**) phage Φ5.

The genome size of the phage isolates was above 20 kb. The genomic material of the isolated phages was not digested by Mung bean nuclease and RNase A. Since Mung bean nuclease specifically cuts single-stranded nucleic acids of both DNA and RNA, it was concluded that the genomic DNA of both phages was double-stranded. RNA nucleic acids are degraded by RNase A, therefore, the nucleic acids of Φ2 and Φ5 were determined as double-stranded DNA (dsDNA) (Figure 2). The phages Φ2 and Φ5 belong to the Myoviridae family.

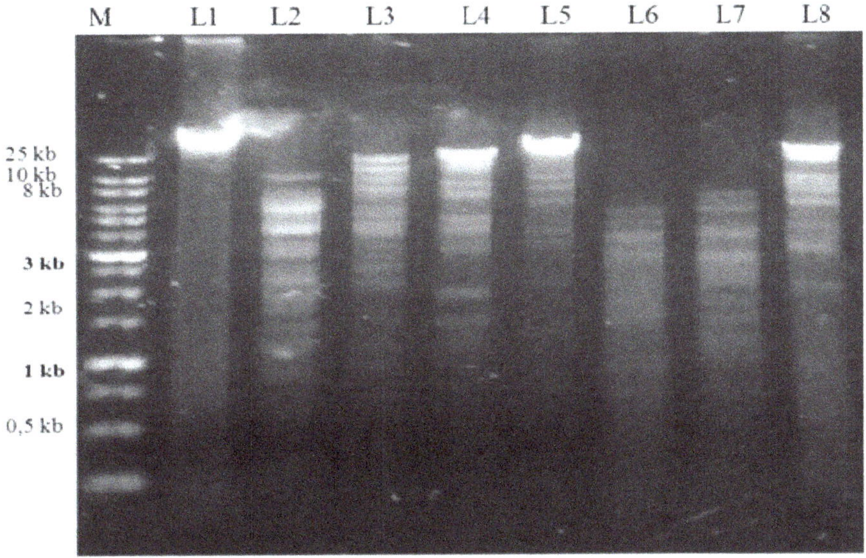

Figure 2. Restriction enzyme-digested fragments of the genomic DNA of *A. hydrophila*-phage 2. Footnote: Lane M: 1kb Plus Opti-DNA Marker (ABM, Canada); Lane L1: genomic DNA of Φ2; Lanes L2–L8: genomic DNA of Φ2 digested with EcoRV; EcoRI; Ncol; SalI; MspI; XmnI; KpnI, restriction enzymes respectively.

2.4. Host Range

Phage 2 and phage 5 were found to inhibit the growth of all *A. hydrophila* strains tested. None of the other 27 species was found to be susceptible to these phages (Table S2, Supplementary Materials).

2.5. Adsorption Rate of Phages and One-Step Growth Curve

The number of free phages in suspension decreased over time, as illustrated in the adsorption curve (Figure 3a). At 40 min, the percentage of Φ2-infected bacteria was over 90%.

The one-step growth experiment (Figure 3b) results revealed that the latent period and burst size of Φ2 were 10 and 213 PFU per infected host cell, respectively.

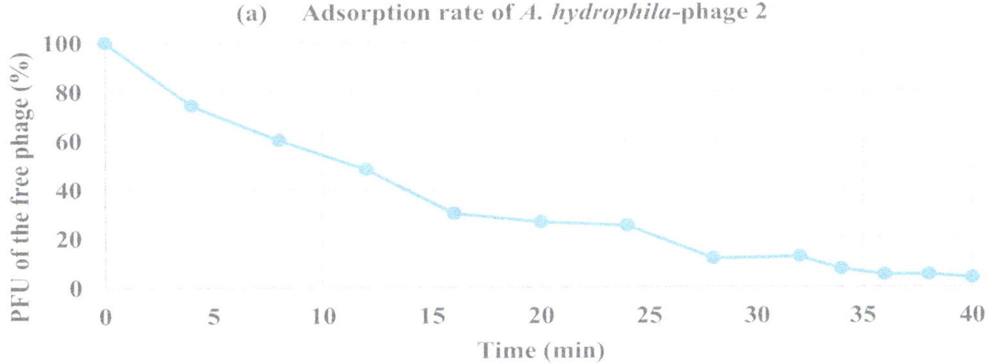

Figure 3. *Cont.*

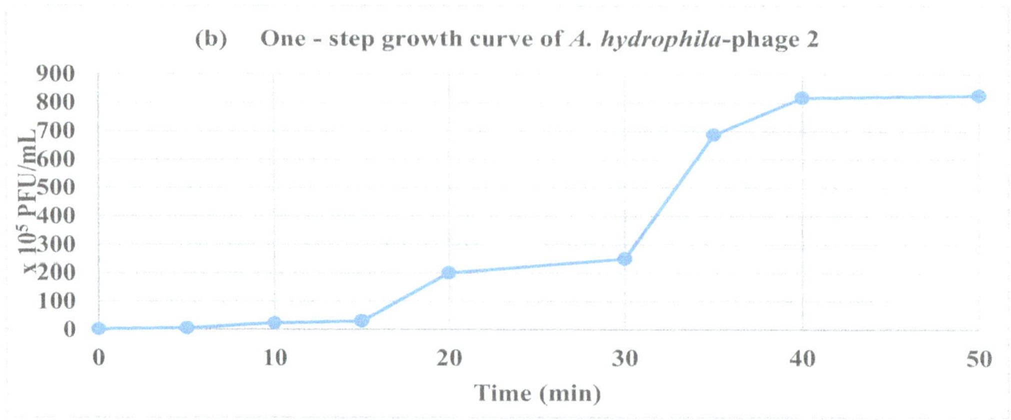

Figure 3. (**a**) Adsorption rate and (**b**) one-step growth curves of Φ2.

2.6. Inactivation of Aeromonas Species in Vitro

The bacterial concentration (OD_{550nm} values) of the uninfected control (only *A. hydrophila* N17) increased continuously during 18 h of incubation. In contrast, during the infection with Φ2 at MOI 1, MOI 0.1, and MOI 0.01 bacterial growth began to be inhibited at 1, 2, and 2.5 h, respectively, and the inhibition was maintained up to 8 h (Figure 4a). Then, the bacterial concentration increased as a consequence of the development of phage-resistant *A. hydrophila* cells.

The lowest OD_{550nm} value was 0.177 ± 0.023 after 4 h of incubation of Φ5 at MOI 0.1. There was a significant decline in the bacterial concentration (MOI 0.01, 0.1, and 1) in the first 3 h, followed by low level stabilization in the next 1, 2, and 4 h for MOI 1, 0.1, and 0.01, respectively (Figure 4b). Then, the bacterial concentration underwent a turnaround because of the development of phage-resistant *A. hydrophila* cells.

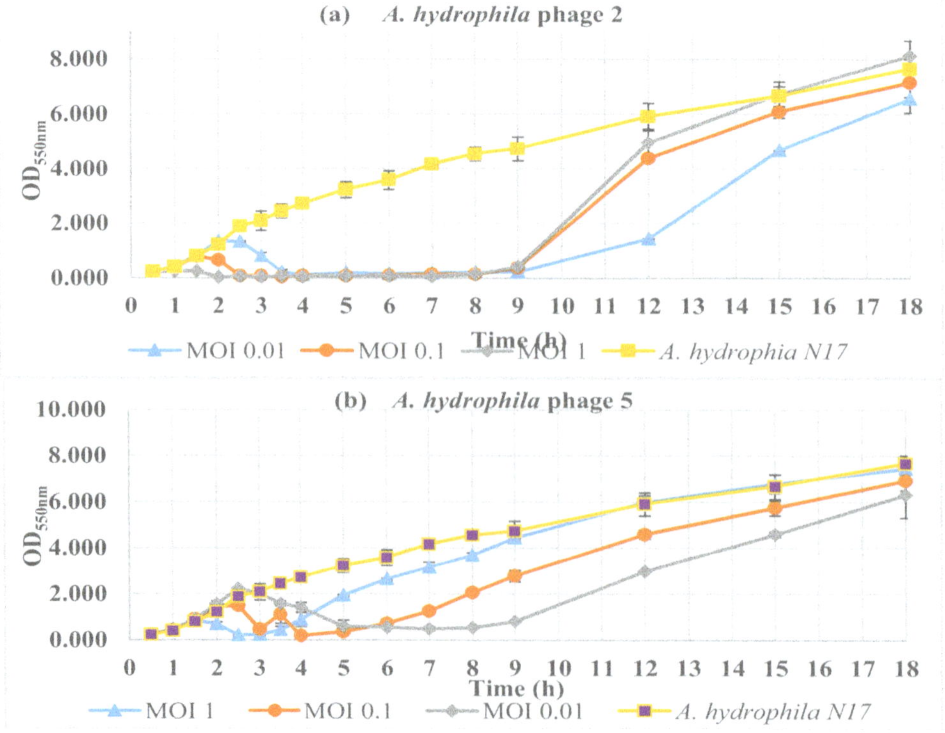

Figure 4. Inactivation of *A. hydrophila* N17 by the phages (**a**) Φ2 and (**b**) Φ5 at different MOI (0.01, 0.1 and 1).

2.7. Phage Treatment of Infected Fish

The negative control 1 (fishes with no injection) and negative control 2 (fishes injected with the growth medium filtered to remove bacterial cells) showed no mortality of catfish (Figure 5), indicating that the uninfected, control medium did not have any detrimental effect on fish health.

Catfish in the positive control groups (infected with *A. hydrophila* N17) that were not treated with bacteriophages started to die at a constant rate starting from post-infection day two, with a cumulative mortality rate of 81.67 ± 2.36% (Figure 5).

In contrast, the fish treated with the phages showed lower mortality rates at each different MOI ($p < 0.01$). While no mortality was observed in the groups treated with MOI 100, the cumulative mortalities in the other groups were 45% (MOI 1) and 68.33 ± 2.36% (MOI 0.01) at the end of the eight-day experiment (Figure 5).

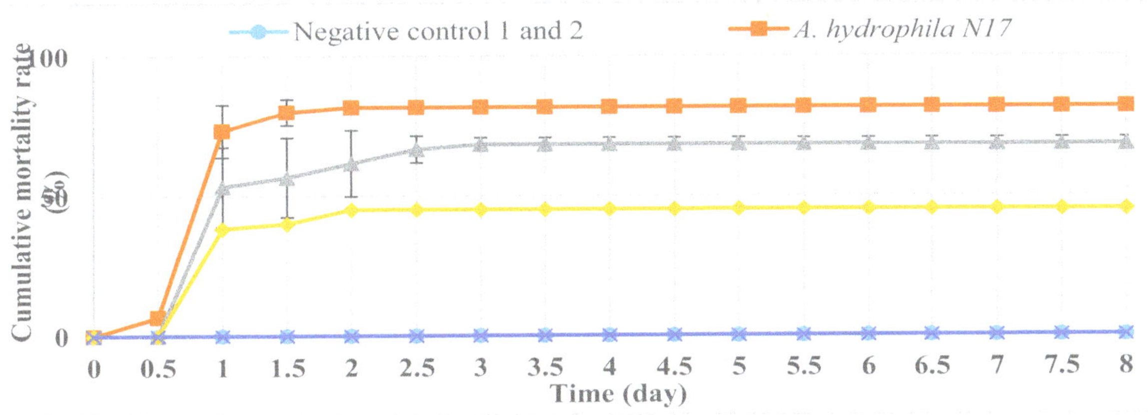

Figure 5. Cumulative mortality rates (%) of striped catfishes obtained in challenging experiments using *A. hydrophia* N17 and the phage cocktail at the different MOIs (0.01, 0.1, and 1). The ratio of Φ2 to Φ5 in a phage cocktail was 1:1.

3. Discussion

The findings of this study demonstrate that the examined *Aeromonas* spp. were resistant to multiple antibiotics and were thus able to cause high mortality rates in catfish in Vietnam, in spite of the use of various antibiotic treatments. In the bacteriophage treatments, however, Φ2 and Φ5 were able to lyse all tested *A. hydrophila* strains, displaying strong inhibition also of the virulent *A. hydrophila* strains carrying many virulence genes. Therefore, Φ2 and Φ5 are promising candidates for the application of a phage therapy to control *Aeromonas* infection in catfish.

Phage Φ2 and Φ5 were found to belong to the *Myoviridae* family, and our findings are in line with those of Ackermann [10] who indicated that 33 of a total of 43 *Aeromonas* phages he investigated were tailed and belonged to the *Myoviridae* family. Recently, other *Aeromonas* phage studies against different *Aeromonas* species by Haq et al. [11], Jun et al. [12], and Kim et al. [13] also reported that all phages they identified belonged to the *Myoviridae* family. Therefore, *Myoviridae* family members are most likely to be abundant in natural environments.

There was a correlation between the diameter of the plaques observed and the latent period and burst size for the *A. hydrophila* phage. The Φ2 had a short latent period (10 min), and these findings are in line with another study conducted by Anand et al. [14] who found that *Aeromonas* phage BPA 6 had a latent period of 10 min and a burst size of 244 PFU/cell.

The different MOI of Φ2 and Φ5 caused different bacterial growth patterns. The higher the MOI value, the sooner phage-resistant bacterial cells appeared. A similar result was noted by Kim et al. [13] for the phage PAS 1 against an *Aeromonas salmonicida* strain, indicating that bacterial resistance appeared after 3, 6, and 24 h at MOIs 10, 1, and 0.1, respectively.

Several *Aeromonas* phages, such as Aeh1, Aeh2, AH1 have also been reported [12,15,16]. However, there have been few reports demonstrating the successful use of phages for the treatment of *Aeromonas* infections in catfish. The treatment of catfish by an intraperitoneal (IP) injection illustrated significant protective effects, which increased the relative percentages of the survival rates observed for fish compared to the controls when the MOI increased. Our study revealed that in the MOI-100 experiment the relative percentage survival was 100%. The study of Jun et al. [12] showed that the relative percentage survival of fish treated with *A. hydrophila* phages pAh6-C and pAh1-C was 16.67 ± 3.82% and 43.33 ± 2.89%, respectively, when the fish were injected with the bacterium (2.6×10^7 CFU/fish). However, the labour-intensive and time-consuming mode of delivery of bacteriophages can constitute a disadvantage for the treatment of fish by IP injection in catfish farms. Therefore, further studies should be conducted into whether phage treatments are effective when an on-farm oral method of administration is evaluated. With the use of bioreactors, large volumes of bacteriophages can be produced for bacteriophage incorporation into fish feed. Moreover, the survival of phages and their persistent survival on or in fish, as well as in phage-coated feed preparations should be studied under different environmental factors (e.g., temperature, salt concentration) to determine whether phages are able to persist and effectively reduce *Aeromonas* spp. levels in fish farms. In conclusion, this study demonstrates that phage treatment of *Aeromonas* spp. might be an effective tool to improve the survival of farmed catfish affected by MAS.

4. Materials and Methods

4.1. Aeromonas Species

Bacterial isolates stored at the Research Institute for Aquaculture No. 2 (Ho Chi Minh City, Vietnam) and the ATCC type strains of the pathogens are listed in Table S2. Isolates were previously obtained from diseased catfish in farms in the south of Vietnam (Table S2).

4.2. Prophage Induction

In order to choose an *Aeromonas* species as a propagation host for phage isolation, *A. hydrophila* N17 was subjected to a prophage induction test. The *Aeromonas* species was cultured in 10 mL fresh Luria-Bertani (or LB) broth (Sigma-Aldrich, St. Louis, MO, USA) and incubated at 30 °C on an orbital shaker operating at 150 rpm until reaching an OD_{550nm} of 0.2. Mitomycin C (Sigma-Aldrich) was added to a final concentration of 1 μg/mL and 5 μg/mL, and again the bacterial suspension was incubated at 30 °C on an orbital shaker operating at 150 rpm. The cell density of the bacteria (OD_{550nm}) was monitored every 1 h for a 6 h period. At the end of the incubation, the bacterial suspension was centrifuged at 10,000 g for 15 min and filtered through a nitrocellulose filter (0.45 μm, Merck Millipore, Burlington, MA, USA) before spotting the filtrate onto an agar plate seeded with the host bacterium to confirm the presence of viable phage particles. A significant decrease in the cell density (OD_{550nm}) suggested that prophages were released [17,18].

4.3. Antibiotic Susceptibility

Antibiotic susceptibility tests of six *A. hydrophila* strains [3] were conducted against 10 different antimicrobial susceptibility discs (OXOID, Hampshire, UK) by the method recommended by the Clinical and Laboratory Standards Institute [19]. The antimicrobial agents tested included tetracycline (30 μg), doxycycline (30 μg), oxytetracycline (30 μg), bactrim (SMX/TMP) (23.75/1.25 μg), gentamycin (40 μg), kanamycin (30 μg), ciprofloxacin (10 μg), enrofloxacin (10 μg), ampicillin (33 μg), and amoxicillin-clavulanic acid (20/10 μg).

The antimicrobial susceptibility of *Aeromonas* species is usually recorded using Enterobacteriaceae breakpoints [20]. Susceptible (S), intermediate resistance (I), and resistant (R) were evaluated according the criteria given in the Performance Standards for Antimicrobial Susceptibility Testing M100-S21

(2017, Table 2A-1, pages 33–39) [19]. Multi-antibiotic resistance (MAR) was recorded when the bacteria resisted to three or more antibiotics [21].

4.4. Isolation and Characterization of Bacteriophages

Phages were isolated from water samples from the Saigon River in the south of Vietnam against *A. hydrophila* N17 and they were purified following the methods described by Jun et al. [12].

Phage titres were determined using both surface spread [22,23] and double-layer [24] agar plaque assay techniques where agar plates were previously seeded with the *Aeromonas* sp. ($\times 10^6$ CFU/mL).

For transmission electron microscopy (TEM): A 200 mesh copper grid was immersed in 40 μL of phage solution for five min before fixing the phage with glutaraldehyde solution (1%) for five min. Then, the phage samples were negatively stained with 5% (*w/v*) uranyl acetate and observed by TEM (JEOL JEM-1010) operating at a voltage of 80 kV at the Vietnam National Institute of Hygiene and Epidemiology. The phage morphology was determined using the criteria of the International Committee on Taxonomy of Viruses (ICTV) (http://www.ictvonline.org/) and Ackermann et al. [25].

Phage genomic DNA extraction and restriction analyses: Phage genomic DNA was extracted using the Phage DNA Isolation Kit (Norgen Biotek Corp, Thorold, Canada). The nature of the nucleic acids was determined by digestion with Mung bean nuclease and RNase A (ThermoFisher Scientific, Waltham, MA, USA) as per the manufacturer's protocols. The genomic DNA phages were digested using the restriction enzymes: EcoRV, EcoRI, Ncol, SalI, MspI, XmnI, and KpnI, as per the manufacturer's instruction (ThermoFisher Scientific). The DNA fragments were then electrophoresed at 120 V for 40 min.

4.5. Host Range

The method was adapted from Le et al. [23] and Goodridge et al. [26] with some modifications described below. The *Aeromonas* spp. (Table S2) were incubated overnight. Then, a 100 μL aliquot of each *Aeromonas* spp. culture (optical density of 0.5 at 550 nm) was spread on brain heart infusion agar (BHIA) (OXOID, UK) and dried for 20 min in a biological safety cabinet Class II. The host range of the phage was determined by pipetting 10 μL of phage preparation (~10^8 PFU/mL) on lawn cultures of the strains. The plates were observed for the appearance of clear zones after incubation at 30 °C after 18 h.

4.6. Adsorption Rate of Phages

Phage adsorption was studied using the method described previously [27]. A phage solution was added to 100 mL of log-phase growing *Aeromonas hydrophila* N17 culture ($\times 10^7$ CFU/mL) in LB broth to get a final MOI of 0.1. The mixture was incubated at 30 °C. An aliquot of 1 mL was collected from the sample every two min over a period of 60 min. The sample was then centrifuged at 4000 g for 15 min, and then the supernatant was diluted with SM buffer + 1% chloroform (http://cshprotocols.cshlp.org/content/2006/1/pdb.rec8111.full?text_only=true). Then, the titers of unabsorbed free phages in the supernatant were determined by the double-layer agar technique, and the results were recorded as percentages of the initial phage counts. The percentages of free phages and the adsorption rates were calculated following the formula of Haq et al. [11].

4.7. One-Step Growth Curve

The phage and bacteria were prepared in the same way as in the adsorption method described above. At 40 min, when the adsorption rate was maximal, the mixture was further incubated at 30 °C with 150 rpm. Samples were collected every 5 min for 120 min and phage titers were determined by the double-layer agar technique. Then, the latent period and burst size were calculated [28].

4.8. Inactivation of *Aeromonas hydrophila* N17 in Vitro

The method used in this study was adapted from Jun et al. [12] and Le et al. [23] with some modifications described below. *A. hydrophila* N17 was streaked onto sheep blood agar (OXOID, UK), incubated at 30 °C overnight, and harvested on LB to have a final concentration of 10^7 CFU/mL. A 10 mL suspension of the *Aeromonas* sp. in LB (around 10^7 CFU/mL) was then mixed with same volume of a phage preparation (concentration of 10^5 to 10^7 PFU/mL) to reach multiplicity of infection (MOI) of 0.01, 0.1, 1 (http://www.bio-protocol.org/e1295). A 20 mL sample of *Aeromonas* sp. in LB ($\sim\times 10^7$ CFU/mL) was used as a control. The mixture was incubated at 30 °C and 150 rpm. Samples were taken every 30 min for 8 h to determine the exact time of the appearance of phage-resistant bacteria, and every 60 min for the next 6 h to determine the increase in the concentration of phage-resistant bacteria. Then, samples were withdrawn every 3 h to the end of the experiment. The concentration of the *Aeromonas* sp. was measured by optical density determination at 550 nm using a spectrophotometer (Thermo Scientific Genesys 20, Waltham, MA, USA).

4.9. Phage Treatment of Infected Fish

A total of 360 healthy catfish (*Pangasianodon hypophthalmus*) (30 g/fish) were divided into 12 groups in 50 L plastic tanks at 30 ± 1 °C. All treatment fishes were infected intraperitoneally with *A. hydrophila* N17 (final concentration: 3.2×10^6 CFU/fish) and were then immediately injected with a phage cocktail (MOI 0.01, 1 and 100). A positive control was composed of fishes injected with *A. hydrophila* N17 only. Negative controls 1 and 2 were fishes with no injection and fishes injected with fluid separated from the broth containing bacteria and medium, respectively. The mixed phage preparation consisted of Φ2 and Φ5.

The mortality rates of the fishes were recorded every 12 h for eight days, and the kidneys of both the dead and surviving fishes were subjected to a bacterial isolation study [3]. Bacteria isolation was carried out from all dead fishes, indicating that the deaths were caused by *A. hydrophila* [3]. All treatments were performed in duplicates.

The animal experiment was conducted according to the animal ethical guidelines of the Vietnamese government (project supported by Vietnam Ministry of Agriculture and Rural Development, 2016–2018, number: 04/TCTS-KHCN-HTQT-DT 2016).

4.10. Statistical analysis

IBM SPSS Statistics 20 software was used to analyze the data. Single factor ANOVA was applied to test for differences in the fish numbers in the *Aeromonas*-infected fishes receiving or not the phage therapy ($p < 0.05$). Standard deviations were calculated in all experiments.

5. Conclusions

The phages Φ2 and Φ5, belonging to the *Myoviridae* family, were successfully isolated and displayed inhibition of the growth of the *A. hydrophila* strains tested. The results obtained from the use of a phage cocktail indicate that phages can be used successfully for the treatment of *Aeromonas* infections in catfish via intraperitoneal injection. Phages may therefore be considered as potential biocontrol agents to combat *Aeromonas* infections in fish farms.

Acknowledgments: Authors would like to acknowledge the financial support from the Vietnam Ministry of Agriculture and Rural Development (2016–2018, number: 04/TCTS-KHCN-HTQT-DT). Son Le Tuan gratefully acknowledges MOET-VIED/USC PhD scholarship.

Author Contributions: Tuan Son Le analysed the data and drafted the manuscript. Thi Hien Nguyen, Hong Phuong Vo, Trong Tuan Tran, Hong Loc Nguyen, Van Cuong Doan, Minh Trung Tran and Tuan Son Le conducted the experiments under the guidance of Ipek Kurtböke, Thi Hien Nguyen, and Hong Phuong Vo, D. Ipek Kurtböke and Paul C. Southgate oversaw the preparation of the manuscript.

References

1. Nguyen, N. Improving Sustainability of Striped Catfish (*Pangasianodon hypophthalmus*) Farming in the Mekong Delta, Vietnam through Recirculation Technology. Ph.D. Thesis, Wageningen University, Wageningen, The Netherlands, 2016.
2. Dung, T.; Ngoc, N.; Thinh, N.; Thy, D.; Tuan, N.; Shinn, A.; Crumlish, M. Common diseases of pangasius catfish farmed in Viet Nam. *GAA* **2008**, *11*, 77–78.
3. Hien, N.T.; Lan, M.T.; Anh, P.V.N.; Phuong, V.H.; Loc, N.H.; Trong, C.Q.; Trung, C.T.; Phuoc, L.H. Report "Genetics of *Aeromonas hydrophila* on Catfish". *Research Institute for Aquaculture No. 2.* 2014. Available online: http://www.sinhhoctomvang.vn/ban-tin/chi-tiet/Phat-hien-gen-gay-doc-cua-vi-khuan-Aeromonas-hydrophila-gay-benh-xuat-huyet-tren-ca-tra-106/ (accessed on 7 August 2017). (in Vietnamese).
4. Vivekanandhan, G.; Savithamani, K.; Hatha, A.; Lakshmanaperumalsamy, P. Antibiotic resistance of *aeromonas hydrophila* isolated from marketed fish and prawn of south India. *Int. J. Food Microbiol.* **2002**, *76*, 165–168. [CrossRef]
5. Guz, L.; Kozinska, A. Antibiotic susceptibility of *Aeromonas hydrophila* and *A. sobria* isolated from farmed carp (*cyprinus carpio l.*). *Bull. Vet. Inst. Pulawy* **2004**, *48*, 391–395.
6. Thi, Q.V.C.; Dung, T.T.; Hiep, D.P.H. The current status antimicrobial resistance in *Edwardsiella ictaluri* and *Aeromonas hydrophila* cause disease on the striped catfish farmed in the mekong delta. *Cantho Univ. J. Sci.* **2014**, *2*, 7–14. (In vietnamese)
7. Pridgeon, J.W.; Klesius, P.H. Major bacterial diseases in aquaculture and their vaccine development. *CAB Rev.* **2012**, *7*, 1–16. [CrossRef]
8. Hsu, C.-H.; Lo, C.-Y.; Liu, J.-K.; Lin, C.-S. Control of the eel (*anguilla japonica*) pathogens, *Aeromonas hydrophila* and *Edwardsiella tarda*, by bacteriophages. *J. Fish. Soc. Taiwan* **2000**, *27*, 21–31.
9. El-Araby, D.; El-Didamony, G.; Megahed, M. New approach to use phage therapy against *Aeromonas hydrophila* induced Motile Aeromonas Septicemia in nile tilapia. *J. Mar. Sci. Res. Dev.* **2016**, *6*. [CrossRef]
10. Ackermann, H.-W. 5500 phages examined in the electron microscope. *Arch. Virol.* **2007**, *152*, 227–243. [CrossRef] [PubMed]
11. Haq, I.U.; Chaudhry, W.N.; Andleeb, S.; Qadri, I. Isolation and partial characterization of a virulent bacteriophage ihq1 specific for *Aeromonas punctata* from stream water. *Microb. Ecol.* **2012**, *63*, 954–963. [CrossRef] [PubMed]
12. Jun, J.W.; Kim, J.H.; Shin, S.P.; Han, J.E.; Chai, J.Y.; Park, S.C. Protective effects of the *Aeromonas* phages pah1-c and pah6-c against mass mortality of the cyprinid loach (*misgurnus anguillicaudatus*) caused by *Aeromonas hydrophila*. *Aquaculture* **2013**, *416*, 289–295. [CrossRef]
13. Kim, J.; Son, J.; Choi, Y.; Choresca, C.; Shin, S.; Han, J.; Jun, J.; Kang, D.; Oh, C.; Heo, S. Isolation and characterization of a lytic *Myoviridae* bacteriophage pas-1 with broad infectivity in *Aeromonas salmonicida*. *Curr. Microbiol.* **2012**, *64*, 418–426. [CrossRef] [PubMed]
14. Anand, T.; Vaid, R.K.; Bera, B.C.; Singh, J.; Barua, S.; Virmani, N.; Yadav, N.K.; Nagar, D.; Singh, R.K.; Tripathi, B. Isolation of a lytic bacteriophage against virulent *Aeromonas hydrophila* from an organized equine farm. *J. Basic Microb.* **2016**, *56*, 432–437. [CrossRef] [PubMed]
15. Chow, M.S.; Rouf, M. Isolation and partial characterization of two *Aeromonas hydrophila* bacteriophages. *Appl. Environ. Microbiol.* **1983**, *45*, 1670–1676. [PubMed]
16. Wu, J.-L.; Lin, H.-M.; Jan, L.; Hsu, Y.-L.; Chang, L.-H. Biological control of fish bacterial pathogen, *Aeromonas hydrophila*, by bacteriophage ah 1. *Fish Pathol.* **1981**, *15*, 271–276. [CrossRef]
17. Fortier, L.-C.; Moineau, S. Morphological and genetic diversity of temperate phages in clostridium difficile. *Appl. Environ. Microbiol.* **2007**, *73*, 7358–7366. [CrossRef] [PubMed]
18. Walakira, J.; Carrias, A.; Hossain, M.; Jones, E.; Terhune, J.; Liles, M. Identification and characterization of bacteriophages specific to the catfish pathogen, *Edwardsiella ictaluri*. *J. Appl. Microbiol.* **2008**, *105*, 2133–2142. [CrossRef] [PubMed]

19. CLSI. Performance standards for antimicrobial susceptibility testing 27th ed. CLSI supplement m100. *Clinical and Laboratory Standards Institute*. 2017. Available online: http://www.facm.ucl.ac.be/intranet/CLSI/CLSI-2017-M100-S27.pdf (accessed on 10 November 2017).
20. Lamy, B.; Laurent, F.; Kodjo, A.; Roger, F.; Jumas-Bilak, E.; Marchandin, H.; Group, C.S. Which antibiotics and breakpoints should be used for *Aeromonas* susceptibility testing? Considerations from a comparison of agar dilution and disk diffusion methods using Enterobacteriaceae breakpoints. *Eur. J. Clin. Microbiol. Infect. Dis.* **2012**, *31*, 2369–2377. [CrossRef] [PubMed]
21. Daka, D.; Yihdego, D. Antibiotic-resistance *Staphylococcus aureus* isolated from cow's milk in the hawassa area, south Ethiopia. *Ann. Clin. Microbiol. Antimicrob.* **2012**, *11*. [CrossRef] [PubMed]
22. Cerveny, K.E.; DePaola, A.; Duckworth, D.H.; Gulig, P.A. Phage therapy of local and systemic disease caused by *Vibrio vulnificus* in iron-dextran-treated mice. *Infect. Immun.* **2002**, *70*, 6251–6262. [CrossRef] [PubMed]
23. Le, T.S.; Southgate, P.C.; O'Connor, W.; Poole, S.; Kurtböke, D.I. Bacteriophages as biological control agents of enteric bacteria contaminating edible oysters. *Curr. Microbiol.* **2017**. [CrossRef] [PubMed]
24. Paterson, W.; Douglas, R.; Grinyer, I.; McDermott, L. Isolation and preliminary characterization of some *Aeromonas salmonicida* bacteriophages. *J. Fish. Board Canada* **1969**, *26*, 629–632. [CrossRef]
25. Ackermann, H.-W.; Dauguet, C.; Paterson, W.; Popoff, M.; Rouf, M.; Vieu, J.-F. *Aeromonas* bacteriophages: Reexamination and classification. *Ann. Inst. Pasteur Virol.* **1985**, *136*, 175–199. [CrossRef]
26. Goodridge, L.; Gallaccio, A.; Griffiths, M.W. Morphological, host range, and genetic characterization of two coliphages. *Appl. Environ. Microbiol.* **2003**, *69*, 5364–5371. [CrossRef] [PubMed]
27. Phumkhachorn, P.; Rattanachaikunsopon, P. Isolation and partial characterization of a bacteriophage infecting the shrimp pathogen *Vibrio harveyi*. *Afr. J. Microbiol. Res.* **2010**, *4*, 1794–1800.
28. Hyman, P.; Abedon, S.T. Practical methods for determining phage growth parameters. *Methods Mol. Boil.* **2009**, *501*, 175–202.

6

Synergistic Action of Phage and Antibiotics: Parameters to Enhance the Killing Efficacy Against Mono and Dual-Species Biofilms

Ergun Akturk [1], Hugo Oliveira [1], Sílvio B. Santos [1], Susana Costa [1], Suleyman Kuyumcu [2], Luís D. R. Melo [1,*] and Joana Azeredo [1,*]

1 LIBRO-Laboratório de Investigação em Biofilmes Rosário Oliveira, Centre of Biological Engineering, University of Minho, Campus de Gualtar, 4700-057 Braga, Portugal

2 Department of Medical Genetics, Medical Faculty, Sifa University, 35535 Izmir, Turkey

* Correspondence: lmelo@deb.uminho.pt (L.D.R.M.); jazeredo@deb.uminho.pt (J.A.)

Abstract: *Pseudomonas aeruginosa* and *Staphylococcus aureus* are opportunistic pathogens and are commonly found in polymicrobial biofilm-associated diseases, namely chronic wounds. Their co-existence in a biofilm contributes to an increased tolerance of the biofilm to antibiotics. Combined treatments of bacteriophages and antibiotics have shown a promising antibiofilm activity, due to the profound differences in their mechanisms of action. In this study, 48 h old mono and dual-species biofilms were treated with a newly isolated *P. aeruginosa* infecting phage (EPA1) and seven different antibiotics (gentamicin, kanamycin, tetracycline, chloramphenicol, erythromycin, ciprofloxacin, and meropenem), alone and in simultaneous or sequential combinations. The therapeutic efficacy of the tested antimicrobials was determined. Phage or antibiotics alone had a modest effect in reducing biofilm bacteria. However, when applied simultaneously, a profound improvement in the killing effect was observed. Moreover, an impressive biofilm reduction (below the detection limit) was observed when gentamicin or ciprofloxacin were added sequentially after 6 h of phage treatment. The effect observed does not depend on the type of antibiotic but is influenced by its concentration. Moreover, in dual-species biofilms it was necessary to increase gentamicin concentration to obtain a similar killing effect as occurs in mono-species. Overall, combining phages with antibiotics can be synergistic in reducing the bacterial density in biofilms. However, the concentration of antibiotic and the time of antibiotic application are essential factors that need to be considered in the combined treatments.

Keywords: *Pseudomonas aeruginosa*; *Staphylococcus aureus*; bacteriophage; dual-species; biofilms; antibiotic; synergy; simultaneous; sequential

1. Introduction

Polymicrobial interactions are widespread in many biofilm-associated infections [1], accounting for a significant higher mortality and considerable high costs to the health-care systems [2,3]. Biofilms are communities of microbial cells adhered to biotic or abiotic surfaces and encased in a self-produced extracellular polymeric matrix that confer protection to the community against adverse environmental conditions and antimicrobials including the presence of antibiotics [4]. In an established polymicrobial biofilm, the co-existence of different species is a clear advantage for the overall biofilm population. These biofilms very often exhibit improved capabilities and functions compared to single-species ones [5,6], such as enhanced degradation of organic compounds [7], increased virulence [8], and increased tolerance against antimicrobials [9].

Pseudomonas aeruginosa and *Staphylococcus aureus* are versatile bacterial pathogens and common etiological agents of polymicrobial associated infections. These two opportunistic pathogens exhibit intrinsic and acquired antibiotic resistance [10]. When co-existing in a biofilm this tolerance largely increases, namely due to the decreased metabolic activity, increased bacterial doubling time, and increased level of mutations and upregulation of efflux pumps [11].

Bacteriophages (or phages), viruses that infect bacteria, are natural antibacterial agents that specifically infect and lyse bacteria. Phages are the most abundant biological entities on our planet and can be used as biocontrol agents targeting bacterial cells either in suspension or in biofilms [12,13]. Due to the phage bacterial host specificity and bacteriolytic activity against antibiotic-resistant strains, phage therapy has been suggested as a valuable approach to control numerous pathogenic bacteria. Phages can penetrate the inner layers of the biofilms and infect dormant cells [14], which is a clear advantage of phages compared to antibiotics in killing biofilms. Therefore, it has been proposed that phages may be a useful combination with antibiotic treatment [15–17]. Several studies demonstrated the efficiency of phage and antibiotic combinations in planktonic cultures of *P. aeruginosa* [17,18] and biofilms [19]. Besides, phages and antibiotics use different mechanisms of action, which make them effective against phage/antibiotic resistance pathogens [17]. Consequently, antibiotic and phage resistance have a low chance of evolving at the same time and, besides, bacteria resistant to one agent will be taken by the other agent. However, to our knowledge, this type of studies was never assessed on dual-species biofilms.

In this study, we report the isolation and characterization of a new *Pakpunavirus* phage, named vB_PaM_EPA1, and the use of several phage-antibiotic combinations against mono and dual-species biofilms of *P. aeruginosa* and *S. aureus*.

2. Results

2.1. Isolation and Characterization of a New *P. aeruginosa*-Infecting Phage

Six clinical strains were used for phage enrichment (Table S1), using raw sewage from Sifa Hospital (Izmir, Turkey) as phage sources. A phage vB_PaM_EPA1 (EPA1) was isolated, and its plaque morphology was characterized by clear and small plaques (0.8 mm in diameter) surrounded by halo rings on the host strain Sifa_Pa_1.5 (Table S1). The morphology of EPA1 particles was observed by Transmission Electron Microscopy (TEM). EPA1 has an icosahedral head with 69 nm in diameter and a contractile tail of 145 × 24 nm. According to Ackermann's classification [20], EPA1 belongs to the *Caudovirales* order and *Myoviridae* family (Figure 1).

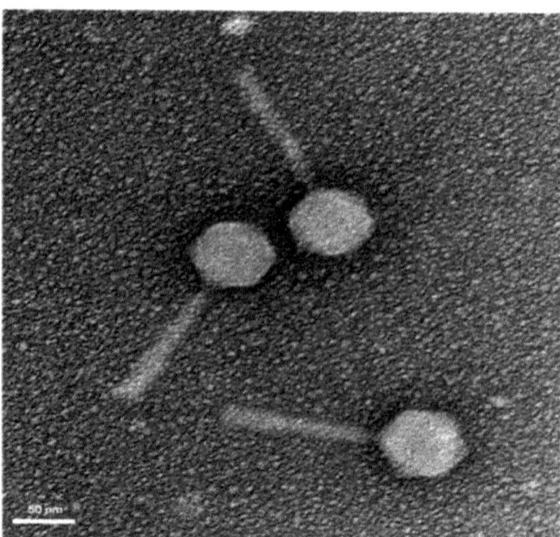

Figure 1. TEM image of *P. aeruginosa* specific phage EPA1 obtained by negative staining with 2% (*w/v*) uranyl acetate. Scale bar represents 50 nm.

2.2. Host range, Efficiency of Plating and One-Step Growth Curve

In total, seventeen drug-resistant clinical isolates (Table S1) and three reference *P. aeruginosa* strains were used to determine the host range and the efficiency of plating (EOP) of EPA1 (Table S1). EPA1 has a broad spectrum of activity (within the panel of strains used) and was able to propagate on 70% (14 out of 20) of the *P. aeruginosa* strains with moderate to high EOP. No lysis from without events were observed. Also, no correlation between phage susceptibility and antibiotic resistance was detected (Table S1). Due to the fact that EPA1 propagates better in *P. aeruginosa* PAO1 strain, we have used this strain to produce the phage for further experiments. Nevertheless, we are aware of the fact that PAO1 encloses filamentous phages that could influence phage production, however no filamentous phages were detected by plating methods or TEM [21]. One-step growth curve (OSGC) experiments were performed to examine the infection parameters of EPA1. The latent period of EPA1 was around 10 min, and the burst size was approximately of 34 progeny phages per infected cell (Figure S1).

2.3. Genome Analysis of EPA1

EPA1 has a linear double-stranded DNA genome containing 91,394 bp with an average 49.2% GC content. This phage encodes 175 putative CDSs, of which 35 have a putative function, and 140 are considered hypothetical/novel (Table S2). Most predicted gene products exhibit homology to phage known proteins belonging to the *Pakpunavirus* (ICTV 2015.029a-dB ratification) genus, mostly *Pseudomonas* phages JG004 (NC_019450.1), PAK_P4 (NC_022986) and vB_PaeM_C2-10_Ab1 (NC_019918). Moreover, seventeen tRNA genes coding for Arg, Asn, Asp, Cys, Gln, Glu, Gly, Ile, Lys, Leu, Met, Phe, Pro, Ser, Thr, Trp and Tyr were found. Regarding regulatory elements, 16 promoters were identified as well as 14 rho-independent terminators. The general characteristics of the phage genome are summarized in Table 1. Whole-genome comparisons through BLASTN show that EPA1 has a high overall nucleotide identity (>90%) with other *P. aeruginosa* phages, such as JG004 (NC_019450.1), vB_PaeM_SCUT-S2 (MK340761.1) and SRT6 (MH370478.1). EPA1 shares >145 proteins with these phages.

Table 1. General features of EPA1 genome.

Feature	vB_PaM_EPA1
Genome size	91,394 bp
G+C content	49,2%
Number of predicted CDSs	175
Number of proteins with assigned functions	35

2.4. Characterisation of Mono and Dual-Species Biofilm Models

In vitro mono and dual-species biofilms were formed in 24-well polystyrene plates for 48 h, and the number of viable bacteria cells were determined by colony forming unit (CFU) counting. It is well documented that *P. aeruginosa* inhibits *S. aureus* proliferation in dual-species biofilms. The reason for the lower density of *S. aureus* population has been attributed to the toxic effect of *P. aeruginosa* exoproducts [22], including LasA protease, 4-hydroxy-2-heptylquinoline-N-oxide (HQNO) [23], the Pel and Psl products [24], and phenazines such as pyocyanin [25]. Therefore, in order to successfully produce dual-species biofilms, biofilm formation has been initiated with an *S. aureus* cell culture, and 24 h later *P. aeruginosa* cells were added on the *S. aureus* biofilm, then incubated for another 24 h. A similar strategy of biofilm formation was also used by DeLeon et al. [26] where biofilms were initiated with *S. aureus*, and 48 h later *P. aeruginosa* cells were added [26]. Our results showed that the number of viable cells of *S. aureus* was 3.77×10^7 CFU/mL and 1.2×10^9 CFU/mL for *P. aeruginosa* in the mono-species biofilms. Regarding the dual-species biofilms, the concentrations were 1.28×10^7 CFU/mL for *S. aureus* and 2×10^8 CFU/mL for *P. aeruginosa*.

2.5. *Biofilm Treatments*

The selected antibiotics (Table 2) and EPA1 were tested individually or in combinations within intact mono, and dual-species 48 h biofilms and treated for 24 h in total. Phage and antibiotics were simultaneously or sequentially added in combined treatments. Twenty-four hours post-treatment, CFUs were enumerated in order to assess the antibiofilm efficacy and to characterize the possible interactions between antimicrobials.

Table 2. List of the antibiotics, MIC values of *P. aeruginosa* and *S. aureus* planktonic cells and their mechanism of action.

Name of Antibiotics	*P. aeruginosa* MIC Values	*S. aureus* MIC Values	Mechanism of Action	
Gentamicin	4 μg/mL	16 μg/mL	Protein Synthesis Inhibitors	30S ribosomal
Kanamycin	10 μg/mL	*	Protein Synthesis Inhibitors	subunit
Tetracycline	8 μg/mL	*	Protein Synthesis Inhibitors	
Chloramphenicol	32 μg/mL	*	Protein Synthesis Inhibitors	50S ribosomal
Erythromycin	128 μg/mL	*	Protein Synthesis Inhibitors	subunit
Ciprofloxacin	<1 μg/mL	<1 μg/mL	DNA Synthesis Inhibitor	
Meropenem	2 μg/mL	2 μg/mL	Cell wall Synthesis Inhibitor	

* These antibiotics were not tested on *S. aureus* biofilm models.

Further, the effects of phage, gentamicin at MIC and phage-gentamicin at MIC combinations (simultaneous and sequential) in mono and dual-species biofilms were also analyzed by confocal laser microscopy (CLSM). For that assessment, fluorescence probes were designed to specifically target differentially both bacterial species. Generally, microscopy analysis corroborated cell counting results.

2.5.1. Antibiotics and Phages Alone cause a Moderate Killing Effect on Biofilms

Three antibiotics were selected (gentamicin, ciprofloxacin and meropenem), and their anti-biofilm ability was tested against *P. aeruginosa* and *S. aureus* mono-species biofilms. These antibiotics were selected depending on their mechanism of action (Table 2): protein synthesis inhibitor (gentamicin), DNA synthesis inhibitor (ciprofloxacin) and cell wall synthesis inhibitor (meropenem). The killing effect of the antibiotics against *P. aeruginosa* biofilms, used in different concentrations, ranged from 0.8 to 5 orders-of-magnitude (Figure 2).

Regarding *S. aureus*, no significant reduction in the number of viable cells was observed when antibiotics were applied at their MIC (Figure S2). However, when gentamicin was applied with 8xMIC, the number of viable cells was reduced approximately 1.4 orders-of-magnitude (Figure S2).

Additionally, EPA1 was individually tested (at multiplicity of infection, MOI, of 1) on *P. aeruginosa* biofilms for 6 h and 24 h. The observed reductions were 3.4 and 0.5 orders-of-magnitude, respectively (Figure 2, Figure 3b,c). The best reduction was observed at 6 h post-treatment; after that, *P. aeruginosa* cells started to regrow (Figure 2). CLSM images corroborated CFUs results. *P. aeruginosa* biofilms after being challenged for 6 h with EPA1 reduced their thickness from 22.4 μm to 7.2 μm, but after 24 h of phage contact an increase in biofilm thickness to 11.7 μm was observed (Figure 3a–c).

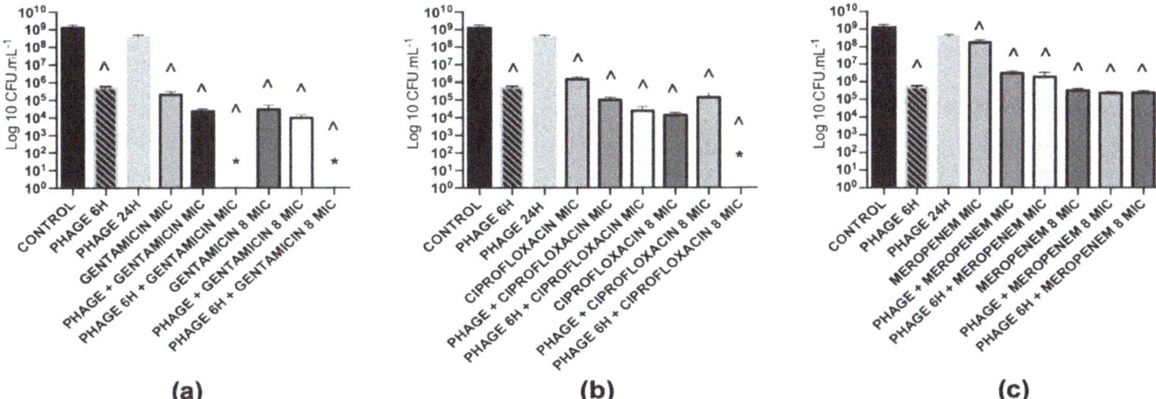

Figure 2. Treatment of *P. aeruginosa* PAO1 48 h biofilms with different antimicrobial agents individually or in combinations; phage EPA1 and (**a**) gentamicin; (**b**) ciprofloxacin; and (**c**) meropenem for 24 h. A prefix PHAGE indicates EPA1 in MOI 1, 6 H and 24 Hindicates treatment time period for 6 and 24 h, MIC indicates the dose of antibiotics with 1-time MIC value of *P. aeruginosa* 8× MIC indicates the dose of antibiotics with 8-times MIC value of *P. aeruginosa*, PHAGE + antibiotic indicates simultaneous treatment, and PHAGE 6 H+ antibiotics indicates phage was added first then antibiotic was added with 6 h delay. * Under detection limit (<10^2). (^) Statistical differences between the control and treated biofilms were determined by two-way repeated-measures analysis of variance (ANOVA) with a Tukey's multiple comparison test.

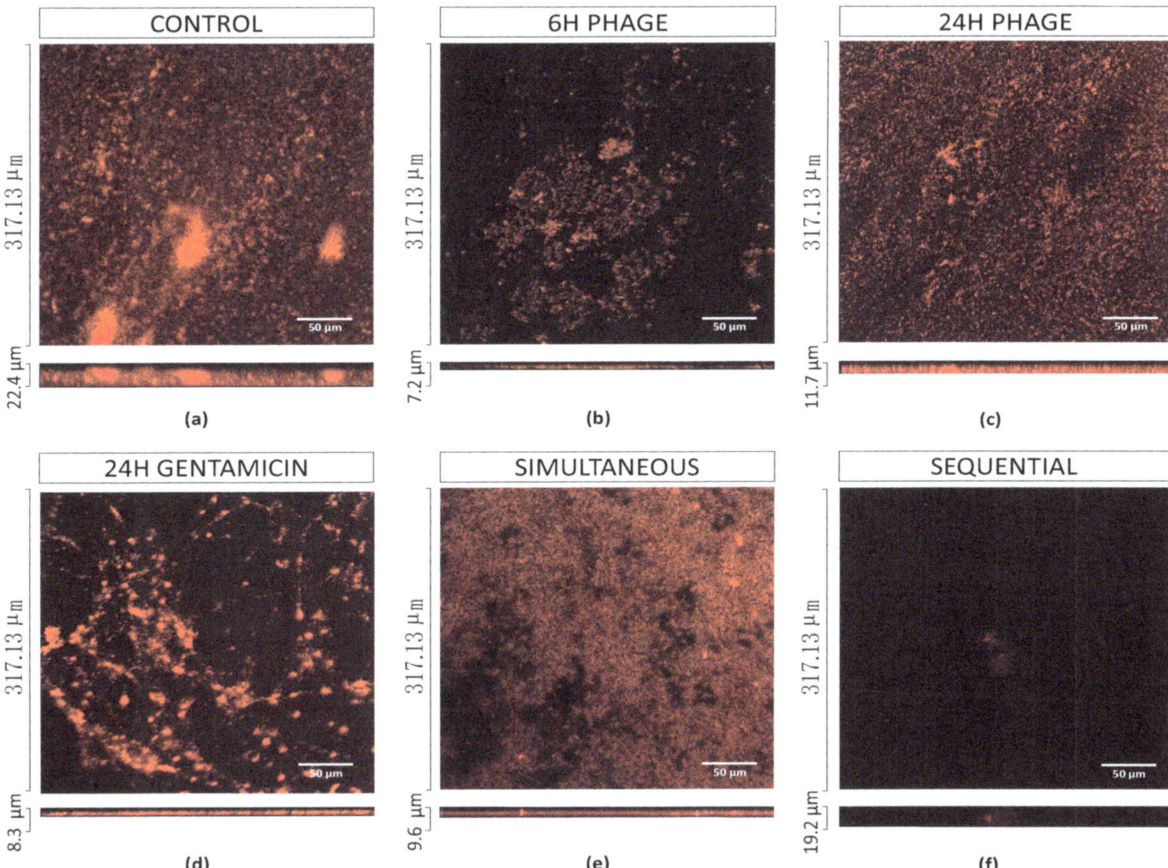

Figure 3. 3D reconstructions of confocal stacks of images of mono-species *P. aeruginosa* biofilms. (**a**) Control, (**b**) 6 h phage treatment, (**c**) 24 h phage treatment, (**d**) 24 h Gentamicin treatment, (**e**) 24 h simultaneous treatment, (**f**) 24 h sequential treatment. All biofilms were stained with EPA1_TFP (with mCherry) recombinant protein. Scale bar represents 50 μm.

2.5.2. Combined Treatments with Simultaneous Application of Phage and Antibiotics have Synergistic Effects for Low Concentrations of Antibiotics

The efficacy of the combinations of phage and antibiotics was also tested on *P. aeruginosa* mono-species biofilms. These maturated intact biofilms were treated in one of two ways; simultaneously (phage and antibiotic were added at the same time) and sequentially (phage was added first, then antibiotic was added with a delay of 6 h).

The combination of phage EPA1 with gentamicin (Figure 3e), ciprofloxacin, or meropenem when applied simultaneously with a lower dose (MIC) resulted in population reductions of 4.7, 4.1 and 2.6 orders-of-magnitudes (Figure 2), respectively. These results show a clear synergistic effect between antimicrobial agents in most cases (Table 3). When the antibiotic concentrations were increased, we were expecting an increase in the killing efficacy of simultaneous combined treatments, however, interestingly 8 × MIC did not increased the overall biofilm killing (in certain cases, we observed an antagonistic effect) (Table 3).

Table 3. General overview of the efficacy of combined treatments in 48 h *P. aeruginosa* mono-species biofilm. Synergistic—the biofilm reduction using phage-antibiotic combinations is greater than the sum of their individual treatments. Additive—the biofilm reduction using phage-antibiotic combination is similar to the sum of their individual treatments. Antagonistic—the biofilm reduction using phage-antibiotic combinations is lower than the sum of their individual treatments.

Treatments	Gentamicin	Ciprofloxacin	Meropenem
Simultaneously MIC	Synergistic	Synergistic	Synergistic
Simultaneously 8 MIC	Additive	Antagonistic	Antagonistic
Sequentially MIC	Synergistic	Synergistic	Synergistic
Sequentially 8 MIC	Synergistic	Synergistic	Antagonistic

2.5.3. Antibiotics that Target Protein and DNA Synthesis Mechanisms Interfere with Phage Replication

In order to understand why increasing the antibiotic concentration did not lead to an increased killing activity, we tested the effect of the antibiotics on phage replication. Phage titer was enumerated after 24 h of simultaneous treatment and compared with the control. Unsurprisingly, the titer of phages, when combined with gentamicin and ciprofloxacin was significantly lower than the titer of phages in control samples (Figure S3). Conversely and as expected, the phage replication was not affected by the presence of meropenem. This antibiotic is affecting bacteria cell wall synthesis and thus does not interfere in phage replication.

2.5.4. Combined Treatments with Sequential Application of Phage and Antibiotics have a better Killing Efficacy than when Applied Simultaneously

The fact that protein and DNA synthesis inhibitors interfere with phage replication, led us to assess a sequential treatment in which the phage was applied first and six hours later the antibiotic. This six hour period was chosen based on previous biofilm/phage interaction studies that refer that after six hours of phage interaction, a regrowth of phage-resistant phenotypes is observed [27]. Our CFU and CLSM results have also corroborated this phenomenon (Figures 2a and 3b,c).

The same phage-drug combinations tested before were applied in sequential treatments. The results showed an almost eradication of the biofilm with gentamicin (MIC, 8× MIC) (Figure 3f) and ciprofloxacin (8xMIC). Besides, other combinations with ciprofloxacin or meropenem (with MIC) also showed an increased killing effect, 4.7 and 2.8 orders-of-magnitudes, respectively. In accordance, increasing the antibiotic concentration of meropenem in sequential treatment (to 8× MIC), resulted in an antagonistic effect (3.7 orders-of-magnitudes), contrarily to what was observed for the other antibiotics (Figure 2). CLSM results also confirmed that almost all biofilm was eradicated except a cluster (Figure 3e). To understand the impact of antimicrobial application order in sequential interaction, the same combinations were applied in the reverse order. Gentamicin was applied first, and then phage was applied six hours after. The collected data showed that killing efficacies of combinations were reduced when gentamicin MIC and 8× MIC were applied first, with reductions of 2.5 and 3.6 orders-of-magnitude, respectively (Figure S4).

The data suggest that biofilm exposure to phage prior to antibiotics is more effective than simultaneous treatment in eliminating biofilm-associated cells. Considering the overall results, when gentamicin was administered at MIC sequentially after six hours of phage addition, it almost eradicated biofilms (Figure 3f).

2.5.5. The Phage Killing Efficacy with the Sequential Treatment of Phage and Gentamicin cannot be Extrapolated to other Protein Synthesis Inhibitors

An impressive biofilm biomass reduction was observed with a protein synthesis inhibitor (gentamicin) at MIC. To understand if this effect can be extrapolated to other antibiotics of the same class, we also tested kanamycin, tetracycline, erythromycin and chloramphenicol (Table 3), in simultaneous and sequential combinations. Contrarily to what we were expecting, the effect observed for gentamicin was not reproduced with the other tested antibiotics (Figure 4). In fact, those antibiotics alone had a low to moderate effect against biofilms, lower than 3 orders-of-magnitude in the overall biomass reduction. Gentamicin alone caused ten times more biomass damage, which could be one of the reasons for the better performance of sequential treatments with gentamicin compared to the other antibiotics.

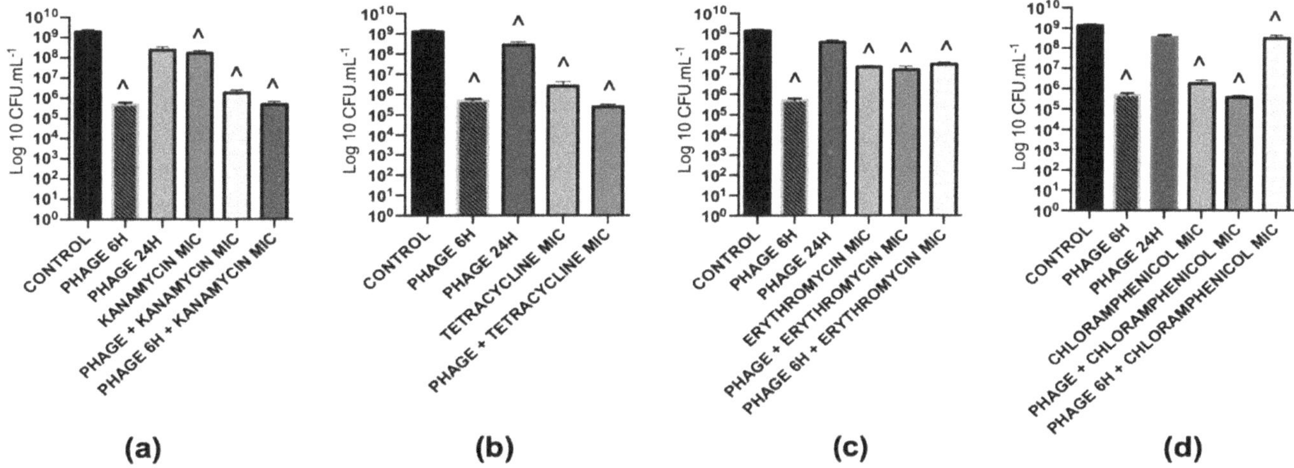

Figure 4. Treatment of *P. aeruginosa* PAO1 48 h biofilms with protein synthesis inhibitor antimicrobial agents individually or in combinations for 24 h. (**a**) Kanamycin is a 30S protein synthesis inhibitor; (**b**) Tetracycline is a 30S protein synthesis inhibitor; (**c**) Erythromycin is a 50S protein synthesis inhibitor; (**d**) Chloramphenicol is a 50Ss protein synthesis inhibitor. A prefix PHAGE indicates EPA1 in MOI 1, 6 H and 24 H indicates treatment time period for 6 and 24 h, MIC indicates the dose of antibiotics with 1-time MIC value of *P. aeruginosa*, PHAGE + antibiotic indicates simultaneous treatment and PHAGE 6 H + antibiotics indicates that phage was added first, then antibiotic was added with 6 h delay. (^) Statistical differences between the control and treated biofilms were determined by two-way repeated-measures analysis of variance (ANOVA) with a Tukey's multiple comparison test.

2.5.6. The Efficacy of Sequential Antibiofilm Treatments is Dependent on the Antibiotic Concentration

We also investigated the effect of the different gentamicin concentrations on the simultaneous and sequential treatment efficacy (Figure 5). A direct correlation was observed between the concentration of gentamicin and the biofilm killing efficacy. An almost complete biofilm eradication (below the detection limits) was observed only when antibiotic concentrations were equal or above the MIC (Table S1).

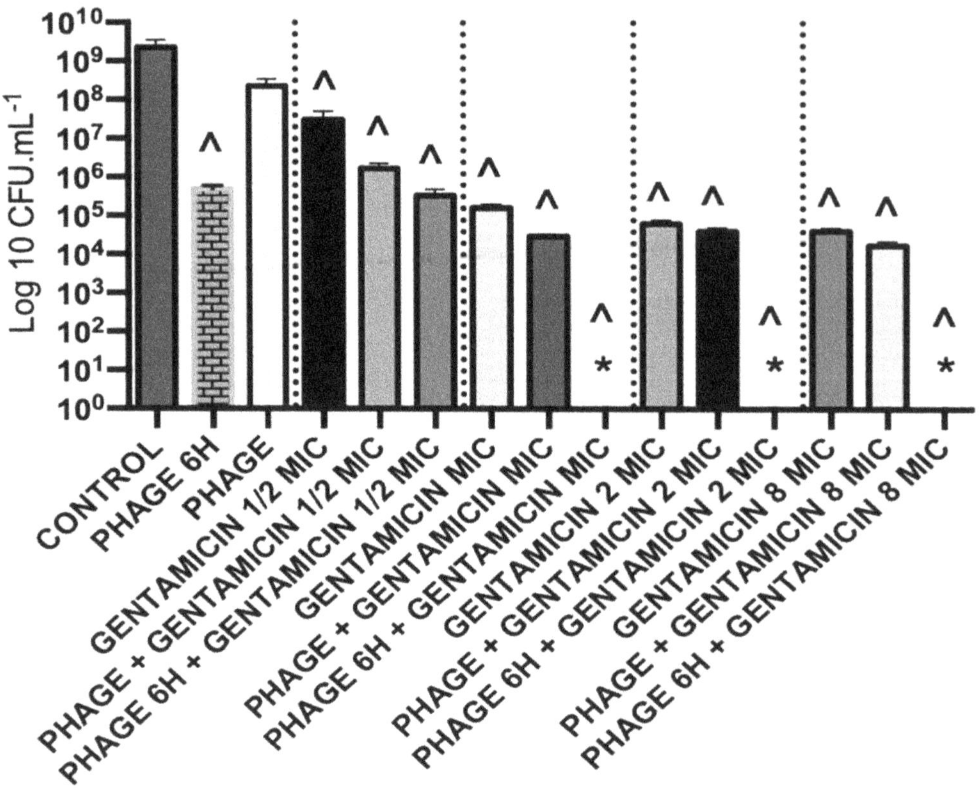

Figure 5. Treatment of *P. aeruginosa* PAO1 48 h biofilms with gentamicin at different concentrations. A prefix PHAGE indicates EPA1 in MOI 1, 1/2 MIC indicates the dose of antibiotics with 1/2× MIC value, MIC indicates the dose of antibiotics with 1× MIC value of *P. aeruginosa*, 2 MIC indicates the dose of antibiotics with 2× MIC value of *P. aeruginosa*, 8 MIC indicates the dose of antibiotics with 8× MIC value of *P. aeruginosa*, PHAGE + antibiotic indicates simultaneous treatment and PHAGE 6 H + antibiotics indicates phage was added first then antibiotic was added with 6 h delay. * Under detection limit (<10^2). (^) Statistical differences between the control and treated biofilms were determined by two-way repeated-measures analysis of variance (ANOVA) with a Tukey's multiple comparison test.

2.5.7. Sequential Application of Phages and Gentamicin have a great Antibiofilm Effect in Dual-Species Biofilms

The killing capacity of gentamicin (MIC) and EPA1 was tested individually and in combination (simultaneous and sequential treatments) in a dual-species biofilm model comprising *P. aeruginosa* and *S. aureus* (Figure 6). Intact biofilms were grown for 48 h and treated for 24 h in total. In the control, it was possible to observe a predominance of *P. aeruginosa* (1.4×10^9 CFU/mL), in comparison with *S. aureus* (2.3×10^5 CFU/mL) (Figure 7). Although *S. aureus* was the first colonizer, CLSM images indicate that both species were randomly distributed throughout the biofilm 3D structures (Figure 6).

The individual treatments with gentamicin with MIC and 8× MIC resulted in a significant reduction of approximately 3.3 orders-of-magnitude and 4.6 orders-of-magnitude of *P. aeruginosa* cells, respectively. Phage treatment was less effective than gentamicin, resulting in a reduction of 0.7 orders-of-magnitude of *P. aeruginosa* cells (Figure 8b). None of the individual treatments showed a significant impact on the *S. aureus* population (Figure 7).

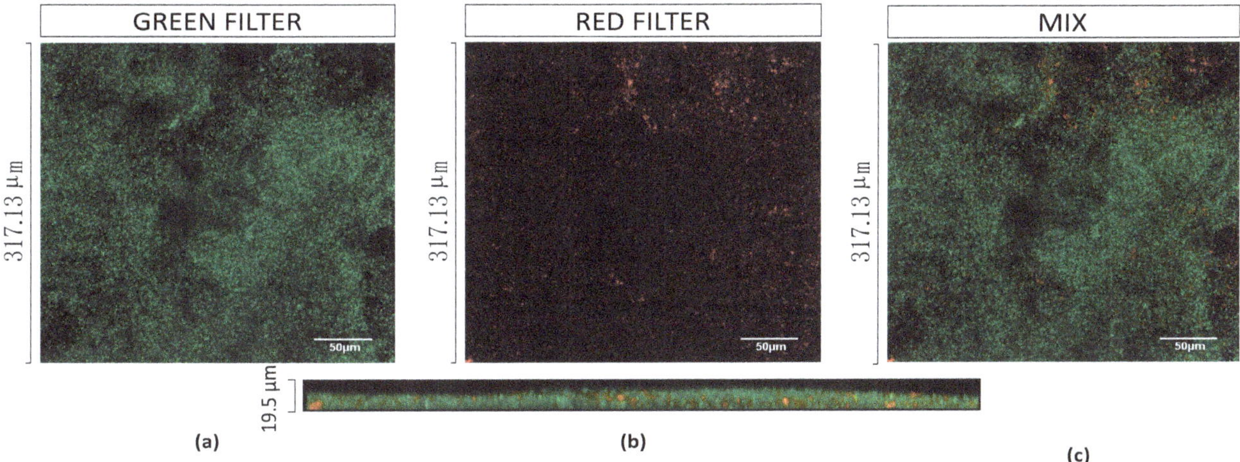

Figure 6. 3D reconstructions of confocal stacks of images of dual-species of *P. aeruginosa* and *S. aureus* biofilms. (**a**) 48 h old intact biofilms were stained by using recombinant proteins, LM12_AMI-SH3 (with GFP) specific for *S. aureus* and (**b**)EPA1_TFP (with mCherry) specific for *P. aeruginosa*. (**c**) 48 h old intact biofilms were stained by using both recombinant proteins. Scale bar represents 50 μm.

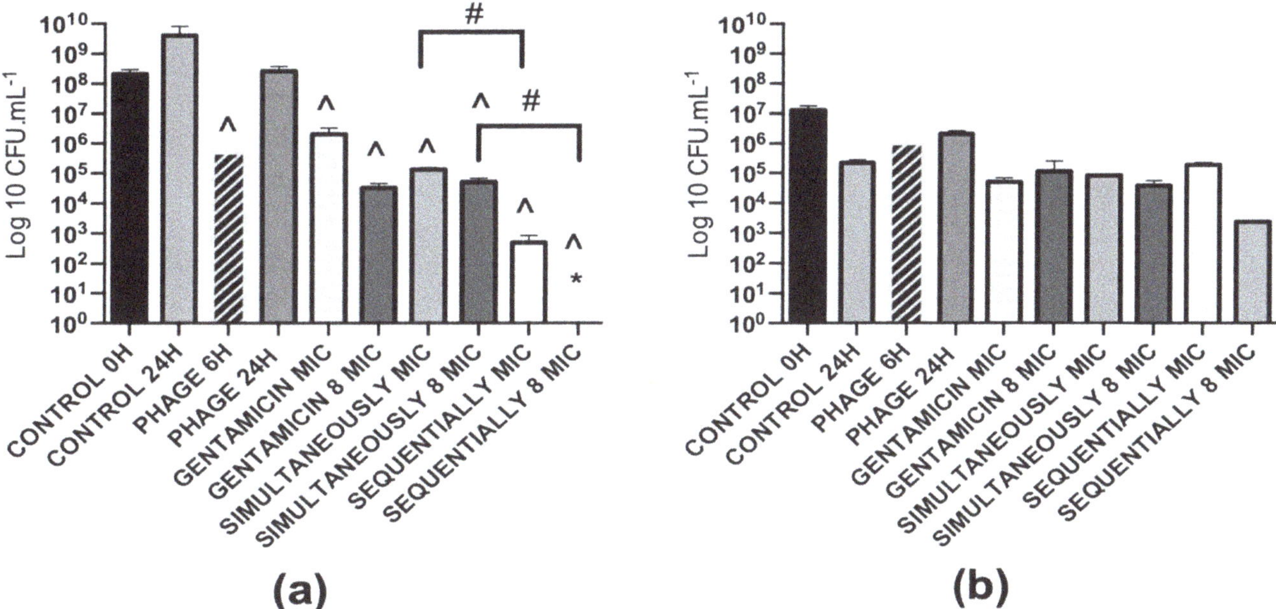

Figure 7. Treatment of 48 h dual-species biofilm. (**a**) *P. aeruginosa* number of viable cells. (**b**) *S. aureus* number of viable cells. A prefix PHAGE indicates EPA1 in MOI 1, 6 H and 24 H indicates treatment time period for 6 and 24 h, MIC indicates the dose of antibiotics with 1× MIC value of *P. aeruginosa*, 8 MIC indicates the dose of antibiotics with 8× MIC value of *P. aeruginosa*, PHAGE + antibiotic indicates simultaneous treatment and PHAGE 6 H + antibiotics indicates phage was added first then antibiotic was added with 6 h delay. * Under detection limit (<10^2). (^) Statistical differences between the control and treated biofilms. (#) Statistical differences between the simultaneously and sequentially treated biofilms. Statistical differences were determined by two-way repeated-measures analysis of variance (ANOVA) with a Tukey's multiple comparison test.

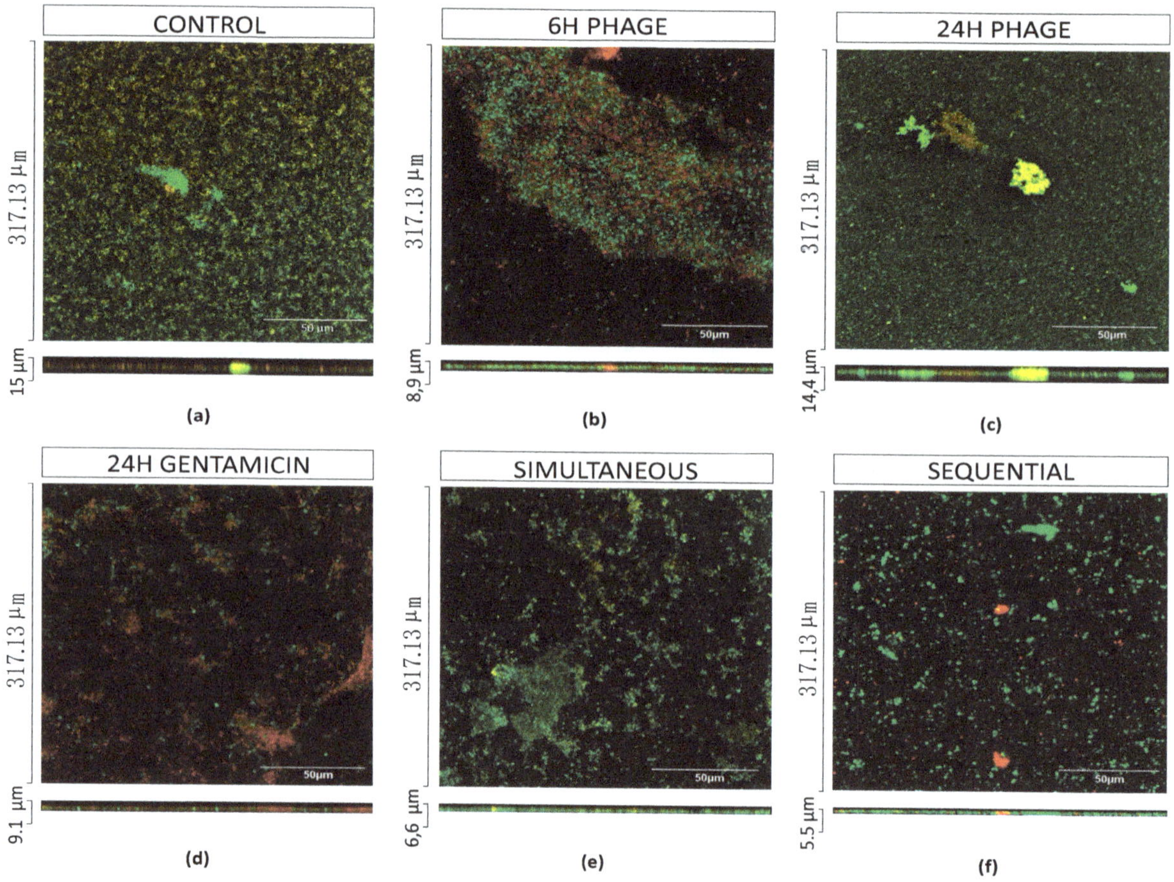

Figure 8. 3D reconstructions of confocal stacks of images of dual-species of *P. aeruginosa* and *S. aureus* biofilms. (**a**) Control, (**b**) 6 h phage treatment, (**c**) 24 h phage treatment, (**d**) 24 h Gentamicin with MIC treatment, (**e**) 24 h simultaneous treatment, (**f**) 24 h sequential treatment. 48 h old intact biofilms were stained by using LM12_AMI-SH3 (with GFP) and EPA1_TFP (with mCherry) recombinant proteins. Scale bar represents 50 µm.

Regarding the simultaneous treatments, no synergy was observed for any combination. On *P. aeruginosa*, phage-gentamicin MIC resulted in 4.1 orders-of-magnitude reduction (additive effect), while the phage-gentamicin 8 × MIC only slightly increased the reduction (4.6 orders-of-magnitude), demonstrating an antagonistic effect (Figure 8d). Both treatments also had a positive effect on *S. aureus* biofilm cell control, significantly reducing CFUs by about 0.4 and 0.8 orders-of-magnitude when using phage-gentamicin MIC and phage-gentamicin 8xMIC treatments, respectively (Figure 7).

Similarly, in mono-species biofilms, a sequential treatment was also tested. Results indicate that a preliminary phage treatment (6 h) before gentamicin application was very effective in biofilm reduction. Phage-gentamicin MIC reduced about 6.3 orders-of-magnitude the *P. aeruginosa* population, while phage-gentamicin 8× MIC almost eradicated *P. aeruginosa* cells (approximately 7orders-of-magnitude reduction) (Figure 8f). Although the phage-gentamicin treatment did not significantly impact the *S. aureus* population, the phage-gentamicin 8× MIC sequential application was also the most efficient treatment in reducing *S. aureus* biofilm cells in about 2 orders-of-magnitude (Figure 7).

In order to infer the impact of combined treatments on the biofilm structure, CLSM observations were performed on dual-species biofilms before and after the treatments. In this case, as in mono-species biofilms, we also observed a reduction of biofilm thickness, from 15 µm to 8.9 µm after 6 h of phage infection, and a biofilm thickness increase to 14.4 µm after 24 h of phage infection. The significant biofilm thickness reductions were observed in simultaneous and sequential combined treatments, after which the remaining biofilms had thicknesses of 6.6 µm and 5.5 µm, respectively.

3. Discussion

EPA1 is a lytic *Pseudomonas* phage, isolated from a hospital sewage, that belongs to the *Myoviridae* family (Figure 1) This phage has no identifiable lysogeny-associated genes or genes coding for toxins (Table S2). Phages from *Pakpunavirus* genus are highly conserved genetically and are described as having a broad host range, being therefore described as good for therapy. Indeed, EPA1 presented similar features and therefore could be considered a good candidate for further phage therapy approaches [28].

Herein, this phage was studied for its potential synergistic activity in combinations (simultaneous and sequential) with different antibiotics (at MIC and 8× MIC) against mono and dual-species biofilms.

Initially, three antibiotics (gentamicin, ciprofloxacin and meropenem) belonging to different classes were tested on mono-species biofilms. The efficacy of antibiotics ranged from 0.8 to 5 orders-of-magnitude (Figure 2) on *P. aeruginosa* biofilms, and no significant reductions were observed for *S. aureus*, except when gentamicin was applied with 8× MIC which reduced the biofilm density by approximately 1.4 orders-of-magnitude (Figure S2). The reductions were of 3.4 and 0.5 orders-of-magnitude when EPA1 was applied individually for 6 h and 24 h on *P. aeruginosa* biofilms, respectively.

To augmenting the effect of antimicrobials, combined therapies were applied. Interestingly, a synergistic effect of phages and antibiotics in simultaneous combinations was only observed when antibiotics were applied at MIC (Figure 2). Surprisingly, the increased concentration of antibiotics (8xMIC) in simultaneous combinations have not resulted in a higher biofilm efficacy (Figure 2). The fact that the increase in antibiotic concentrations did not lead to an increase of the antibiofilm efficacy might be related to phage replication inhibition phenomena [18]. As phage particles are constituted mainly by proteins, protein synthesis inhibitors and DNA synthesis inhibitors might affect the formation of new phage particles and therefore have an antagonistic effect on phage replication [18,29]. Our results (Figure S3) corroborate that phage titers obtained after phage infection in combination with antibiotic treatments were significantly lower than the titer of phage in the control (phage infection without antibiotic treatment).

Phage-antibiotic sequential approaches were already reported as a promising antibiofilm strategy [30]. In this study, an impressive biofilm biomass reduction was obtained when antibiotics were added to biofilms after 6 h of phage treatment. This was the time point where phages caused the maximum biofilm reduction. Similar observations were already reported elsewhere [27]. When phages interact with *P. aeruginosa* biofilms an initial population reduction is observed up to 6 h of phage contact and after that period the biofilm regrows. Biofilm regrowth was attributed to the emergence of phage-resistant variants that were equally well adapted to the biofilm phenotype [27].

On sequential treatments, we observed a synergistic effect with all combinations, when antibiotics were applied at their MICs. However, the antibiotic that showed the best antibiofilm efficacy was gentamicin. The combined treatment with this antibiotic was enough to eliminate all detectable biofilm cells in a concentration-dependent manner. The same phenomenon was not observed when other four protein synthesis inhibitors were used (Figure 4).

The antimicrobial synergy between phages has been in part explained by a more efficient penetration of both antibiotics and phages into the biofilm. In fact, it has been described that phages can degrade the biofilm matrix using depolymerases [31,32], enhancing their penetration into the deep layers of the biofilm. In the case of EPA1, no depolymerase was identified in its genome, therefore we have no evidence that this phenomenon might have been responsible for a synergistic action of the combined therapy. We have previously reported that phages can access the bottom layers of the biofilm migrating through the biofilm void spaces [33]. This might be the case in our study, since both mono and dual-species biofilms appeared to be heterogeneous structures with plenty of void spaces (Figures 3 and 6). This phenomenon leads phages to replicate in the deeper-layer of biofilm, reaching high titers and interrupting the biofilm matrix. The addition of antibiotics following this interruption results in an enhanced bacterial reduction due to the deeper penetration of these agents. When phages are applied prior to the antibiotic, they also avoid the antagonistic effect of antibiotics on phage replication, as was previously described [18]. After determining the best-case scenario to treat *P. aeruginosa* biofilms, it was our intention to study the impact of this treatment on dual-species biofilms. The relevance of studying polymicrobial communities has gained more interest on the last decade, mainly due to the fact that the vast majority of biofilms are formed by more than one species of bacteria and in some case also fungi, protozoa and algae [34]. This reason triggered the design of this study, and to our knowledge, this is the first time that this strategy is reported in dual-species biofilms.

The establishment of dual-species biofilm models was difficult, due to the inhibitory effect of *P. aeruginosa* on *S. aureus* cells, which is widely reported [9,10,35,36]. It is described that polymicrobial biofilms of chronic wounds are first colonized by small numbers of resident Gram-positive aerobic cocci, including *S. aureus*, after which there is a shift on wound microbiome, and Gram-negative bacilli are predominant on this environment [37]. As previously performed by DeLeon et al. [26], in our experiments, dual-species biofilms were established in two-steps. Colonization by *S. aureus* and a further addition of *P. aeruginosa* led to the establishment of stable biofilms.

In general, dual-species biofilms were more tolerant to all treatments than mono-species *P. aeruginosa* biofilms. Nevertheless, the sequential treatment at 8× MIC almost eradicated *P. aeruginosa* biofilm cells, but it did not increase the antimicrobial effect on *S. aureus*.

The presence of external selective pressures, like antibiotics or phages, can stimulate a cell response that can lead to increased tolerance to antibiotics, namely as a result of EPS production by *P. aeruginosa*. Alginate, Pel, and Psl, which are part of the biofilm extracellular matrix have a structural and protective function [38,39]. More specifically, Psl is described as creating a protective barrier against aminoglycosides [40]. Also, quorum-sensing molecules can justify the weaker effect of these approaches on dual-species biofilms [41].

The data collected herein showed that the concentration of gentamicin needs to be increased (8× MIC) to eliminate *P. aeruginosa* cells successfully in dual-species biofilms in comparison with mono-species biofilms. This can result in an overdose of antibiotics that can lead to toxicity in treatments [42].

Overall, from this study, two main conclusions emerge. First, the combined treatment with a sequential application of phages and then antibiotic is the most promising approach to combat infectious biofilms when compared with their individual and simultaneous treatments. Second, the majority of the studies of antibiofilm approaches are conducted in mono-species biofilms, and as demonstrated herein, the treatment outcomes are completely different when a second species is added. So, to achieve success, a phage cocktail comprising different *P. aeruginosa* and *S. aureus* phages targeting different bacterial receptors should be tested prior to antibiotic addition.

4. Material and Methods

4.1. Bacterial Strains and Culture Conditions

The biofilm-forming strains *P. aeruginosa* PAO1 and *S. aureus* (ATCC®25923™) were obtained from LPhage Laboratory in the Centre of Biology (CEB) strain collection (Braga, Portugal). Additional one *P. aeruginosa* clinical isolate and one Spanish Type Culture Collection (CECT) strain were obtained from Lphage Laboratory in CEB strain collection and Sifa Hospital Strain collection (Izmir, Turkey). In total, this accounts for a total of 20 strains used (Table S1) for isolating and characterizing the phage. The antibiogram profile of the clinical strains was previously established by the provider institutes. All strains were grown in Tryptic Soy Broth (TSB, VWR Chemicals, Randor, PA, USA), Tryptic Soy Agar (TSA; VWR Chemicals) or in TSA soft overlays (TSB with 0.6% agar) at 37 °C. In addition, mannitol salt agar (MSA; VWR Chemicals) was used to enumerate *S. aureus* cells in dual-species biofilms, while *P. aeruginosa* cells were counted in non-selective media (TSA).

4.2. Phage Isolation and Production

Phage was isolated from effluent samples of raw sewage from Sifa Hospitals in Izmir, Turkey. The phage enrichment method was applied to isolate the phage [43]. Briefly, 100 mL of the effluent were mixed with 100 mL of double-strength TSB and with 10 µL of each of the exponentially grown *P. aeruginosa* strains. The obtained suspensions were incubated at 37 °C and 120 rpm (BIOSAN ES-20/60, Riga, Latvia) overnight. Suspensions were further centrifuged (15 min, 9000× *g*, 4 °C), and the supernatants were filtered through a 0.22 µm polyethersulfone (PES) membrane (ThermoFisher Scientific, Massachusetts, USA). The presence of phages was confirmed by performing spot assays on bacterial lawns. The prepared plates were further incubated overnight at 37 °C, and the presence of inhibition halos observed. When phage plaques appeared, successive rounds of single plaque purification were carried out until purified plaques were observed, reflected by a single plaque morphology.

The purified phage was produced by using the double agar layer method, as described before [43]. Briefly, 100 µL of a phage suspension at 10^8 PFU/mL were spread on *P. aeruginosa* PAO1 lawns for overnight incubation at 37 °C. If full lysis was observed, plates were further incubated at 4 °C for 6 h at 120 rpm (BIOSAN PSU-10i), with 2 mL of SM Buffer (100 mM NaCl, 8 mM MgSO4, 50 mM Tris/HCl, pH 7.5) to resuspend the phage particles. The liquid phase was collected and centrifuged (15 min, 9000× *g*, 4 °C), and the supernatants were filtered through a 0.22 µm PES membrane. Purified phages were stored at 4 °C for further use.

4.3. Electron Microscopy

Phage suspension was sedimented by centrifugation (25,000× *g*, 60 min, 4 °C) using a ScanSpeed 1730R centrifuge (Labogene, Lillerød, Denmark). The pellet was further washed in tap water by repeating the centrifugation step. Subsequently, phage suspension was deposited on copper grids with a carbon-coated Formvar carbon film on a 200 square mesh nickel grid, stained with 2% uranyl acetate (pH 4.0) and examined using a Jeol JEM 1400 transmission electron microscope (TEM) (Tokyo, Japan).

4.4. Phage Host Range and Efficiency of Plating Determination

Phage host range was determined on the strains listed in Table 3, using the spot test method [43]. Briefly, 100 µL of each host-growing culture were added to 3 mL of TSB-soft agar and poured onto TSB agar plates. The bacterial lawns were spotted with 10 µL of serial 10-fold dilutions of the phage suspension and incubated at 37 °C for overnight and results were analyzed. The EOP was calculated by dividing the titer of the phage (PFU/mL) obtained in each isolate by the titer determined in the propagating host. EOP was recorded as high (>10%), moderate (0.01–9%) or low (<0.01%) [43].

4.5. Genome Sequencing and in Silico Analysis

P. aeruginosa EPA1 genomic DNA was extracted according to the standard methods with phenol-chloroform-isoamyl alcohol, as described elsewhere [44]. The genome was sequenced using the genome sequencer FLX Instrument (Roshe Life Science), *de novo* assembled using Geneious R9 and manually inspected. The genome was annotated using MyRAST algorithm [45]. The CDSs putative functions were assigned using BLASTP [46] with tRNAs being predicted with tRNAscan-SE [47] and ARAGORN [48]. HHPRED [49] was used to detect protein homology and structure prediction. N-terminal signal peptides with SignalP 3.0. [50] Transcriptional factors were determined by MEME [51] and ARNold [52] for the promoter and rho-independent terminators, respectively. For comparative studies, genomic comparisons were made using BLASTN and OrthoVenn [53], for DNA and protein sequence similarities.

4.6. *Minimal Inhibitory Concentration Determination*

Seven different antibiotics were selected to use in the study: gentamicin, kanamycin, tetracycline, chloramphenicol, erythromycin, ciprofloxacin and meropenem. MIC values were determined by the microdilution method for *P. aeruginosa* PAO1 according to the described method [54] (Table 2).

4.7. *Establishing Mono and Dual-Species Biofilms*

Mono and dual-species biofilm formation was performed in 24 polystyrene well plates (Orange Scientific, Braine-l'Alleud, Belgium). For initiating the biofilms, one bacterial colony (*P. aeruginosa* or *S. aureus)* was incubated in TSB overnight in an orbital shaker (120 rpm, BIOSAN ES-20/60) at 37 °C.

For establishing mono-species biofilms, 10 μL of the starter culture were transferred into 24-well plates containing 990 μL of fresh TSB media. The plates were incubated for 24 h in an orbital shaker incubator (120 rpm, BIOSAN ES-20/60) at 37 °C. After 24 h, half of the growth media (500 μL TSB, 1:1, *v:v*) was replaced with fresh TSB then, incubated for more 24 h.

For dual-species biofilms, the procedure was similar with some differences. *S. aureus* cells were inoculated prior to *P. aeruginosa* addition. Thus, biofilms were initiated with 10 μL of the overnight culture of *S. aureus* (~10^8 CFU/mL) in 990 μL TSB and incubated for 24 h in an orbital shaker (120 rpm) at 37 °C. After that, half of the growth media (500 μL TSB, 1:1, *v:v*) was replaced with TSB including 10 μL of the starter culture of *P. aeruginosa* (~10^8 CFU/mL, 1:49, *v/v*) and incubated for additional 24 h.

In mono and dual-species biofilms, the liquid part was aspirated, and the wells were washed twice with saline solution (0.9% NaCl (*w/v*)) to remove planktonic bacteria. Biofilms were further scraped in saline solution (1 mL) using a micropipette tip, and the number of viable cells was determined using the microdrop method [43]. Three independent experiments were performed in duplicate.

4.8. *Biofilm Challenge*

Forty-eight hours old mono and dual-species biofilms were treated with the antimicrobials; individually, in simultaneous or sequential combinations for 24 h post-treatment. Briefly, biofilms were washed twice with the saline solution and antibiotics (MIC or 8× MIC) and phage (MOI 1) were applied in TSB, individually. Also, the efficacy of two combinations was tested. In simultaneous combination, one of the selected antibiotics with MIC or 8× MIC combined with phage at MOI 1 in TSB solution was added into biofilm-bearing wells for 24 h post-treatment. In sequential combination, phage at MOI 1 was added into biofilm-bearing wells for 6 h, and then one of the antibiotics (final concentration of MIC or 8× MIC) was added into the well plates for additional 18 h. The reverse sequential combination, gentamicin at MIC and 8× MIC were added into biofilm wells for 6 h, and then phage EPA1 with MOI 1 was added into the well plates for additional 18 h. The number of viable cells was enumerated using the microdrop method [43].

The potential interaction of treatments with biofilms is described as synergistic when the biofilm reduction in combinations is greater than the sum of individual treatments of antimicrobials, as described by Chaudhry et al. [18]. An interaction is described as an additive when the biofilm reduction in combinations is similar/equal to the sum of individual treatments of antimicrobials. An interaction is described as antagonistic when the biofilm reduction in combinations is lower than the sum of individual treatments of antimicrobials. The efficacy of treatment can be defined according to the result of the following equations:

$$\log(AP) - ((\log(A) + \log(P))$$

$$=0, \text{ additive interaction}$$

$$>0, \text{ Synergistic interaction}$$

$$<0, \text{ Antagonistic interaction}$$

In which P is the reduction in the number of viable biofilm cell in individual phage treatment; A the reduction in the number of viable biofilm cell in individual antibiotic treatment; AP the reduction in the number of viable biofilm cell in combined treatment.

4.9. Development of Probes for Biofilm Imaging

To assess the structure of biofilm models, bacteria-specific fluorescent probes were constructed using phage proteins. Given the expertise of our laboratory on phage-based protein construction, this method was selected instead of the use of commercial probes in the biofilm imaging process.

The red fluorescent mCherry gene derived from the DsRed of *Discosoma* sea anemones was inserted into the plasmid pET28a (+) (Novagen, Merck, Darmstady, Germany), between the *Sac*I and *Xho*I restriction sites conserving the plasmid N-terminal hexahistidine (His)-tag sequence and originating the pET_mCherry plasmid. Primers were designed to obtain fragments of the EPA1_gp81 tail fiber C-terminus (further referred to as the EPA1_TFP with mCherry). The fragments were amplified with Phusion DNA Polymerase (ThermoFisher Scientific) with the EPA1 genome as DNA template and digested with the restriction enzymes *Sac*I and *Xho*I. The digested fragments were inserted into pET28a(+) and ligated with the T4 ligase (ThermoFisher Scientific) to obtain the construction (pET_ EPA1_TFP), further used to transform *E. coli* TOP10 competent cells (Invitrogen, California, USA). Colonies were screened through colony PCR and positives used for plasmid extraction and further confirmation through Sanger sequencing. A correct pET_EPA1_TFP plasmid was used to transform competent *E. coli* BL21. Besides, the *S. aureus* phage vB_SauM-LM12 [43] endolysin truncated at its N-terminus and fused with GFP (LM12_AMI-SH3 with GFP) was constructed by our group [55].

Expression of the different peptides was performed as described before [56]. Briefly, the cells harboring recombinant plasmids were grown at 37 °C in Lysogeny Broth (LB) supplemented with 50 μg/mL of kanamycin until reaching an optical density at 620 nm (OD_{620nm}) of 0.6. Recombinant protein expression induced with isopropyl-β-D-thiogalactopyranoside (IPTG; Thermo Fisher Scientific) at 1 mM final concentration was carried overnight at 16 °C, 150 rpm. Cells were collected by centrifugation (9000× *g*, 15 min, 4 °C) and further resuspended in lysis buffer (20 mM NaH_2PO_4, 500 mM sodium chloride, 10 mM imidazole, pH 7.4). Cell disruption was made by thaw-freezing (3 cycles, from −80 °C to room temperature) followed by a 5 min sonication (Cole-Parmer Ultrasonic Processor) for 10 cycles (30 s ON, 30 s OFF), 40% amplitude. Soluble cell-free extracts were separated by centrifugation, filtered, and loaded on a 1 mL HisPur™Ni-NTA Resin (Thermo Fisher Scientific) stacked into a Polypropylene column (Qiagen). After two washing steps with protein-dependent imidazole concentrations (lysis buffer supplemented with 20 mM imidazole in the first wash, and 40 mM imidazole in the second wash), the protein was eluted with 300 mM imidazole. Protein fractions were observed through SDS-PAGE. The purified proteins were quantified using the Pierce™ BCA Protein Assay Kit (Thermo Ficher).

4.10. CLSM Analysis

CLSM was performed as described before [56] with some modifications. Briefly, the 13 mm in diameter Thermanox® Plastic Coverslip (Rochester, New York, USA) were placed in 24-well plates, and mono and dual-biofilms were formed as mentioned before. Coverslips were further washed twice with saline solution, and treatments were applied. After the treatment, the suspension was aspirated, and the wells were washed twice with 0.9% saline solution. The fluorescence probes, EPA1_TFP with mCherry (laser excitation line 635nm and emissions filters BA 655–755, red channel) and LM12_AMI-SH3 with GFP (laser excitation line 488 nm and emissions filters BA 505–605, green channel) were used for detection of cells in biofilms. The coupons were stained with 15 μL of probes in a final concentration of 20 mM for 15 min. After, the images were acquired in a Confocal Scanning Laser Microscope (Olympus B × 61, Model FluoView 1000) with the program FV10-Ver4.1.1.5 (Olympus). For each condition, three independent biofilms were used.

4.11. Statistical Analysis

The results of assays were compared using two-way analysis of variance (ANOVA) by applying the Tukey's multiple comparisons test using Prism 6 (GraphPad, La Jolla, CA, USA). Means and standard deviations (SD) were calculated with the software. Differences among conditions were considered statistically significant when $p < 0.001$.

4.12. Nucleotide Sequence Accession Number

The genome sequence of *Pseudomonas* phage vB_PaM_EPA1 was deposited in the GenBank database under the accession number MN013356.

Supplementary Materials:
Figure S1. One-step growth curve of phage vB_PaM_EPA1 in *P. aeruginosa* Sifa_Pa_1.5 at 37 °C. Shown are the PFU per infected cell; Figure S2. Treatment of *S. aureus* 48 h biofilms population with different antimicrobial agents (gentamicin, ciprofloxacin and meropenem) for 24 h; Figure S3. The effect of the antibiotics (gentamicin, ciprofloxacin and meropenem) on phage replication for 24 h post-treatment; Figure S4. Treatment of *P. aeruginosa* PAO1 48 h biofilms population with reverse sequential combinations. Table S1. Bacterial strains feature and susceptibility to phage EPA1; Table S2. The genome annotation of phage vB_PaM_EPA1.

Author Contributions: J.A., L.M. and E.A. conceived and designed the experiments; E.A. and S.C. performed the experiments; E.A., L.M., S.S., H.O., S.K. and J.A. analyzed the data; E.A. wrote the paper. The overall editing was performed by L.M. and J.A. All authors read and approved the final manuscript.

References

1. Røder, H.L.; Sørensen, S.J.; Burmølle, M. Studying Bacterial Multispecies Biofilms: Where to Start? *Trends Microbiol.* **2016**, *24*, 503–513. [CrossRef] [PubMed]
2. Wolcott, R.D.; Rhoads, D.D.; Bennett, M.E.; Wolcott, B.M.; Gogokhia, L.; Costerton, J.W.; Dowd, S.E. Chronic wounds and the medical biofilm paradigm. *J. Wound Care* **2014**, *19*, 45–53. [CrossRef] [PubMed]
3. Römling, U.; Balsalobre, C. Biofilm infections, their resilience to therapy and innovative treatment strategies. *J. Intern. Med.* **2012**, *272*, 541–561. [CrossRef]
4. Hall, C.W.; Mah, T.-F. Molecular mechanisms of biofilm-based antibiotic resistance and tolerance in pathogenic bacteria. *FEMS Microbiol. Rev.* **2017**, *41*, 276–301. [CrossRef] [PubMed]
5. Lopes, S.P.; Ceri, H.; Azevedo, N.F.; Pereira, M.O. Antibiotic resistance of mixed biofilms in cystic fibrosis: Impact of emerging microorganisms on treatment of infection. *Int. J. Antimicrob. Agents* **2012**, *40*, 260–263. [CrossRef] [PubMed]
6. Hotterbeekx, A.; Kumar-Singh, S.; Goossens, H.; Malhotra-Kumar, S. In vivo and In vitro Interactions between *Pseudomonas aeruginosa* and *Staphylococcus* spp. *Front. Cell. Infect. Microbiol.* **2017**, *7*, 1–13. [CrossRef]
7. Yoshida, S.; Ogawa, N.; Fujii, T.; Tsushima, S. Enhanced biofilm formation and 3-chlorobenzoate degrading activity by the bacterial consortium of *Burkholderia sp.* NK8 and *Pseudomonas aeruginosa* PAO1. *J. Appl. Microbiol.* **2009**, *106*, 790–800. [CrossRef]
8. Pastar, I.; Nusbaum, A.G.; Gil, J.; Patel, S.B.; Chen, J.; Valdes, J.; Stojadinovic, O.; Plano, L.R.; Tomic-Canic, M.; Davis, S.C. Interactions of Methicillin Resistant *Staphylococcus aureus* USA300 and *Pseudomonas aeruginosa* in Polymicrobial Wound Infection. *PLoS ONE* **2013**, *8*, e56846. [CrossRef]
9. Kart, D.; Tavernier, S.; Van Acker, H.; Nelis, H.J.; Coenye, T. Activity of disinfectants against multispecies biofilms formed by *Staphylococcus aureus*, *Candida albicans* and *Pseudomonas aeruginosa*. *Biofouling* **2014**, *30*, 377–383. [CrossRef]
10. Radlinski, L.; Rowe, S.E.; Kartchner, L.B.; Maile, R.; Cairns, B.A.; Vitko, N.P.; Gode, C.J.; Lachiewicz, A.M.; Wolfgang, M.C.; Conlon, B.P. *Pseudomonas aeruginosa* exoproducts determine antibiotic efficacy against *Staphylococcus aureus*. *PLoS Biol.* **2017**, *15*, 1–25. [CrossRef]

11. Nguyen, A.T.; Oglesby-Sherrouse, A.G. Interactions between *Pseudomonas aeruginosa* and *Staphylococcus aureus* during co-cultivations and polymicrobial infections. *Appl. Microbiol. Biotechnol.* **2016**, *100*, 6141–6148. [CrossRef] [PubMed]
12. Fong, S.A.; Drilling, A.; Morales, S.; Cornet, M.E.; Woodworth, B.A.; Fokkens, W.J.; Psaltis, A.J.; Vreugde, S.; Wormald, P.-J. Activity of Bacteriophages in Removing Biofilms of *Pseudomonas aeruginosa* Isolates from Chronic Rhinosinusitis Patients. *Front. Cell. Infect. Microbiol.* **2017**, *7*, 418. [CrossRef]
13. Ozkan, I.; Akturk, E.; Yeshenkulov, N.; Atmaca, S.; Rahmanov, N.; Atabay, H.I. Lytic Activity of Various Phage Cocktails on Multidrug-Resistant Bacteria. *Clin. Investig. Med.* **2016**, *39*, S66–S70. [CrossRef]
14. Pires, D.P.; Melo, L.D.R.; Vilas Boas, D.; Sillankorva, S.; Azeredo, J. Phage therapy as an alternative or complementary strategy to prevent and control biofilm-related infections. *Curr. Opin. Microbiol.* **2017**, *39*, 48–56. [CrossRef] [PubMed]
15. Knezevic, P.; Curcin, S.; Aleksic, V.; Petrusic, M.; Vlaski, L. Phage-antibiotic synergism: A possible approach to combatting *Pseudomonas aeruginosa*. *Res. Microbiol.* **2013**, *164*, 55–60. [CrossRef] [PubMed]
16. Torres-Barceló, C.; Arias-Sánchez, F.I.; Vasse, M.; Ramsayer, J.; Kaltz, O.; Hochberg, M.E. A window of opportunity to control the bacterial pathogen *Pseudomonas aeruginosa* combining antibiotics and phages. *PLoS ONE* **2014**, *9*, e106628. [CrossRef] [PubMed]
17. Torres-Barceló, C.; Hochberg, M.E. Evolutionary Rationale for Phages as Complements of Antibiotics. *Trends Microbiol.* **2016**, *24*, 249–256. [CrossRef] [PubMed]
18. Chaudhry, W.N.; Concepcion-Acevedo, J.; Park, T.; Andleeb, S.; Bull, J.J.; Levin, B.R. Synergy and order effects of antibiotics and phages in killing *Pseudomonas aeruginosa* biofilms. *PLoS ONE* **2017**, *12*, e0168615. [CrossRef] [PubMed]
19. Danis-Wlodarczyk, K.; Vandenheuvel, D.; Jang, H.B.; Briers, Y.; Olszak, T.; Arabski, M.; Wasik, S.; Drabik, M.; Higgins, G.; Tyrrell, J.; et al. A proposed integrated approach for the preclinical evaluation of phage therapy in *Pseudomonas infections*. *Sci. Rep.* **2016**, *6*, 28115. [CrossRef] [PubMed]
20. Ackermann, H.W. 5500 Phages examined in the electron microscope. *Arch. Virol.* **2007**, *152*, 227–243. [CrossRef] [PubMed]
21. Knezevic, P.; Voet, M.; Lavigne, R. Prevalence of Pf1-like (pro)phage genetic elements among *Pseudomonas aeruginosa* isolates. *Virology* **2015**, *483*, 64–71. [CrossRef] [PubMed]
22. Palmer, K.L.; Aye, L.M.; Whiteley, M. Nutritional cues control *Pseudomonas aeruginosa* multicellular behavior in cystic fibrosis sputum. *J. Bacteriol.* **2007**, *189*, 8079–8087. [CrossRef] [PubMed]
23. Hoffman, L.R.; Deziel, E.; D'Argenio, D.A.; Lepine, F.; Emerson, J.; McNamara, S.; Gibson, R.L.; Ramsey, B.W.; Miller, S.I. Selection for *Staphylococcus aureus* small-colony variants due to growth in the presence of *Pseudomonas aeruginosa*. *Proc. Natl. Acad. Sci. USA* **2006**, *103*, 19890–19895. [CrossRef] [PubMed]
24. Qin, Z.; Yang, L.; Qu, D.; Molin, S.; Tolker-Nielsen, T. *Pseudomonas aeruginosa* extracellular products inhibit *staphylococcal* growth, and disrupt established biofilms produced by *Staphylococcus epidermidis*. *Microbiology* **2009**, *155*, 2148–2156. [CrossRef] [PubMed]
25. Dietrich, L.E.P.; Price-Whelan, A.; Petersen, A.; Whiteley, M.; Newman, D.K. The phenazine pyocyanin is a terminal signalling factor in the quorum sensing network of *Pseudomonas aeruginosa*. *Mol. Microbiol.* **2006**, *61*, 1308–1321. [CrossRef] [PubMed]
26. DeLeon, S.; Clinton, A.; Fowler, H.; Everett, J.; Horswill, A.R.; Rumbaugh, K.P. Synergistic Interactions of *Pseudomonas aeruginosa* and *Staphylococcus aureus* in an In Vitro Wound Model. *Infect. Immun.* **2014**, *82*, 4718–4728. [CrossRef] [PubMed]
27. Pires, D.P.; Dötsch, A.; Anderson, E.M.; Hao, Y.; Khursigara, C.M.; Lam, J.S.; Sillankorva, S.; Azeredo, J. A Genotypic Analysis of Five *P. aeruginosa* Strains after Biofilm Infection by Phages Targeting Different Cell Surface Receptors. *Front. Microbiol.* **2017**, *8*, 1229. [CrossRef]
28. Essoh, C.; Latino, L.; Midoux, C.; Blouin, Y.; Loukou, G.; Nguetta, S.-P.A.P.A.; Lathro, S.; Cablanmian, A.; Kouassi, A.K.; Vergnaud, G.; et al. Investigation of a Large Collection of *Pseudomonas aeruginosa* Bacteriophages Collected from a Single Environmental Source in Abidjan, Côte d'Ivoire. *PLoS ONE* **2015**, *10*, 1–25. [CrossRef]
29. Sturino, J.M.; Klaenhammer, T.R. Inhibition of bacteriophage replication in *Streptococcus thermophilus* by subunit poisoning of primase. *Microbiology* **2007**, *153*, 3295–3302. [CrossRef]
30. Torres-Barceló, C.; Gurney, J.; Gougat-Barberá, C.; Vasse, M.; Hochberg, M.E. Transient negative effects of antibiotics on phages do not jeopardise the advantages of combination therapies. *FEMS Microbiol. Ecol.* **2018**, *94*, fiy107. [CrossRef]

31. Gutiérrez, D.; Briers, Y.; Rodríguez-Rubio, L.; Martínez, B.; Rodríguez, A.; Lavigne, R.; García, P. Role of the Pre-neck Appendage Protein (Dpo7) from Phage vB_SepiS-phiIPLA7 as an Anti-biofilm Agent in *Staphylococcal* Species. *Front. Microbiol.* **2015**, *6*, 1315. [CrossRef] [PubMed]
32. Lin, D.M.; Koskella, B.; Lin, H.C. Phage therapy: An alternative to antibiotics in the age of multi-drug resistance. *World J. Gastrointest. Pharmacol. Ther.* **2017**, *8*, 162. [CrossRef] [PubMed]
33. Vilas Boas, D.; Almeida, C.; Sillankorva, S.; Nicolau, A.; Azeredo, J.; Azevedo, N.F. Discrimination of bacteriophage infected cells using locked nucleic acid fluorescent in situ hybridization (LNA-FISH). *Biofouling* **2016**, *32*, 179–190. [CrossRef] [PubMed]
34. Burmølle, M.; Ren, D.; Bjarnsholt, T.; Sørensen, S.J. Interactions in multispecies biofilms: Do they actually matter? *Trends Microbiol.* **2014**, *22*, 84–91. [CrossRef] [PubMed]
35. Smith, A.C.; Rice, A.; Sutton, B.; Gabrilska, R.; Wessel, A.K.; Whiteley, M.; Rumbaugh, K.P. Albumin Inhibits *Pseudomonas aeruginosa* Quorum Sensing and Alters Polymicrobial Interactions. *Infect. Immun.* **2017**, *85*, 1–12. [CrossRef] [PubMed]
36. Filkins, L.M.; Graber, J.A.; Olson, D.G.; Dolben, E.L.; Lynd, L.R.; Bhuju, S.; O'Toole, G.A. Coculture of *Staphylococcus aureus* with *Pseudomonas aeruginosa* Drives *S. aureus* towards Fermentative Metabolism and Reduced Viability in a Cystic Fibrosis Model. *J. Bacteriol.* **2015**, *197*, 2252–2264. [CrossRef] [PubMed]
37. Mendes, J.J.; Neves, J. Diabetic Foot Infections: Current Diagnosis and Treatment. *J. Diabet. Foot Complicat.* **2012**, *4*, 26–45.
38. Leid, J.G.; Willson, C.J.; Shirtliff, M.E.; Hassett, D.J.; Parsek, M.R.; Jeffers, A.K. The exopolysaccharide alginate protects *Pseudomonas aeruginosa* biofilm bacteria from IFN-gamma-mediated macrophage killing. *J. Immunol.* **2005**, *175*, 7512–7518. [CrossRef]
39. Ryder, C.; Byrd, M.; Wozniak, D.J. Role of polysaccharides in *Pseudomonas aeruginosa* biofilm development. *Curr. Opin. Microbiol.* **2007**, *10*, 644–648. [CrossRef]
40. Colvin, K.M.; Irie, Y.; Tart, C.S.; Urbano, R.; Whitney, J.C.; Ryder, C.; Howell, P.L.; Wozniak, D.J.; Parsek, M.R. The Pel and Psl polysaccharides provide *Pseudomonas aeruginosa* structural redundancy within the biofilm matrix. *Environ. Microbiol.* **2012**, *14*, 1913–1928. [CrossRef]
41. Rémy, B.; Mion, S.; Plener, L.; Elias, M.; Chabrière, E.; Daudé, D. Interference in Bacterial Quorum Sensing: A Biopharmaceutical Perspective. *Front. Pharmacol.* **2018**, *9*, 203. [CrossRef] [PubMed]
42. Koban, Y.; Genc, S.; Bilgin, G.; Cagatay, H.H.; Ekinci, M.; Gecer, M.; Yazar, Z. Toxic Anterior Segment Syndrome following Phacoemulsification Secondary to Overdose of Intracameral Gentamicin. *Case Rep. Med.* **2014**, *2014*, 143564. [CrossRef] [PubMed]
43. Melo, L.D.R.; Brandão, A.; Akturk, E.; Santos, S.B.; Azeredo, J. Characterization of a new *Staphylococcus aureus* Kayvirus harboring a lysin active against biofilms. *Viruses* **2018**, *10*, 182. [CrossRef] [PubMed]
44. Oliveira, H.; Pinto, G.; Oliveira, A.; Oliveira, C.; Faustino, M.A.; Briers, Y.; Domingues, L.; Azeredo, J. Characterization and genome sequencing of a *Citrobacter freundii* phage CfP1 harboring a lysin active against multidrug-resistant isolates. *Appl. Microbiol. Biotechnol.* **2016**, *100*, 10543–10553. [CrossRef] [PubMed]
45. Aziz, R.K.; Bartels, D.; Best, A.; DeJongh, M.; Disz, T.; Edwards, R.A.; Formsma, K.; Gerdes, S.; Glass, E.M.; Kubal, M.; et al. The RAST Server: Rapid annotations using subsystems technology. *BMC Genom.* **2008**, *9*, 75. [CrossRef] [PubMed]
46. Altschul, S.F.; Gish, W.; Miller, W.; Myers, E.W.; Lipman, D.J. Basic local alignment search tool. *J. Mol. Biol.* **1990**, *215*, 403–410. [CrossRef]
47. Schattner, P.; Brooks, A.N.; Lowe, T.M. The tRNAscan-SE, snoscan and snoGPS web servers for the detection of tRNAs and snoRNAs. *Nucleic Acids Res.* **2005**, *33*, W686–W689. [CrossRef]
48. Laslett, D.; Canback, B. ARAGORN, a program to detect tRNA genes and tmRNA genes in nucleotide sequences. *Nucleic Acids Res.* **2004**, *32*, 11–16. [CrossRef]
49. Söding, J. Protein homology detection by HMM-HMM comparison. *Bioinformatics* **2005**, *21*, 951–960. [CrossRef]
50. Bendtsen, J.D.; Nielsen, H.; Von Heijne, G.; Brunak, S. Improved prediction of signal peptides: SignalP 3.0. *J. Mol. Biol.* **2004**, *340*, 783–795. [CrossRef]
51. Bailey, T.L.; Boden, M.; Buske, F.A.; Frith, M.; Grant, C.E.; Clementi, L.; Ren, J.; Li, W.W.; Noble, W.S. MEME Suite: Tools for motif discovery and searching. *Nucleic Acids Res.* **2009**, *37*, 202–208. [CrossRef] [PubMed]

52. Naville, M.; Ghuillot-Gaudeffroy, A.; Marchais, A.; Gautheret, D. ARNold: A web tool for the prediction of rho-independent transcription terminators. *RNA Biol.* **2011**, *8*, 11–13. [CrossRef] [PubMed]
53. Wang, Y.; Coleman-Derr, D.; Chen, G.; Gu, Y.Q. OrthoVenn: A web server for genome wide comparison and annotation of orthologous clusters across multiple species. *Nucleic Acids Res.* **2015**, *43*, W78–W84. [CrossRef] [PubMed]
54. Cui, H.; Ma, C.; Lin, L. Co-loaded proteinase K/thyme oil liposomes for inactivation of *Escherichia coli* O157:H7 biofilms on cucumber. *Food Funct.* **2016**, *7*, 4030–4040. [CrossRef] [PubMed]
55. Costa, S. Development of a Phage-Based Lab-on-Chip for the Detection of Foodborne Pathogens. Master's Thesis, University of Minho, Braga, Portugal, 2016.
56. Cerca, N.; Gomes, F.; Pereira, S.; Teixeira, P.; Oliveira, R. Confocal laser scanning microscopy analysis of *S. epidermidis* biofilms exposed to farnesol, vancomycin and rifampicin. *BMC Res. Notes* **2012**, *5*, 244. [CrossRef] [PubMed]

7

Bacteriophages: Protagonists of a Post-Antibiotic Era

Pilar Domingo-Calap [1,2,*] and Jennifer Delgado-Martínez [1]

1 Department of Genetics, Universitat de València, 46100 Burjassot, Valencia, Spain; jendel@alumni.uv.es
2 Institute for Integrative Systems Biology (I2SysBio), Universitat de València-CSIC, 46980 Paterna, Valencia, Spain
* Correspondence: domingocalap@gmail.com

Abstract: Despite their long success for more than half a century, antibiotics are currently under the spotlight due to the emergence of multidrug-resistant bacteria. The development of new alternative treatments is of particular interest in the fight against bacterial resistance. Bacteriophages (phages) are natural killers of bacteria and are an excellent tool due to their specificity and ecological safety. Here, we highlight some of their advantages and drawbacks as potential therapeutic agents. Interestingly, phages are not only attractive from a clinical point of view, but other areas, such as agriculture, food control, or industry, are also areas for their potential application. Therefore, we propose phages as a real alternative to current antibiotics.

Keywords: bacteriophages; phage therapy; antibiotic resistance; phage display; enzybiotics

---

1. Introduction

Viruses can infect all types of cells, including bacteria and archaea [1]. Specifically, bacteriophages (phages) are natural killers of bacteria and they were discovered a century ago by Frederick Twort and Félix d'Hérelle, independently [2,3]. In 1915, Twort thought that pathogenic bacteria required an essential substance to grow [4]. By analyzing in detail cultures of *Staphylococcus* sp. from vaccinia virus vaccines, he observed bacteria-free regions in the culture. Although he was unaware of what kind of substance produced those halos, after observing it under the lens, he confirmed that it was bacterial debris and defined it as a bacteriolytic agent [5]. In 1917, Félix d'Hérelle designated as "bacteriophages" some entities that were able to lyse bacterial cells after examining the effect of phages against *Salmonella gallinarum* in the feces of chickens [6–8]. In addition, d'Hérelle was the first to apply phages as a therapy to successfully treat children with severe dysentery.

In 1923, d'Hérelle and his assistant George Eliava established the George Eliava Institute of Bacteriophages, Microbiology, and Virology (Eliava Institute) in Tbilisi, present-day Georgia. During the Second World War, the Eliava Institute's experts provided combinations (cocktails) of different phages to soldiers, especially to treat wounds, gangrene, and diseases, such as cholera. Nowadays, the Eliava Institute carries out clinical trials with patients from all over the world, which often result in high success rates after treatment. Different phage applications in fields, such as human therapy, illness prevention, veterinary, environmental control, and food safety are investigated there [9]. This institute is responsible for the identification of more than 4000 phages, and a large number of phage-related studies have been done there. Because of this, the Eliava Institute is nowadays an important reference center for phages. Due to the discovery of antibiotics and the widespread use of penicillin in the 1940s, the use of phages fell out of favor, and, as a consequence of the Second World War, they were quickly reduced to only being used in Eastern countries, which had no access to antibiotics. Therefore, only Eastern countries (in particular, those of the former USSR), were (and are) using phages to treat bacterial infections, such as *Salmonella* and *Shigella* diseases, among others [10].

In spite of the rapid success of antibiotics, the emergence of multiresistant bacteria is a general concern. Nowadays, some bacterial strains are resistant to almost all available antibiotics. Routinely, surgical interventions can lead to serious complications due to the emergence of resistant bacterial strains that cannot be treated with conventional antibiotics [11]. Regarding the origin of this resistance, horizontal genetic transfer has been thought of as a key factor in the acquisition of antibiotic-resistant genes [7]. Moreover, spontaneous mutations can also occur in some genes under the action of antibiotics, and therefore contribute to its emergence [12]. High mutation and gene flow rates allow for bacteria to evolve quickly under the strong selection pressures that are exerted by antibiotics. In addition, the use of broad-spectrum antibiotics and their misuse promote this problem [13]. As a consequence, bacteria have developed several mechanisms to prevent antibiotic function, such as changes in receptors through enzymes or mutation, removal of the antibiotic by membrane pumps, or antibiotic modification to escape its effect [12–14]. For these reasons, it is important to propose alternative methods to fight against bacterial resistance. Here, we demonstrate how bacteriophages can be useful in this battle, and a wide variety of interesting phage applications are also reviewed.

Bacteriophages can be classified according to their genome, morphology, biological cycle, or the environment where they live [15–17]. Concerning the biological cycles of phages, there are two main types—lytic and lysogenic cycles (Figure 1). The lytic cycle implies bacterial death, which generates virion output. For this, they take advantage of the replication system of the host cell, and when their proteins and viral components are formed, they induce cell lysis [18,19]. In contrast, lysogenic cycles are based in the integration of the genetic material of the phage into the genome of the host cell. At the end of the replication cycle, no new virions are obtained, but bacterial cells with phage genetic material are created, as temperate phages [18]. Due to the variability between phages, it is important to determine which are the most appropriate bacteriophages for each potential application [20].

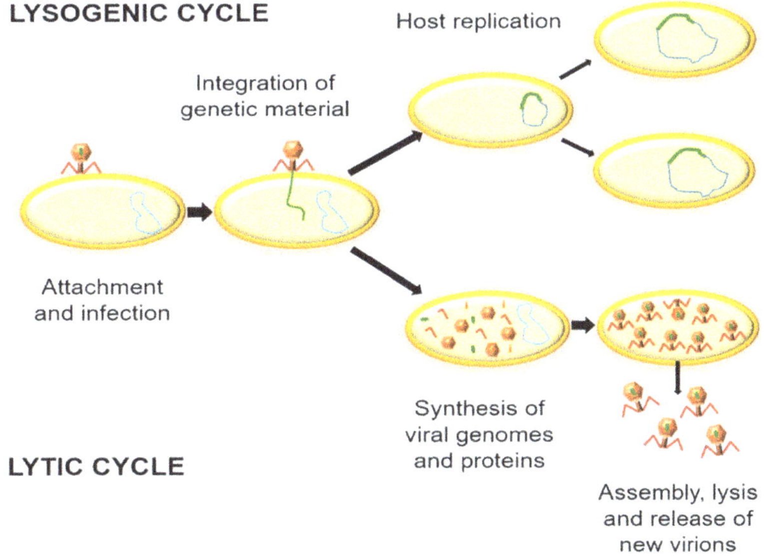

Figure 1. Biological cycles of phages. Firstly, the virus binds to the bacterial cell and injects its genetic material. In the lysogenic cycle, the integration of viral genetic material into the genome of the host occurs, and the bacterial cell replicates without producing virions. In the lytic cycle, viral genetic material is replicated and viral proteins are synthesized. Then, an assembly of virions is achieved, followed by the lysis of the bacteria and the release of new virions.

2. Phages in the Biosphere

Viruses are ubiquitous in the biosphere and can be found in all environments, being the most abundant biological entity [21]. It is believed that there are 10^{31}–10^{32} virions in the biosphere, approximately distributed as 2.6×10^{30} virions in soils, 1.2×10^{30} virions in the ocean, 3.5×10^{30} virions in the oceanic subsurface, and 0.25–2.5 $\times$ 10^{31} virions in the terrestrial subsurface [22]. In addition, significant viral quantities have been found in extreme environments, with between nearly 9.0 $\times$ 10^6 and 1.3 $\times$ 10^8 virions mL^{-1} in sea ice and approximately 5.6–8.7 $\times$ 10^{10} virions cm^{-3} in algal flocks [16]. Other extreme conditions in which viruses have been found include high-temperature environments (thermal waters, geothermal springs, volcanoes, hydrothermal vents, etc.), cold environments (lakes of polar areas, sea ice, etc.), and hypersaline zones [22]. Although few studies have focused on their presence in soils and the rhizosphere, around 1.5 $\times$ 10^8 virions g^{-1} are estimated to be present there [16]. Bacteria can be found in almost any environment, such as seawater, fresh water, and soils [23], so phages are expected to be found in any place where a host is located (Table 1). In addition, some of them may be specifically localized, whilst others can be widely distributed throughout the biosphere [24]. Indeed, only around 6000 different bacteriophage species are known, hiding a great diversity that is still unknown [25]. It is theorized that, in the ocean, there are at least 10^7 phages mL^{-1} [17], and the number of soil phages could be as great as 10^8 virions g^{-1} [26], representing a large proportion of the total amount of viruses in the biosphere.

Phages and bacterial cells have been coevolving for a long time, showing dynamic interactions between them [27]. Experimentally, it has been shown that coevolution between phages and bacteria can increase the rate of molecular evolution. This has been studied in *Pseudomonas fluorescens* SBW25 infected with the phage Φ2, and it has been shown that not all genes evolve equally in the phage. Interestingly, those that evolve quickly are related to the infection of the bacterium, coding for proteins that are related to host attachment [28]. In addition, coevolution leads to the maintenance of bacterial diversity and is responsible for changes in the physiology, abundance, abilities, and virulence of bacteria [29]. Similarly, phages are also influenced by their interaction with bacteria, especially in their defense strategies [30]. Although phages are highly specific, some of them show a wide host range. Moreover, due to phage-bacteria interactions, phages can participate in the biogeochemical cycles of biotic and abiotic environments. When bacterial lysis occurs, bacteria debris remains in the medium, being a nutritional source, and carbon, nitrogen, and phosphorus cycles are enriched or modified [31]. Therefore, phages play an important role in their environment. For example, they participate in nutrient acquisition in marine ecosystems and improve carbon transfer through phage lysis [32].

As with bacteria, we can find phages living in higher organisms, mostly in the digestive tract, vagina, respiratory and oral tract, skin, and mucosal epithelium, forming the so-called "phageome" [33]. Due to the great diversity and quantity of phages in the body, it is possible that they participate in human homeostasis. For example, gut phages are lytic and temperate, and both types are important for avoiding bacterial imbalance. It is suggested that the introduction of viruses in the gut occurs during the first four days of life and that they undergo changes with the development of the body [34].

Thanks to metagenomics, it is possible to determine phage variability and their abundance in each environment. Epifluorescence microscopy and transmission electron microscopy can help to identify new phages [22]. Before these techniques, counts were made in bacterial cultures and by obtaining plaque forming units (PFU), which may lead to difficulties mainly because not all bacteria are cultivable under artificial conditions, and not all phages make lysis plaques [35]. For these reasons, the real abundance and diversity of phages are higher than observed.

Phages can also be found in artificial places or infrastructures that humans inhabit, such as hospitals, showing that natural places are not the only source of phages [36]. Hospital sewage is an especially good reservoir of phages. As explained by numerous articles about multiresistant bacteria, phages that were isolated from the wastewater of medical centres are used in applications against resistant bacteria that cause diseases. Additionally, clinical materials or medical devices can be a source of phages [37,38].

Remarkably, wastewater treatment plants (WWTPs) are the habitat of many types of microorganisms, which makes them interesting considering that many interactions among bacteria and phages take place in them. More than 1000 different types of viruses have been found in WWTPs and a large proportion of them are bacteriophages. The water of WWTPs undergoes several debugging and cleaning processes to obtain potable water, and these physical and chemical methods manage to eliminate many bacterial cells, although they usually fail to remove phages. Therefore, this affords an opportunity to isolate bacteriophages [39].

Accordingly, phages are a ubiquitous ecological solution to develop new treatments against bacteria, although further studies should be done to better understand the relationship between them and bacteria before their application.

Table 1. Summary of the main places where phages can be found: nature, urbanized places, and the human body.

Phages in nature	Soil Terrestrial subsurface Fresh water Ocean Oceanic subsurface Extreme environments: sea ice, algal flocks, hypersaline zones, etc.
Artificial places	Hospital and similar places Wastewater treatment plants Some areas under human impact
Body of animals	Digestive tract Vagina Respiratory and oral tract Skin Mucosal epithelium

3. Potential Application of Phages

Phages should be considered as great potential tools due to their multiple benefits. Since their discovery, phages have been used as models to understand fundamental genetic processes and as great tools in molecular biology. Phage products, such as ligases, polymerases, or recombinant phages, are commonly used in research laboratories. Here, we place an emphasis on the potential application of phages against pathogenic bacteria. The emergence of multidrug-resistant bacteria has led to the need for new treatments. To this end, we assess how phages can help to overcome this critical situation by coming up with potential applications of phages that may be of interest in different areas. Different approaches using phages are proposed, and some of the most relevant ones in the fight against bacterial resistance are described in detail.

3.1. Phage Therapy

Phage therapy is based on the therapeutic use of phages to treat pathogenic bacterial infections [40]. Lytic phages are preferably chosen in phage therapy for two main reasons. Firstly, because lytic phages will destroy their host bacteria, whilst temperate ones will not. Secondly, because temperate phages can transfer virulence and resistance genes due to their life cycle, in which the genome of the phage is integrated into and replicates together with the bacterial genetic material [8,19]. The intrinsic characteristics of lytic phages, such as high host-receptor specificity and bacterial cell lysis to release virions, make them highly suitable for clinical applications [7,41]. Some remarkable features of the use of phages include their short replication time and their ability to obtain a large number of viral progeny only in their specific hosts, the specificity to prevent damage in nonpathogenic bacteria (they are ecologically safe and have no known side effects), and their fast and low-cost production. In addition, their short genomes allow for us to understand the molecular mechanisms implicated in controlling resistant cells [7]. Another significant feature of phages is their ability to coevolve with their host, in a hit-and-run response, to counteract possible resistant mutants, with higher mutation rates being described for viruses than for bacteria [30].

3.1.1. Main Applications of Phage Therapy

As previously mentioned, phage therapy has been used since a century ago. However, their use is restricted to Eastern countries, which have different guidelines for clinical trials and research articles are mainly published in Russian or other non-English languages. Because of that, phage therapy is not currently used in European and North American countries. Researchers are now making efforts to follow clinical trials guidelines to use phages in clinics. An interesting European project under human clinical trial is called Phagoburn, which was funded in 2013 by the European Commission. This project is based in the use of phage cocktails for burn injuries infected with *Escherichia coli* or *Pseudomonas aeruginosa* [42].

The main application of phage therapy is its use as a therapeutic agent to eliminate pathogenic bacteria involved in disease or infection as well as those that form biofilm. Another interesting approach is the use of phages as a preventive disinfectant, especially in medical areas or clinical devices. Additionally, current technology or the combination of phages with other techniques can improve these clinical applications. Despite the effectiveness of a single type of bacteriophage against a bacterial strain due to its high specificity, phage cocktails are an interesting strategy to solve issues relating to resistance and a low range of action [43]. They are normally composed of different phages that attack different bacterial strains or species. In this way, phage cocktails can play a decisive role in biofilms by allowing for the phages' effects to last longer by delaying the emergence of resistance to all the phages that are part of the cocktail. Furthermore, it has been proven that these cocktails have other benefits, such as decontaminating food by removing *E. coli*, *Salmonella enterica* or *Listeria* [44].

Outside medicine, phage therapy plays an important role in other fields, such as food production and cattle raising. Phages are useful to ensure food safety because they allow for the removal of bacterial infections in animals and thus prevent the consumption of contaminated food. Some interesting examples are the use of phages to control typical food infections that are caused by *Salmonella* (salmonellosis), *Campylobacter* (campylobacteriosis in poultry), *Listeria monocytogenes*, or *E. coli* [2].

3.1.2. Benefits and Drawbacks of Phage Therapy

Bacteriophages present many benefits that make them excellent tools to treat bacterial diseases and to contribute to the fight against the emergence of bacterial resistance. One of the greatest concerns regarding antibiotics is their side effects, since they can damage the microbiome, which is related to many types of imbalances or diseases. In this regard, the specificity of phages can solve this problem, since they will only replicate inside their specific host (phages cannot infect eukaryotic cells). In contrast to antibiotics, phages can proliferate quickly inside the host (and only if they find their host), can be administered in small doses and with long intervals of time between them, and they are removed once their population is eliminated [2,23]. The action of phages inside the host is very specific, as phage replication only occurs inside bacteria. On the contrary, antibiotics are less precise and they reach more areas without the presence of bacteria in the organism [11]. Another benefit of phages is that they can be used in difficult-to-reach parts of the body, such as treating central nervous system infections, which commonly poses a serious problem [8]. A remarkable feature of phages is that they can evolve, whilst antibiotics are static substances that cannot change even if their environment changes. Another interesting feature of phages is their isolation and production costs, as previously mentioned. The cost of antibiotic production is high, both economically and because antibiotics are not natural and have to be synthesized in a laboratory [23].

It is worth noting that the great specificity of phages is both an advantage and a limitation of phage therapy. Phages avoid damage to the microbiome, but prior to their application, it is necessary to determine in vitro which bacteria are causing the disease. This can be a difficult process because identification must take place quickly in order to apply the treatment to the patient [45,46]. A way to solve this setback is the use of phage cocktails, as this widens the range of action [2]. However, it is possible that in vitro and in vivo phage behavior may be different, and as a result of the lack of in vivo studies, their effectiveness cannot be fully assured [47].

The pharmacology of phages can be very complex, for both the action of phages inside the body (pharmacodynamics) and the body's function on the phages (pharmacokinetics) [33]. In phage therapy, the interactions between phage and bacteria are related to pharmacodynamics. Regarding pharmacokinetics, it is believed that this is linked to the density of phages within the hosts. In the event of a small bacteria population, a large dose of phages must be used in order for them to replicate faster than bacteria. Furthermore, if the bacterial density is small, the phages might not replicate quickly enough and they will not perform the desired action [48]. This can depend on the phage dose, which in turn depends on the bacterial density, the size of phage particles, and the phage virulence, as the more virulent the phage, the better it will attack its host. The resolution of this point is based on a virulent phage with a great burst size (producers of large progenies in a short time) and that is specifically administrated at the infection site.

In addition, it is possible that phages or their products can be recognized by the immune system and induce immune responses. Nevertheless, phage lysis is usually faster than the action of neutralizing antibodies phages. However, some researchers suggest that it is possible that an immune response occurs, owing to the products and enzymes that are released from bacterial lysis. Noteworthy, recent studies showed that phage T4 is highly immunogenic and can be used as potential vaccine candidates [49]. In addition, in many cases immune responses can be avoided by modifying the mode of phage administration [33]. The immune mechanisms that detect phages and subsequently take action are not well understood. Thus, it is necessary to investigate these matters to evaluate phages' effect on the body. On the other hand, different studies are in agreement that the application of phage therapy has no direct consequences on the patient [50]. Despite the fact that phage safety must be confirmed, phages are consumed indirectly by means of fermented foods, breathing, or every time we accidentally drink sea water. For that reason, it seems that bacteriophages do not pose a potential risk [51]. Apart from the route that phages naturally use to arrive in their bacterial host, there are new strategies to improve the lifespan of bacteriophages in an organism. Biomaterials that do not interfere in phage activity should be used, as liposomes or capsules around phages that are made of alginate are accompanied by different ions. One question that needs to be dealt with is the physical limitations of these structures, and the most appropriate way of encapsulating phages must be chosen according to their future function [52].

Above all, the most urgent point that should be solved is the scarcity of basic information related to doses, forms of administration, protocols, and the correct mode of application of this therapy in the specific case of each phage [2,45]. This question, together with the difficulties of patenting phages (since they are natural entities), is an impediment for pharmaceutical companies to accept this therapy [42]. Legal regulations must be established to define limitations and the safe use of phage therapy. Lastly, ethical and social acceptance of phage therapy is a great impediment, since it is difficult to believe that viruses not only are not dangerous for humans, but that they have also the potential to treat diseases.

3.1.3. Emergence of Bacterial Resistance against Phages

Another controversial topic is the emergence of bacterial resistance against phages. Bacteria present natural mechanisms to prevent viral infection (Figure 2). Some of these mechanisms are associated with phages' receptors, e.g., bacteria can hide, change, or even lose phage receptors [8]. Each of these mechanisms is activated in response to a stimulus, for example, receptor loss usually occurs when there is a change in the composition of the bacterium's cell surface, as is seen in *Bordetella* spp. and *Shigella flexneri* [8,41]. If the loss of the receptor occurs, the phage cannot recognize the bacteria, and, subsequently, no new phages will be generated. This occurs, for example, in *E. coli* and *Staphylococcus aureus* as a consequence of membrane protein modifications. Some bacteria even have the ability to secrete extracellular polymeric substances (EPS), glycoconjugates, or alginates in order to prevent the adhesion of the phage to the bacteria. These secretions have been observed in *Pseudomonas* spp., which ejects EPS, and *Enterobacteriaceae*, which secretes glycoconjugates [41].

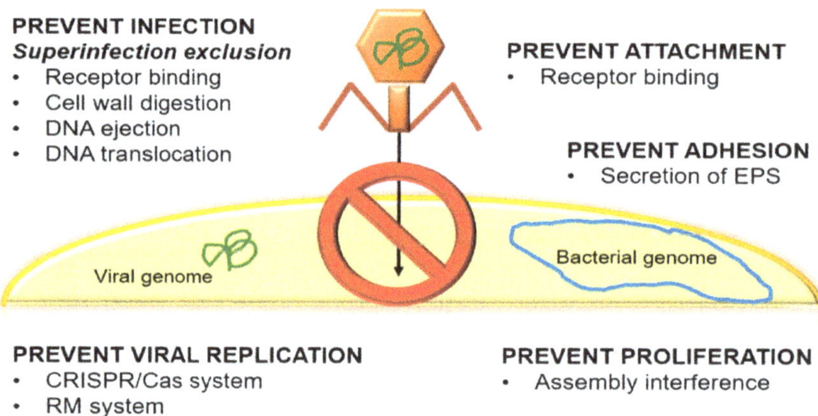

Figure 2. Principal natural mechanisms to prevent viral infection in bacteria. EPS: extracellular polymeric substances, CRISPR/Cas: Clustered Regularly Interspaced Short Palindromic Repeats/Caspase, RM: restriction modification.

There are others systems to escape phages, such as by viral DNA removal by different methods, Clustered Regularly Interspaced Short Palindromic Repeats (CRISPR)-associated proteins, or the superinfection exclusion (Sie) system [9,41]. CRISPR is considered to be the immune system of bacteria to protect the genetic material of the cell against possible attacks of viruses or plasmids [53]. To counteract the CRISPR system, phages have been co-evolving with bacteria thanks to phage-anti-CRISPR [54]. On the other hand, Sie is based on membrane-associated proteins. These proteins interact with proteins that are related to DNA injection when the phage is bound to a membrane receptor. Through this process, it is possible to interrupt the injection of DNA and thus reduce phage virulence, preventing the infection from spreading [55]. Another process is based on the abortive infection (Abi) system, which is responsible for interfering with the replication, transcription, or translation of the phage or in virions formation [41]. This mechanism is activated when the phage has managed to enter the cell because it has evaded the restriction systems and the CRISPR system of the host. The objective of Abi is to destroy the infected cell so that it does not transmit the invasion to the rest of the cells [30]. An interesting way to increase phage fitness against bacteria and to reduce the emergence of resistance is experimental evolution. This method consists of preadapting a phage to its host in vitro for several generations. In addition, experimental evolution produces benefits for phage therapy, since the bacteria–phage coevolution over many generations can make the bacteria diminish their ability to adapt to the environment [56].

The combination of phages with antibiotics is another strategy to apply phages as therapeutic agents. It is possible to reduce resistance because phages can kill antibiotic-resistant variants and vice versa [57]. Owing to these combinations, the phage-antibiotic synergy (PAS) effect usually takes place, which consists of an increase in phage virulence as a result of the administration of sublethal concentrations of antibiotics and it can be convenient to remove pathogenic cells quickly [43]. In addition, additive effects of the components can occur and they can be beneficial. Through animal studies, it has been proven that these treatments have preventive action for bacteria resistance [45], for example, decreasing mutations that confer resistance to bacteria [46]. On the other hand, some of these antibiotics block the cellular cycle of bacteria, and as a result, bacterial cells undergo an increase in volume that facilitates the division of phages and their release at a faster pace [58]. Some studies have confirmed the effectiveness of this method, like the combination of phage SBW25ϕ2 with kanamycin antibiotic against *P. fluorescens* SBW25 [57]. The success of combinations depends on the target cell and phage and antibiotic types. Moreover, it is important that phages and antibiotics detect different regions of union of pathogenic bacteria to ensure the effectiveness of the treatment. These deductions arise from experiments with different phages and antibiotics to decrease *E. coli* in urinary tract infections. Specifically, the best results were obtained from the combination of phages and the antibiotic ciprofloxacin (at a sublethal concentration) against *E. coli* [57]. This synergy has been shown using cefotaxime combined with phage T4 against biofilm formations of *E. coli* [59]. Furthermore, because of the lack of information about the safety of phages, and sometimes the ignorance of phages' effects, it is estimated that the combination of both provides more support than the use of individual bacteriophages only [45]. It is thought that this therapy can be better than phage cocktails because phages and antibiotics act in different ways inside bacterial cells, while all the phages in a phage cocktail may have similar modes of action, which might be a problem for the emergence of resistance [60]. Nevertheless, this association presents some defects. As a consequence of the PAS effect, and mainly due to antibiotics in sublethal concentrations, an SOS (emergency repair) response can arise, which consists of bacterial responses to stress as a consequence of damage to bacterial DNA, causing serious effects by increasing the antibiotic resistance. Other side effects can be the appearance of double resistant mutants, the potentiation of antibiotic resistant bacteria due to the phages preference to infect sensitive variants, or the interference between the action of the phage and the antibiotic resulting in an action that is less effective than the sum of both [45]. It is also important to know when to apply each treatment (phages and antibiotics). It seems that to prevent resistance, an intermediate interval of time between phage and antibiotic applications is better than the simultaneous application of both or their use after a very long period of time between them [60].

3.2. Phage-Derived Enzymes

An alternative to the use of phages against bacterial diseases is the use of phage-derived enzymes. Phages produce several enzyme types, each one being suitable for attacking specific bacteria [61]. Phage enzymes were discovered in 1986 when investigating an enzyme secreted by *Streptococcus* after being infected by a bacteriophage. The activity of this enzyme was the rupture of the cell wall and it was called lysin [62–64]. In nature, these enzymes are found inside phages and help them to penetrate into the host to assure phage replication, among other functions. In general, they degrade peptidoglycan, thereby producing bacterial lysis by osmotic imbalance. Lysins can be used as enzybiotics because, applied exogenously as recombinant proteins, they can remove bacteria. This approach has been used for more than 20 years, especially against Gram-positive bacteria. It was thought that Gram-negative bacteria could physically block the passage of lytic enzymes due to the presence of its outer membrane, but it was later discovered that some phage enzymes can cross this layer. Although it is postulated that these enzymes may cause unwanted immune responses, several studies have shown no serious side effects after their use [65].

Despite their success in killing bacteria, they present some problems of stability and lack of solubility, which may be solved by enzyme engineering. Sometimes, the use of recombinant enzymes is recommended. The great progress in enzyme engineering and synthetic biology, in addition to their low cost of production, makes this technique one of the most effective against antibiotic resistance in its application in clinics. Moreover, lytic enzymes are interesting in other areas, such as agriculture, food industry, diagnostics, environmental control, and bioluminescence [65].

As previously mentioned, one type of phage-derived enzyme is lysins. Within them, we can find endolysins, which are derived from the lytic cycle, and virion-associated lysins (VALs), which are implicated in the entrance to the host cell. Some of them can suffer changes upon the modifications of their host cell and are very specific to species or bacterial serotype [61]. VALs can be part of the phage tail or be inside the capsid. Once the phage is recognized by its receptors in the host, a conformational change in the phage allows entrance into the bacteria thanks to the degradation of peptidoglycan carried out by VALs. The mode of action of VALs against bacteria consists of allowing for the injection of the phage. This fact is possible thanks to the rupture of the peptidoglycan layer of the bacteria through the hydrolysis of chemical bonds. In its clinical application to treat bacterial diseases, this ability is used to induce the osmotic lysis of the bacteria [61]. Differently, endolysins must cross the cell membrane to reach the cell wall and cause lysis, since they are synthesized in the cytoplasm of infected cells at the end of the viral cycle. They are classified into canonical endolysins (the most interesting as enzybiotics) and exported endolysins. Canonical endolysins need other specific phage enzymes, called holins, which will form holes through which the endolysins will leave the cytoplasm [65]. Endolysins are useful as alternatives to antibiotics due to their bactericidal function. This ability has been proven by applying these purified enzymes on bacteria. Endolysins usually have two domains: one is catalytic active (N-terminal), whilst the other attaches to the cell wall (C-terminal). Additionally, some laboratories are creating chimeric endolysins in order to improve bacterial lysis. One example is the chimera Cpl-711, which combines the endolysins Cpl-1 and Cpl-7S from Cp-1 and Cp-7 pneumococcal bacteriophages against *Streptococcus pneumoniae* and their multiresistant strains [66]. An interesting feature of lysins is their high specificity, which reduces the probability of developing bacterial resistance, making resistance an extremely rare event [61].

Holins are proteins derived from phages acting at the end of the lytic process in order to trigger and control the degradation of the cell wall from the bacterial cells. These small membrane proteins control lysis time and are diverse. They are commonly small, have a positive and hydrophobic C terminal domain, and include one to three hydrophobic transmembrane domains by which they can be classified [67]. Membrane channels or pores are created when the concentration of holins exceeds a threshold, and then endolysins will perform their function. The canonical holins form large pores at one side of the host and locally expose the peptidoglycans to cytoplasmic canonical endolysins. Pinholins, another group, form small pores that depolarize the membrane, triggering signal-anchor-release (SAR) endolysin activation and inducing degradation of peptidoglycans in the whole cellular periplasmic space [68]. They can be combined with other enzymes to amplify the host range of endolysins. Since holins have a large strain spectrum, they are interesting against multiresistant strains such as *S. aureus* or *S. suis* [19].

Polysaccharide depolymerases are very useful due to their ability to attack carbohydrates of bacterial membranes [19,69]. Depolymerases present two different forms, as part of the phage particle that is attached to the base plate (in the phage membrane or capsid) or as a protein resulting from cell lysis after phage replication. They also differ in the mode to remove carbohydrate polymers on the membrane of the host bacteria. They are called hydrolases when they are able to hydrolyse the glycosyl–oxygen bond and turn it into a glyosidic bond. In contrast, lyases add a double linkage into uronic acid particles, thanks to the β-elimination system, after the disruption of the glycosidic linkage between a monosaccharide and the C4 of the acid. An example of lyases are the hyaluronan lyases [67]. Lyases would be an indirect way of dealing with bacteria because these enzymes act on bacteria that are encapsulated by weakening the polymer structure that makes up the capsule. This process helps to decrease bacterial virulence by allowing for the immune system to perform its action [70]. One interesting property of depolymerases is their wide bacterial range. In contrast to lysins, resistance against phage depolymerases can emerge due to modifications in polysaccharide composition of capsule, exopolysaccharides, or lipopolysaccharide [61]. New studies are currently emerging to ensure their safety and efficacy against capsulated *E. coli* in mice [69]. Moreover, it seems that some depolymerases eliminate biofilms, such as a depolymerase derived from a phage against *Staphylococcus epidermis*, which is an interesting application due to the difficulties of removing these formations. Depolymerases favor the penetration of the phage into the biofilm and the host cells due to its capacity for degradation of capsular polysaccharides [43]. Another group is the virion-associated peptidoglycan hydrolases (VAPGHs) as lysozymes, lytic transglycosylases, endopeptidases, or glucosaminidases. In contrast to endolysins that act in the final step of viral replication, VAPGHs can favour phage entry to the host by creating a hole through the cell wall of the host cell. With this, the phage can insert its tail and carry out the injection of its genetic material. An interesting example is gp49 from *S. aureus* phage phi11. Under normal conditions, gp49 is not necessary, but when the temperature or density fluctuates, this enzyme can improve infection. These enzymes are located almost anywhere in the phage, as they have been found in the tail, the head, the capsid, and the viral membrane [69,71]. Hydrolases are suitable to carry out their function in Gram-positive and Gram-negative cells because they are encoded by phages that attack both bacterial groups [19]. VAPGHs present several benefits that make them suitable as antimicrobial agents in therapeutic fields and also as food control or food decontaminants, especially in foods that undergo processes at high temperatures during manufacturing, as in dairy products. In addition, it has been shown that they can be useful against multiresistant bacterial strains [71]. Recent research proposed VAPGHs activity to treat plant diseases, such as those provoked by *Agrobacterium tumefaciens* [72]. Finally, to improve their bactericidal capacities, chimeric proteins can be created by combining several enzymes or by exchanging their functional domains. Some of these chimeric proteins have been used to treat diseases that are caused by *S. aureus*. Although few studies have been done to determine bacterial resistance emergence under VAPGHs treatment, bacterial resistance has not been reported so far [71].

Phage-derived enzymes are very useful and an attractive solution against bacterial infections. Synthetic biology allows for creating and modifying phage proteins to improve bacterial range spectrum, reduce bacterial resistance, and reduce immunogenicity. In addition, enzybiotics can be a great tool to be used against intracellular pathogens, where phages have difficulties to reach due to the lack of receptors for eukaryotic cells. Besides, phage-derived enzymes can be easily delivered into specific infection sites, acting locally in the infection and reducing side effects.

3.3. Phage Display

Despite the fact that natural bacteriophages have been studied to diminish bacterial resistance with success, some researchers have gone beyond this to find alternative antibacterial methods based on phages. This leads to phage modifications by gene engineering, the principal advantage of which is greater accuracy capacity [73]. However, there are more benefits of phage engineering, such as obtaining phage elements which are able to detect bacterial hosts, changing phage hosts, or promoting their action [74].

Phage display was developed in 1985 by George P. Smith [75]. It is a technique that is based on the expression of the phage cover of foreign peptides. The phage is exposed to the target (natural or synthetic) of interest until some of the peptides exposed in the phage bind specifically to that target. To carry out these processes, libraries of phage particles are commonly created by means of random peptides. These peptides are bound to components of the phage coat. Random oligonucleotides must be introduced at a specific location within the phage. The function of the library is to facilitate the search for the appropriate peptides through several screenings of ligands for each target. In addition, once the specific peptide has been recognized, it is possible to maximize its specificity and affinity. To check if the proteins that are expressed by the phage bind to the chosen target, a "biopanning" process is performed three to six times. This method consists of the immobilization of the target and its exposure to randomly selected peptide libraries. Then, less to more rigorous washes are made to eliminate phages that are bound nonspecifically to the target. Finally, once the phage has correctly attached to that target, different methods are used to separate it from the target and to sequence it until finding the specific peptide. It is usually said that phage display is a link between phenotype and genotype [76,77].

It is possible to use different types of bacteriophages for phage display, but the most advantageous are the filamentous ones, since they allow for genetic material expansion simply by increasing their filament size. The process of introducing genetic material into the phage does not damage its internal structures. These phages, which are usually temperate, do not kill bacterial cells to carry out their biological cycle and release new virions. Phage M13 is a typical bacteriophage used for this technology. In general, the most interesting gene in phage display is gene VIII, which codes for major structural proteins and is suitable for displaying short peptides and obtaining a high number of desirable molecules. In contrast, gene III codes for minor proteins and is more appropriate for expressing large peptides, although few copies of them will be obtained [78].

Phage display is an excellent tool for vaccine production, the development of new drugs, the study of protein–protein interactions, the selection and modification of substances of interest, the development of monoclonal antibodies with the desired specificity for therapeutic use, the creation of libraries of peptides and other substances, in epitope mapping (as antivenom), or the production of food as biocontrol. In the same way, it is a very useful technique to choose and isolate antibodies against desirable antigens or other targets, and to then create an antibody library [3,77,78]. Related to our subject of study, one application is the use of phage display against bacterial resistance. A typical response of bacteria when they are exposed to antibiotics is the secretion of enzymes. Particularly, they express β-lactamases, which hydrolyses the β-lactam ring with the aim of stopping antibiotic attacks, thus rendering the bacterial cells resistant to them. This resistance is generated as a result of the contact between bacteria and antibiotics presenting a β-lactam ring. β-lactam antibiotics have been widely used since their discovery. As a result, bacteria have been evolving, and, consequently, resistance has emerged. Through the implementation of phage display, this technique can be used to find peptides against β-lactamases enzymes by testing different peptide libraries [79]. Another example is the use of phage display against multiresistant strains of *L. monocytogenes*. These bacteria are usually transmitted by food and cause diseases such as arthritis and infections called listeriosis, which affect the central nervous system. As a result of the increase in antibiotic resistance, alternative methods have been sought to combat these diseases. One of these methods is the use of phage display and peptide libraries. After finding peptides that bind to the bacteria of interest (*L. monocytogenes*), peptides were isolated and it was checked if they presented microbicidal activities [80].

Similarly, the creation of new drugs opens many possibilities for future medicine. This is achieved by following the basic protocol of phage display but against therapeutic targets (e.g., specific points on which to act against pathogenic bacterial diseases). In addition, people under immunosuppression, such as HIV patients, transplant recipients, and pregnant women, are very susceptible to pathogenic infections. It is expected that more than 50% of patients with HIV will develop resistance to many of the current treatments [81]. Therefore, new alternative treatments should be proposed in order to solve this problem.

Moreover, phage display allows for the production of two main types of vaccines: phage display vaccines and phage DNA vaccines. On the one hand, phage display vaccines are based on a virion inside of which is the gene that codes for the antigen that is displayed, and they are more stable than phage DNA vaccines, when considering that the virion protects them. On the other hand, in phage DNA vaccines, inside of the virion there is DNA with the antigen gene that has been cloned in a eukaryotic cassette. As a result of these vaccines, there is a greater immune response than with conventional vaccines. Some of the investigations with these types of vaccines are directed against bacteria, autoimmune diseases, cancer, fungi, parasites, or even contraceptive vaccines [82]. There are also studies to use vaccines with the aim of preventing or reducing antimicrobial resistance. This could be innovative because they produce an immune response if the patient is exposed to a pathogen; as a result, the disease is avoided or weakened. In addition, if vaccination rates increase among the population, it can produce herd immunity, which protects unvaccinated people [13].

Like others methods, phage display presents some drawbacks that should be analysed. In the passage to a soluble medium, the binding capacity of the peptide to its target may be lost. In addition, peptide functions in vitro and in vivo can be different, with the risk of producing side effects in the patient. Peptides are also unstable due to proteolysis, and their ability to develop immune responses can be a problem for their application. Nevertheless, there are some techniques that are being developed to overcome these setbacks. Many of them are related to protein engineering or nanotechnology and are aimed at decreasing immunogenicity and increasing peptide affinity and half-life [83].

4. Conclusions

Multidrug-resistant bacteria are currently emerging for almost all the present-day antibiotics. Antibiotics are stable molecules exerting a selective pressure that allows for bacteria to evolve in order to escape, and new treatments should be proposed. Bacteriophages are a real alternative solution to this problem. Phages have different potential applications, starting from their use as bacterial killers in phage therapy, the use of their derivative enzymes, or their use in phage display. Phage therapy has been used for almost a century and it looks like a safe and effective treatment, although it is necessary to do more research to guarantee its safety in the short and long term. Very interesting and useful variants of phage therapy are emerging to enhance phage functions and to take advantage of them in many different areas. The large amount of possibilities due to the great diversity of phages, the use of phage cocktails, the combination with antibiotics, or promising phage display techniques allows for taking the most convenient approach for each scenario and to open new research areas to determine its advantages and disadvantages in each case. Surprisingly, there are also many new applications derived from phage therapy from which other fields can benefit.

Phages appear to be a great solution not only as an alternative treatment against bacterial diseases (phage therapy or use of phage-derived enzymes) but also as interesting tools in the prevention (phage-delivered enzymes) and diagnosis (bacterial detection and typing). Despite the success that these phage-based treatments are expected to have, we are also facing a big concern: the lack of regulation in developed countries and the acceptance of the general public. Further research in this field will help to create regulatory and safety protocols that will lead to the general use of phages in the clinical and pharmaceutical fields.

Author Contributions: Conceptualization, P.D.-C. Writing-Original Draft Preparation, J.D.-M. and P.D.-C. Writing-Review & Editing, P.D.-C.

Acknowledgments: We thank Rafael Sanjuán for previous discussions.

References

1. Domingo-Calap, P.; Georgel, P.; Bahram, S. Back to the future: Bacteriophages as promising therapeutic tools. *HLA* **2016**, *87*, 133–140. [CrossRef] [PubMed]
2. El-Shibiny, A.; El-Sahhar, S. Bacteriophages: The possible solution to treat infections caused by pathogenic bacteria. *Can. J. Microbiol.* **2017**, *63*, 865–879. [CrossRef] [PubMed]
3. Cisek, A.; Dąbrowska, I.; Gregorczyk, K.; Wyżewski, Z. Phage therapy in bacterial infections treatment: One hundred years after the discovery of bacteriophages. *Curr. Microbiol.* **2016**, *74*, 277–283. [CrossRef] [PubMed]
4. Guzmán, M. El bacteriófago, cien años de hallazgos trascendentales. *Biomédica* **2015**, *35*, 159–161. [PubMed]
5. Trudil, D. Phage lytic enzymes: A history. *Virol. Sin.* **2015**, *30*, 26–32. [CrossRef] [PubMed]
6. Sadava, D.; Heller, G.; Orians, G.; Purves, W.; Hillis, D. *Life: The Science of Biology*, 8th ed.; Médica Panamericana: México, Mexico, 2008; pp. 286–287, ISBN 9789500682695.
7. Gelman, D.; Eisenkraft, A.; Chanishvili, N.; Nachman, D.; Coppenhagem Glazer, S.; Hazan, R. The history and promising future of phage therapy in the military service. *J. Trauma Acute Care Surg.* **2018**, *85*, S18–S26. [CrossRef] [PubMed]
8. Wittebole, X.; De Roock, S.; Opal, S. A historical overview of bacteriophage therapy as an alternative to antibiotics for the treatment of bacterial pathogens. *Virulence* **2013**, *5*, 226–235. [CrossRef] [PubMed]
9. Kutateladze, M. Experience of the Eliava Institute in bacteriophage therapy. *Virol. Sin.* **2015**, *30*, 80–81. [CrossRef] [PubMed]
10. Haddad Kashani, H.; Schmelcher, M.; Sabzalipoor, H.; Seyed Hosseini, E.; Moniri, R. Recombinant endolysins as potential therapeutics against antibiotic-resistant *Staphylococcus aureus*: Current status of research and novel delivery strategies. *Clin. Microbiol. Rev.* **2017**, *31*. [CrossRef] [PubMed]
11. Golkar, Z.; Bagasra, O.; Pace, D. Bacteriophage therapy: A potential solution for the antibiotic resistance crisis. *J. Infect. Dev. Ctries.* **2014**, *8*, 129–136. [CrossRef] [PubMed]
12. Martínez, J. General principles of antibiotic resistance in bacteria. *Drug Discov. Today Technol.* **2014**, *11*, 33–39. [CrossRef] [PubMed]
13. Jansen, K.; Knirsch, C.; Anderson, A. The role of vaccines in preventing bacterial antimicrobial resistance. *Nat. Med.* **2018**, *24*, 10–19. [CrossRef] [PubMed]

14. Bassegoda, A.; Ivanova, K.; Ramón, E.; Tzanov, T. Strategies to prevent the occurrence of resistance against antibiotics by using advanced materials. *Appl. Microbiol. Biotechnol.* **2018**, *102*, 2075–2089. [CrossRef] [PubMed]
15. Ackermann, H. 5500 Phages examined in the electron microscope. *Arch. Virol.* **2006**, *152*, 227–243. [CrossRef] [PubMed]
16. Weinbauer, M. Ecology of prokaryotic viruses. *FEMS Microbiol. Rev.* **2004**, *28*, 127–181. [CrossRef] [PubMed]
17. Ofir, G.; Sorek, R. Contemporary phage biology: From classic models to new insights. *Cell* **2018**, *172*, 1260–1270. [CrossRef] [PubMed]
18. Furfaro, L.; Chang, B.; Payne, M. Applications for bacteriophage therapy during pregnancy and the perinatal period. *Front. Microbiol.* **2018**, *8*. [CrossRef] [PubMed]
19. Criscuolo, E.; Spadini, S.; Lamanna, J.; Ferro, M.; Burioni, R. Bacteriophages and their immunological applications against infectious threats. *J. Immunol. Res.* **2017**, *2017*. [CrossRef] [PubMed]
20. Nilsson, A. Phage therapy—Constraints and possibilities. *Ups. J. Med. Sci.* **2014**, *119*, 192–198. [CrossRef] [PubMed]
21. Viertel, T.; Ritter, K.; Horz, H. Viruses versus bacteria—Novel approaches to phage therapy as a tool against multidrug-resistant pathogens. *J. Antimicrob. Chemother.* **2014**, *69*, 2326–2336. [CrossRef] [PubMed]
22. Parikka, K.; Le Romancer, M.; Wauters, N.; Jacquet, S. Deciphering the virus-to-prokaryote ratio VPR: Insights into virus-host relationships in a variety of ecosystems. *Biol. Rev.* **2016**, *92*, 1081–1100. [CrossRef] [PubMed]
23. Matsuzaki, S.; Uchiyama, J.; Takemura-Uchiyama, I.; Daibata, M. Perspective: The age of the phage. *Nature* **2014**, *509*. [CrossRef] [PubMed]
24. Clokie, M.; Millard, A.; Letarov, A.; Heaphy, S. Phages in nature. *Bacteriophage* **2011**, *1*, 31–45. [CrossRef] [PubMed]
25. De Vos, D.; Pirnay, J. Phage therapy: Could viruses help resolve the worldwide antibiotic crisis? In *AMR Control 2015: Overcoming Global Antibiotic Resistance*; Carlet, J., Upham, G., Eds.; Global Health Dynamics Limited: Ipswich, UK, 2015; pp. 110–114, ISBN 9780957607231.
26. Ashelford, K.; Day, M.; Fry, J. Elevated abundance of bacteriophage infecting bacteria in soil. *Appl. Environ. Microbiol.* **2003**, *69*, 285–289. [CrossRef] [PubMed]
27. Sharma, S.; Chatterjee, S.; Datta, S.; Prasad, R.; Dubey, D.; Prasad, R.K.; Vairale, M.G. Bacteriophages and its applications: An overview. *Folia Microbiol.* **2016**, *62*, 17–55. [CrossRef] [PubMed]
28. Buckling, A.; Rainey, P. Antagonistic coevolution between a bacterium and a bacteriophage. *Proc. R. Soc. B Biol. Sci.* **2002**, *269*, 931–936. [CrossRef] [PubMed]
29. Paterson, S.; Vogwill, T.; Buckling, A.; Benmayor, R.; Spiers, A.J.; Thomson, N.R.; Quail, M.; Smith, F.; Walker, D.; Libberton, B.; et al. Antagonistic coevolution accelerates molecular evolution. *Nature* **2010**, *464*, 275–278. [CrossRef] [PubMed]
30. Stern, A.; Sorek, R. The phage-host arms race: Shaping the evolution of microbes. *BioEssays* **2010**, *33*, 43–51. [CrossRef] [PubMed]
31. Díaz-Muñoz, S.; Koskella, B. Bacteria–phage interactions in natural environments. *Adv. Appl. Microbiol.* **2014**, *89*, 135–183. [PubMed]
32. Srinivasiah, S.; Bhavsar, J.; Thapar, K.; Liles, M.; Schoenfeld, T.; Wommack, K.E. Phages across the biosphere: Contrasts of viruses in soil and aquatic environments. *Res. Microbiol.* **2008**, *159*, 349–357. [CrossRef] [PubMed]
33. Forde, A.; Hill, C. Phages of life-the path to pharma. *Br. J. Pharmacol.* **2018**, *175*, 412–418. [CrossRef] [PubMed]
34. Manrique, P.; Dills, M.; Young, M. The human gut phage community and its implications for health and disease. *Viruses* **2017**, *9*, 141. [CrossRef] [PubMed]
35. Van Geelen, L.; Meier, D.; Rehberg, N.; Kalscheuer, R. Some current concepts in antibacterial drug discovery. *Appl. Microbiol. Biotechnol.* **2018**, *102*, 2949–2963. [CrossRef] [PubMed]
36. Hua, Y.; Luo, T.; Yang, Y.; Dong, D.; Wang, R.; Wang, Y.; Xu, M.; Guo, X.; Hu, F.; He, P. Phage therapy as a promising new treatment for lung infection caused by carbapenem-resistant *Acinetobacter baumannii* in mice. *Front. Microbiol.* **2017**, *8*, 2659. [CrossRef] [PubMed]

37. Jeon, J.; Ryu, C.M.; Lee, J.Y.; Park, J.H.; Yong, D.; Lee, K. In vivo application of bacteriophage as a potential therapeutic agent to control OXA-66-like carbapenemase-producing Acinetobacter baumannii strains belonging to sequence type 357. *Appl. Environ. Microbiol.* **2016**, *82*, 4200–4208. [CrossRef] [PubMed]
38. Peng, F.; Mi, Z.; Huang, Y.; Yuan, X.; Niu, W.; Wang, Y.; Hua, Y.; Fan, H.; Bai, C.; Tong, Y. Characterization, sequencing and comparative genomic analysis of vB_AbaM-IME-AB2, a novel lytic bacteriophage that infects multidrug-resistant *Acinetobacter baumannii* clinical isolates. *BMC Microbiol.* **2014**, *14*, 181. [CrossRef] [PubMed]
39. Lood, R.; Ertürk, G.; Mattiasson, B. Revisiting antibiotic resistance spreading in wastewater treatment plants–bacteriophages as a much neglected potential transmission vehicle. *Front. Microbiol.* **2017**, *8*. [CrossRef] [PubMed]
40. Phage Therapy Center. Available online: http://www.phagetherapycenter.com/pii/PatientServlet?command=static_phagetherapy&secnavpos=1&language=0 (accessed on 29 June 2018).
41. Drulis-Kawa, Z.; Majkowska-Skrobek, G.; Maciejewska, B.; Delattre, A.; Lavigne, R. Learning from bacteriophages-advantages and limitations of phage and phage-encoded protein applications. *Curr. Protein Pept. Sci.* **2012**, *13*, 699–722. [CrossRef] [PubMed]
42. Reardon, S. Phage therapy gets revitalized. *Nature* **2014**, *510*, 15–16. [CrossRef] [PubMed]
43. Pires, D.; Melo, L.; Vilas Boas, D.; Sillankorva, S.; Azeredo, J. Phage therapy as an alternative or complementary strategy to prevent and control biofilm-related infections. *Curr. Opin. Microbiol.* **2017**, *39*, 48–56.
44. Knoll, B.; Mylonakis, E. Antibacterial bioagents based on principles of bacteriophage biology: An overview. *Clin. Infect. Dis.* **2013**, *58*, 528–534. [CrossRef] [PubMed]
45. Torres-Barceló, C.; Hochberg, M. Evolutionary rationale for phages as complements of antibiotics. *Trends Microbiol.* **2016**, *24*, 249–256. [CrossRef] [PubMed]
46. Kutateladze, M.; Adamia, R. Bacteriophages as potential new therapeutics to replace or supplement antibiotics. *Trends Biotechnol.* **2010**, *28*, 591–595. [CrossRef] [PubMed]
47. Ghannad, M.; Mohammadi, A. Bacteriophage: Time to re-evaluate the potential of phage therapy as a promising agent to control multidrug-resistant bacteria. *Iran. J. Basic Med. Sci.* **2012**, *15*, 693–701.
48. Levin, B.; Bull, J. Opinion: Population and evolutionary dynamics of phage therapy. *Nat. Rev. Microbiol.* **2004**, *2*, 166–173. [CrossRef] [PubMed]
49. Tao, P.; Zhu, J.; Mahalingam, M.; Batra, H.; Rao, V.B. Bacteriophage T4 nanoparticles for vaccine delivery against infectious diseases. *Adv. Drug Deliv. Rev.* **2018**, *6*. [CrossRef] [PubMed]
50. Roach, D.; Debarbieux, L. Phage therapy: Awakening a sleeping giant. *Emerg. Top. Life Sci.* **2017**, *1*, 93–103. [CrossRef]
51. Sarker, S.; McCallin, S.; Barretto, C.; Berger, B.; Pittet, A.C.; Sultana, S.; Krause, L.; Huq, S.; Bibiloni, R.; Bruttin, A.; et al. Oral T4-like phage cocktail application to healthy adult volunteers from Bangladesh. *Virology* **2012**, *434*, 222–232. [CrossRef] [PubMed]
52. Cortés, P.; Cano-Sarabia, M.; Colom, J.; Otero, J.; Maspoch, D.; Llagostera, M. Nano/Micro formulations for bacteriophage delivery. *Methods Mol. Biol.* **2018**, *1693*, 271–283.
53. Makarova, K.; Haft, D.H.; Barrangou, R.; Brouns, S.J.; Charpentier, E.; Horvath, P.; Moineau, S.; Mojica, F.J.; Wolf, Y.I.; Yakunin, A.F.; et al. Evolution and classification of the CRISPR–Cas systems. *Nat. Rev. Microbiol.* **2011**, *9*, 467–477. [CrossRef] [PubMed]
54. Yosef, I.; Manor, M.; Kiro, R.; Qimron, U. Temperate and lytic bacteriophages programmed to sensitize and kill antibiotic-resistant bacteria. *Proc. Natl. Acad. Sci. USA* **2015**, *112*, 7267–7272. [CrossRef] [PubMed]
55. Seed, K. Battling phages: How bacteria defend against viral attack. *PLoS Pathog.* **2015**, *11*, e1004847. [CrossRef] [PubMed]
56. Scanlan, P.; Buckling, A.; Hall, A. Experimental evolution and bacterial resistance: Coevolutionary costs and trade-offs as opportunities in phage therapy research. *Bacteriophage* **2015**, *5*. [CrossRef] [PubMed]
57. Valério, N.; Oliveira, C.; Jesus, V.; Branco, T.; Pereira, C.; Moreirinha, C.; Almeida, A. Effects of single and combined use of bacteriophages and antibiotics to inactivate Escherichia coli. *Virus Res.* **2017**, *240*, 8–17. [CrossRef] [PubMed]
58. Comeau, A.; Tétart, F.; Trojet, S.; Prère, M.; Krisch, H. La «synergie phages-antibiotiques». *Med. Sci.* **2008**, *24*, 449–451. [CrossRef] [PubMed]
59. Ryan, E.; Alkawareek, M.; Donnelly, R.; Gilmore, B. Synergistic phage-antibiotic combinations for the control of *Escherichia coli* biofilms in vitro. *FEMS Immunol. Med. Microbiol.* **2012**, *65*, 395–398. [CrossRef] [PubMed]

60. Torres-Barceló, C.; Arias-Sánchez, F.I.; Vasse, M.; Ramsayer, J.; Kaltz, O.; Hochberg, M.E. A window of opportunity to control the bacterial pathogen *Pseudomonas aeruginosa* combining antibiotics and phages. *PLoS ONE* **2014**, *9*, e106628. [CrossRef] [PubMed]
61. Maciejewska, B.; Olszak, T.; Drulis-Kawa, Z. Applications of bacteriophages versus phage enzymes to combat and cure bacterial infections: An ambitious and also a realistic application? *Appl. Microbiol. Biotechnol.* **2018**, *102*, 2563–2581. [CrossRef] [PubMed]
62. Maxted, W. The active agent in nascent phage lysis of streptococci. *J. Gen. Microbiol.* **1957**, *16*, 584–595. [CrossRef] [PubMed]
63. Krause, R. Studies on the bacteriophages of *hemolytic streptococci*: II. Antigens released from the streptococcal cell wall by a phage-associated lysin. *J. Exp. Med.* **1958**, *108*, 803–821. [CrossRef] [PubMed]
64. Fischetti, V. Purification and physical properties of group C streptococcal phage-associated lysin. *J. Exp. Med.* **1971**, *133*, 1105–1117. [CrossRef] [PubMed]
65. São-José, C. Engineering of phage-derived lytic enzymes: Improving their potential as antimicrobials. *Antibiotics* **2018**, *7*. [CrossRef] [PubMed]
66. Diez-Martínez, R.; De Paz, H.D.; García-Fernández, E.; Bustamante, N.; Euler, C.W.; Fischetti, V.A.; Menendez, M.; García, P. A novel chimeric phage lysin with high in vitro and in vivo bactericidal activity against Streptococcus pneumoniae. *J. Antimicrob. Chemother.* **2015**, *70*, 1763–1773. [CrossRef] [PubMed]
67. Drulis-Kawa, Z.; Majkowska-Skrobek, G.; Maciejewska, B. Bacteriophages and phage-derived proteins—Application approaches. *Curr. Med. Chem.* **2015**, *22*, 1757–1773. [CrossRef] [PubMed]
68. Wang, I.N.; Smith, D.L.; Young, R. Holins: The protein clocks of bacteriophage infections. *Annu. Rev. Microbiol.* **2000**, *54*, 799–825. [CrossRef] [PubMed]
69. Lin, H.; Paff, M.; Molineux, I.; Bull, J. Therapeutic application of phage capsule depolymerases against K1.; K5.; and K30 capsulated E. coli in mice. *Front. Microbiol.* **2017**, *8*, 2257. [CrossRef] [PubMed]
70. Pires, D.; Oliveira, H.; Melo, L.; Sillankorva, S.; Azeredo, J. Bacteriophage-encoded depolymerases: Their diversity and biotechnological applications. *Appl. Microbiol. Biotechnol.* **2016**, *100*, 2141–2151. [CrossRef] [PubMed]
71. Rodríguez-Rubio, L.; Martínez, B.; Donovan, D.; Rodríguez, A.; García, P. Bacteriophage virion-associated peptidoglycan hydrolases: Potential new enzybiotics. *Crit. Rev. Microbiol.* **2012**, *39*, 427–434. [CrossRef] [PubMed]
72. Attai, H.; Rimbey, J.; Smith, G.; Brown, P. Expression of a peptidoglycan hydrolase from lytic bacteriophages Atu_ph02 and Atu_ph03 triggers lysis of *Agrobacterium tumefaciens*. *Appl. Environ. Microbiol.* **2017**, *83*. [CrossRef] [PubMed]
73. Olsen, I. Modification of phage for increased antibacterial effect towards dental biofilm. *J. Oral Microbiol.* **2016**, *8*. [CrossRef] [PubMed]
74. Hauser, A.; Mecsas, J.; Moir, D. Beyond antibiotics: New therapeutic approaches for bacterial infections. *Clin. Infect. Dis.* **2016**, *63*, 89–95. [CrossRef] [PubMed]
75. Smith, G.P. Filamentous fusion phage: Novel expression vectors that display cloned antigens on the virion surface. *Science* **1985**, *228*, 1315–1317. [CrossRef] [PubMed]
76. Pande, J.; Szewczyk, M.; Grover, A. Phage display: Concept, innovations, applications and future. *Biotechnol. Adv.* **2010**, *28*, 849–858. [CrossRef] [PubMed]
77. Christensen, D.; Gottlin, E.; Benson, R.; Hamilton, P. Phage display for target-based antibacterial drug discovery. *Drug Discov. Today* **2001**, *6*, 721–727. [CrossRef]
78. Ebrahimizadeh, W.; Rajabibazl, M. Bacteriophage vehicles for phage display: Biology, mechanism and application. *Curr. Microbiol.* **2014**, *69*, 109–120. [CrossRef] [PubMed]
79. Muteeb, G.; Rehman, M.T.; Ali, S.Z.; Al-Shahrani, AM.; Kamal, M.A.; Ashraf, G.M. Phage display technique: A novel medicinal approach to overcome antibiotic resistance by using peptide-based inhibitors against β-lactamases. *Curr. Drug Metab.* **2017**, *18*, 90–95. [CrossRef] [PubMed]
80. Flachbartova, Z.; Pulzova, L.; Bencurova, E.; Potocnakova, L.; Comor, L.; Bednarikova, Z.; Bhide, M. Inhibition of multidrug resistant *Listeria monocytogenes* by peptides isolated from combinatorial phage display libraries. *Microbiol. Res.* **2016**. [CrossRef] [PubMed]
81. Kovacs, J.; Masur, H. Prophylaxis against opportunistic infections in patients with human immunodeficiency virus infection. *N. Engl. J. Med.* **2000**, *342*, 1416–1429. [CrossRef] [PubMed]

82. Bazan, J.; Całkosiński, I.; Gamian, A. Phage display—A powerful technique for immunotherapy. *Hum. Vaccin. Immunother.* **2012**, *8*, 1829–1835. [CrossRef] [PubMed]
83. Omidfar, K.; Daneshpour, M. Advances in phage display technology for drug discovery. *Expert Opin. Drug Discov.* **2015**, *10*, 651–669. [CrossRef] [PubMed]

8

Fighting Fire with Fire: Phage Potential for the Treatment of *E. coli* O157 Infection

Cristina Howard-Varona [1,†], Dean R. Vik [1,†], Natalie E. Solonenko [1], Yueh-Fen Li [1], M. Consuelo Gazitua [1], Lauren Chittick [1], Jennifer K. Samiec [1], Aubrey E. Jensen [1], Paige Anderson [1], Adrian Howard-Varona [1], Anika A. Kinkhabwala [2], Stephen T. Abedon [1,*] and Matthew B. Sullivan [1,3,*]

1 Department of Microbiology, The Ohio State University, Columbus, OH 43210, USA; howard-varona.2@osu.edu (C.H.-V.); vik.1@buckeyemail.osu.edu (D.R.V.); solonenko.2@osu.edu (N.E.S.); li.918@osu.edu (Y.-F.L.); consuelogazitua@gmail.com (M.C.G.); chittick.3@osu.edu (L.C.); Jennifer.Samiec@osumc.edu (J.K.S.); aubrey.jensen9@gmail.com (A.E.J.); anderson.2805@buckeyemail.osu.edu (P.A.); ahowardv11@gmail.com (A.H.-V.)
2 EpiBiome, Inc., 29528 Union City blvd, Union City, CA 94587, USA; anikaak@gmail.com
3 Department of Civil, Environmental and Geodetic Engineering, The Ohio State University, Columbus, OH 43210, USA
* Correspondence: abedon.1@osu.edu (S.T.A.); sullivan.948@osu.edu (M.B.S.)
† The author contributed equally to this work.

Abstract: Hemolytic–uremic syndrome is a life-threating disease most often associated with Shiga toxin-producing microorganisms like *Escherichia coli* (STEC), including *E. coli* O157:H7. Shiga toxin is encoded by resident prophages present within this bacterium, and both its production and release depend on the induction of Shiga toxin-encoding prophages. Consequently, treatment of STEC infections tend to be largely supportive rather than antibacterial, in part due to concerns about exacerbating such prophage induction. Here we explore STEC O157:H7 prophage induction in vitro as it pertains to phage therapy—the application of bacteriophages as antibacterial agents to treat bacterial infections—to curtail prophage induction events, while also reducing STEC O157:H7 presence. We observed that cultures treated with strictly lytic phages, despite being lysed, produce substantially fewer Shiga toxin-encoding temperate-phage virions than untreated STEC controls. We therefore suggest that phage therapy could have utility as a prophylactic treatment of individuals suspected of having been recently exposed to STEC, especially if prophage induction and by extension Shiga toxin production is not exacerbated.

Keywords: Antibiotic-resistant bacteria; bacteriophage therapy; phage therapy; lysogenic conversion; prophage induction; read recruitment; shiga toxin

---

1. Introduction

Prophages are bacteriophage (phage) genomes that replicate alongside their bacterial host's genome until induced to produce viral particles. This carriage state, termed a lysogenic cycle, is characteristic of temperate phages (as opposed to strictly lytic, or virulent, phages), and the prophage-carrying bacterial host is termed a lysogen. Recent reviews provide information on the diverse and impactful biology and distribution of temperate phages, along with methods for temperate phage detection [1–3]. One impact of temperate phage biology is lysogenic conversion: the modification of a host phenotype by prophage genes, including genes encoding bacterial virulence factors [4–6].

Notable among prophage-encoded virulence factors are exotoxins, such as those associated with the O157:H7 serotype of Shiga-toxigenic *Escherichia coli* (STEC) [7]. STEC O157:H7 is a polylysogenic human pathogen, often derived from ruminant gastrointestinal tracks and known for its capacity to encode two Shiga toxins, dubbed Stx1 and Stx2 [8,9]. These are generally encoded by the Shiga-toxigenic prophages 933V and 933W, respectively [10–12]. Of these, only the lamboid 933W prophage appears capable of inducing, and does so spontaneously [11,13–17]. This induction and the associated lytic cycle are a prerequisite for Shiga toxin production and release [18–20]. Shiga toxin release during STEC O157:H7 infection can lead to hemorrhagic colitis and hemolytic–uremic syndrome (HUS), which damages kidney nephrons of the STEC-infected human patients [20–22], but causes little to no pathogenesis in ruminants [23].

Certain antibiotics that induce the STEC SOS response also can induce Shiga-toxigenic prophages, resulting in new intracellular Shiga toxin production and subsequent phage lysis-associated toxin release [4,11,16,20,24–26]. Thus, prophage induction, in addition to bacterial lysis, drives increases of Shiga toxin within STEC-infected individuals, and prophage-inducing antibiotics therefore are not recommended for STEC treatment. Consequently, STEC killing via other non-prophage inducing methods—even lytic mechanisms, such as through infection by strictly lytic phages—should serve as viable STEC treatment. Treatment using non-Shiga-toxigenic phages (phage therapy) should not in itself give rise to an increased degree of patient exposure to Shiga toxin than would occur without such non-inductive lysis. Furthermore, lysogen killing by means that do not induce prophages should curtail future induction events, which presumably will result in less overall Shiga toxin production.

Based on the above assumptions, we reasoned that lysis of STEC O157:H7 by strictly lytic phages might eliminate STEC O157:H7 without further contributing to Shiga toxin production. If true, then such lytic phages might be employed as a means of anti-STEC treatment, and by extension as anti-Shiga-toxigenic phage agents—in effect an anti-temperate phage form of phage therapy.

Here we test this hypothesis through in vitro experiments designed to explore the use of strictly lytic phages, unrelated to Shiga toxin-encoding prophages, as anti-STEC bactericidal agents, in order to assess the potential impact of phage therapy on the production of Shiga-toxigenic 933W phages by *E. coli* O157:H7.

2. Results

2.1. Detecting Spontaneous Prophage Induction

From the American Type Culture Collection (ATCC—identifier ATCC43895) we acquired the STEC serotype O157:H7 whose genome sequence is published under strain EDL933 [11,12]. In order to have an up-to-date genome sequence (herein termed STEC), we re-sequenced our working strain and identified prophage regions with the online tool PHASTER [27] (Supplementary Materials). This confirmed the working strain as largely identical to the published EDL933 at 100% average nucleotide identity (ANI) with only a ~1% difference in genome length (see Supplementary Materials, Table S1). Predicted prophage content between STEC and EDL933 was also largely congruent, with the small variation observed likely due to differences in sequencing and assembly methodology (Supplementary Materials, Figure S1).

With a fully-sequenced working strain, we then assessed spontaneous prophage induction in STEC as follows. STEC cultures were grown in triplicate for 5 h, treated with chloroform for 2.5 h to lyse the cells and release encapsidated phage DNA, and 0.2 μm-filtered to remove cells and large cellular debris. Samples were then treated with DNase to minimize free DNA and enrich for encapsidated DNA. The DNA was then extracted and sequenced, and the resulting reads were mapped to the STEC genome, including prophage regions. Given that most free bacterial DNA was removed with DNase, elevated read recruitment across the entirety of any prophage region would indicate induction and subsequent encapsidation of the prophage region(s). This read recruitment methodology is especially useful for identifying which prophages are induced within polylysogens, as previously shown [28–30].

Mean read recruitment coverage values were calculated per host or prophage region and normalized by the sequencing depth and the sequence length of either the 933W genomic region (59,338 bp) or the

STEC genome without the 933W prophage (5,499,692 bp). This revealed that prophage 933W, which encodes the Stx2 genes and is responsible for much of STEC's pathogenesis [20,31], had substantially higher mean coverage (4675×) than either the rest of the host genome (0.09×) or other prophage regions (0.12×), and that this elevated read coverage encompassed nearly all (95%) of the 933W genome (Figure 1, Table 1, and Supplementary Materials). We interpret this as evidence for spontaneous induction and encapsidation of 933W in this STEC strain, a finding consistent with prior work that describes prophage 933W as a highly spontaneously inducible prophage [11,13–17].

With this qualitative screening identifying only the 933W prophage as having been induced, we sought to quantify 933W phage production as a product of spontaneous induction via a quantitative PCR (qPCR) approach targeting the Shiga toxin gene *stx2a* encoded by 933W. To this end, we grew and sampled STEC as done for the whole-genome induction screen above, and found that the prophage 933W-encoded *stx2a* copy number increased eight-fold from the start to the end of the aforementioned 7.5 h experiment (~10^5 to 8×10^5 per μL of filtrate) (Figure 2). This corroborates the sequence-based indication of prophage 933W spontaneous induction and implies ongoing induction over the course of culture incubation, since encapsidated DNA was present in somewhat smaller amounts at the start of the incubation. Prophage 933W induction, therefore, should be quantitatively reducible by preventing ongoing lysogen growth, such as may be accomplished in the course of phage therapy.

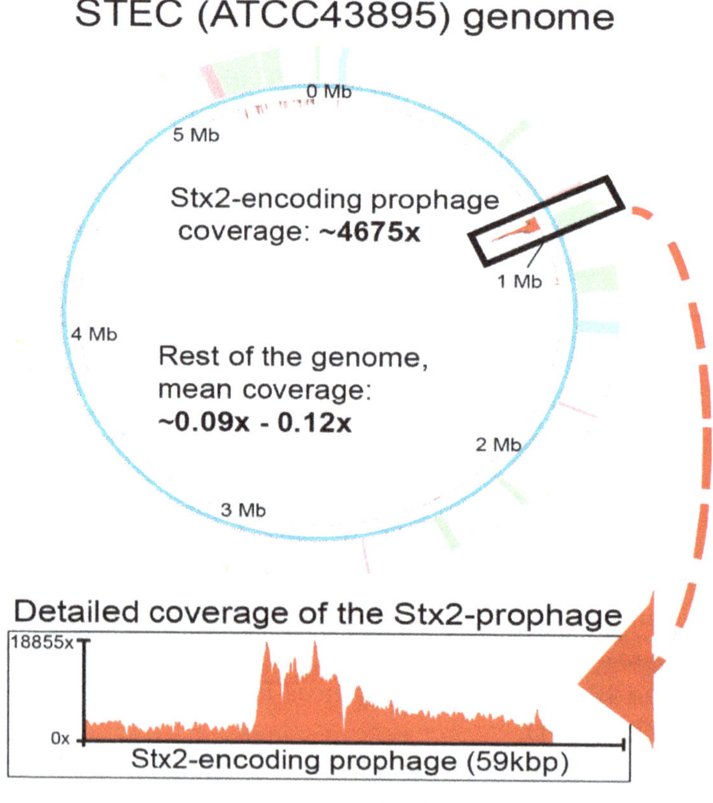

Figure 1. Phage 933W is the only prophage that is spontaneously induced. Shown here is the read mapping from sequenced *Escherichia coli* (STEC) cultures in biological triplicates. The circular plot represents the host genome, with the PHASTER-predicted prophages in colors (pink, red, or blue) in the outer circle, as well as the reads mapped to the entire genome. Prophage 933W is covered ~4675 times on average throughout its entire length, whereas the rest of the non-prophage and prophage genomic regions are covered, on average, 0.09 and 0.12 times, respectively. The prophage 933W region and read-mapping to such a region is amplified below the circular plot to show that the entire prophage length is covered by reads, and their proportion. Detailed information of the reads can be found in Table 1 and in the Supplementary Materials, Dataset.

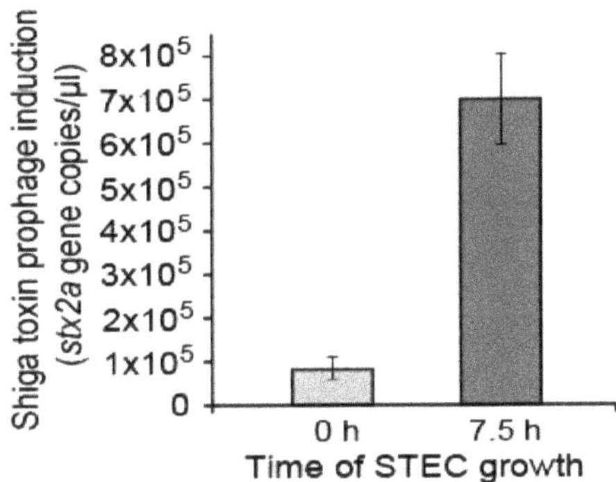

Figure 2. Quantification of prophage 933W induction in uninfected STEC cultures via quantitative PCR (qPCR). Primers are used against the *stx2* subunit *a* gene at 0 and 7.5 h of STEC growth. The former represents a transfer of cells from an overnight growth into fresh media, and the latter represents when cell growth is stopped and the DNA harvesting procedure begins (see Methods). The average of three biological replicates and their error is plotted on the graph. The difference between the two time points is significantly different (*t*-test, $p < 0.05$). Data from this experiment can be found in the Supplementary Materials (see Dataset).

Table 1. Coverage of uninfected ATCC43895 (STEC)'s prophage and non-prophage regions. Represented is the raw coverage, the normalized coverage (to sequencing depth and region length), and the final transformed coverage (multiplied by 10^{11} for better reading) of each of the 17 prophages and the non-prophage regions of STEC, in biological triplicates.

Lysate	Prophage or Not?	Genomic Entity	Raw Coverage	Coverage Normalized by Sequencing Depth and Entity Length	Final Adjusted Coverage (Raised to 10^{11})
No phage control ATCC43895 (STEC)-Replicate 1	Prophages	#1-58370-85143	0.069	5.69×10^{-14}	0.01
		#2-648527-680910	0.067	5.50×10^{-14}	0.01
		#3 and 4-911029-938407 bp	0.835	6.89×10^{-13}	0.07
		#5 (Stx2)-973564-1032902 bp	585.776	4.41×10^{-8}	4407.33
		#6 and 7-1202175-1293616 bp	2.606	2.15×10^{-12}	0.22
		#8-1390536-1436457 bp	0.018	1.47×10^{-14}	0
		#9-1708731-1719671 bp	0.002	1.57×10^{-15}	0
		#10-2054278-2078426 bp	0.167	1.38×10^{-13}	0.01
		#11 (Stx1)-2302225-2335340 bp	8.057	6.65×10^{-12}	0.66
		#12-2579647-2589259 bp	0	0	0
		#13, 14 and 15-5103469-5282316 bp	1.229	1.01×10^{-12}	0.1
		#16-5286283-5348617 bp	0.274	2.26×10^{-13}	0.02
		#17-5449904-5468395 bp	0.24	1.98×10^{-13}	0.02
	Non-prophage	Host genome, non-prophage	0.852	7.04×10^{-13}	0.07
No phage control ATCC43895 (STEC)-Replicate 2	Prophages	#1-58370-85143	0.15	8.91×10^{-14}	0.01
		#2-648527-680910	0.514	3.05×10^{-13}	0.03
		#3 and 4-911029-938407 bp	1.883	1.12×10^{-12}	0.11
		#5 (Stx2)-973564-1032902 bp	881.779	4.77×10^{-8}	4774.17
		#6 and 7-1202175-1293616 bp	4.605	2.74×10^{-12}	0.27
		#8-1390536-1436457 bp	0.118	7.00×10^{-14}	0.01
		#9-1708731-1719671 bp	0.22	1.30×10^{-13}	0.01
		#10-2054278-2078426 bp	0.372	2.21×10^{-13}	0.02
		#11 (Stx1)-2302225-2335340 bp	14.645	8.70×10^{-12}	0.87
		#12-2579647-2589259 bp	0.097	5.73×10^{-14}	0.01
		#13, 14 and 15-5103469-5282316 bp	2.283	1.36×10^{-12}	0.14
		#16-5286283-5348617 bp	0.437	2.59×10^{-13}	0.03
		#17-5449904-5468395 bp	0.562	3.34×10^{-13}	0.03
	Non-prophage	Host genome, non-prophage	1.743	1.04×10^{-12}	0.1

Table 1. *Cont.*

Lysate	Prophage or Not?	Genomic Entity	Raw Coverage	Coverage Normalized by Sequencing Depth and Entity Length	Final Adjusted Coverage (Raised to 10^{11})
No phage control ATCC43895 (STEC)-Replicate 3	Prophages	#1-58370-85143	0.226	1.48×10^{-13}	0.01
		#2-648527-680910	0.299	1.96×10^{-13}	0.02
		#3 and 4-911029-938407 bp	1.379	9.03×10^{-13}	0.09
		#5 (Stx2) 973564-1032902 bp	811.189	4.84×10^{-8}	4844.55
		#6 and 7-1202175-1293616 bp	4.466	2.93×10^{-12}	0.29
		#8-1390536-1436457 bp	0.089	5.82×10^{-14}	0.01
		#9-1708731-1719671 bp	0.117	7.66×10^{-14}	0.01
		#10-2054278-2078426 bp	0.399	2.61×10^{-13}	0.03
		#11 (Stx1)-2302225-2335340 bp	13.974	9.15×10^{-12}	0.92
		#12-2579647-2589259 bp	0.277	1.82×10^{-13}	0.02
		#13, 14 and 15-5103469-5282316 bp	2.031	1.33×10^{-12}	0.13
		#16-5286283-5348617 bp	0.345	2.26×10^{-13}	0.02
		#17-5449904-5468395 bp	0.541	3.54×10^{-13}	0.04
	Non-prophage	Host genome, non-prophage	1.681	1.10×10^{-12}	0.11

2.2. *Fighting Prophage Induction with Phage Treatment*

Given that 933W induction is known to be associated with Shiga toxin production in *E. coli* O157:H7 [20], we next considered whether treatment using exogenously supplied, strictly lytic phages could reduce lysogen numbers without exacerbating prophage induction. We used the T4-like phages p000v and p000y that we previously isolated and sequenced [32], and which we here characterized for their infection of STEC (Supplementary Materials: Figures S2 and S3, Dataset). We then grew and sampled STEC as described above, except we also added either of these exogenous phages to the STEC culture at ratios of roughly 4–6 phages per target bacterium (multiplicity of infection (MOI): ~4–6), where initial infective titers were $\sim 6.4 \times 10^8$ and $\sim 4.6 \times 10^8$ plaque-forming units per ml for phages p000v and p000y, respectively. Indeed, by the end of the experiment, addition of these phages had decreased the levels of 933W prophage induction, as quantified by qPCR. Namely, while the qPCR-measured ratio of *stx2a* copies per μL between 7.5 and 0 h was ~8 without phage (Figure 2), with the addition of phages p000v and p000y it decreased to ~0.3× and ~0.4×, respectively (Figure 3, Table 2). Thus, these results show that exogenous, strictly lytic phages reduce *stx2a* copies (a proxy for 933W prophage induction) and suggest that Shiga toxin production would also be reduced, due to both no further stimulation of prophage induction upon lytic phage infection, on the one hand, and reduction in the number of lysogens present on the other.

Table 2. Summary of the prophage induction quantification obtained by qPCR in uninfected and infected STEC cultures, as presented in Figures 2 and 3.

***Stx2a* Copies Per μL During STEC Growth with and without Phage**				
Phage	**0 h**	**7.5 h**	**Ratio**	**MOI**
None	8.39×10^4	6.97×10^5	8.31	NA
p000v	6.93×10^3	2.09×10^3	0.30	6.43
p000y	8.00×10^3	2.88×10^3	0.36	4.61

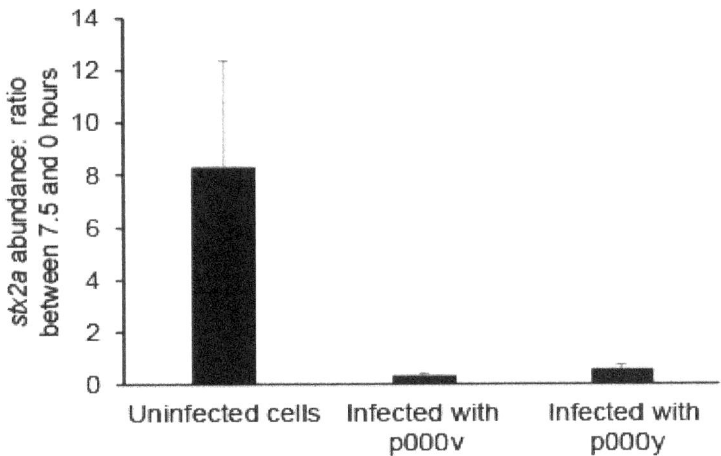

Figure 3. Quantification of prophage 933W induction in phage-infected STEC cultures via qPCR. The Shiga toxin (*stx2* subunit *a*) gene abundance in prophage 933W is measured at 0 and 7.5 h post-phage addition to STEC cell cultures at multiplicities of infection (MOIs) of ~4.6 (for phage p000y) and ~6.4 (for phage p000v). Represented is the ratio of such *stx2a* abundance between 7.5 and 0 h of STEC growth, using the average of the biological replicates and their error, either in the absence (left most bar in the graph) or presence (the other two bars) of phages. The differences between in the absence of phages (uninfected cells) and in the presence of phages (infected with p000v or p000y) are statistically significant ($p < 0.05$).

3. Discussion

The primary question regarding the potential for using phage therapy to treat pathogenic lysogens is whether such treatment might exacerbate patient exposure to toxins produced upon prophage induction. For Shiga-toxigenic *E. coli* O157:H7 in particular, Shiga toxin production and release is associated with prophage induction, mostly prophage 933W [14,19,33–35]. Consequentially, treatment options for STEC infections are largely supportive rather than antimicrobial for tackling Shiga toxin production and patient exposure [36,37].

There are three related routes by which Shiga toxin exposure could occur (Figure 4). First, the standard route (point 1a, Figure 4) is through prophage induction, resulting in Shiga toxin (Stx) gene expression followed by Shiga toxin release via phage-induced bacterial lysis [20,38]. Thus, it is crucial to avoid treatments that can lead to additional prophage induction, which can result from certain antibiotic uses [20,39].

A second route of Shiga toxin release (point 2a, Figure 4) may occur via artificial lysis of induced lysogens by exogenous phages, if such lysogens are capable of becoming infected and sustaining a second bacteriolytic phage infection. This could accelerate cell lysis and thus toxin release if the exogenous phage has a faster replication cycle or is otherwise competitively superior to the prophage. Alternatively, co-infection by an exogenous phage and induced prophage may confound either of the phages' replication cycle, thereby delaying the time to cell lysis. Both instances could reasonably attenuate toxin production overall due to the reduction of either the duration or the efficiency of prophage expression, thus reducing toxin translation.

A third route (points 3a and 3b, Figure 4) may occur when the induced and then released Shiga-toxigenic temperate phage lytically infects other *E. coli* not already lysogenized by Shiga-toxigenic phages, which would consequently enable these non-STEC bacteria to express Shiga toxin [40–42]. This latter route may not be easily blocked if sufficient numbers of these alternative hosts are present and support substantial Shiga-toxigenic phage population growth (point 3b, Figure 4). Based on our results, Shiga-toxin amplification from such infections may, however, be curtailed by intervening with phage treatment prior to lysogen induction and resulting Shiga-toxigenic phage production.

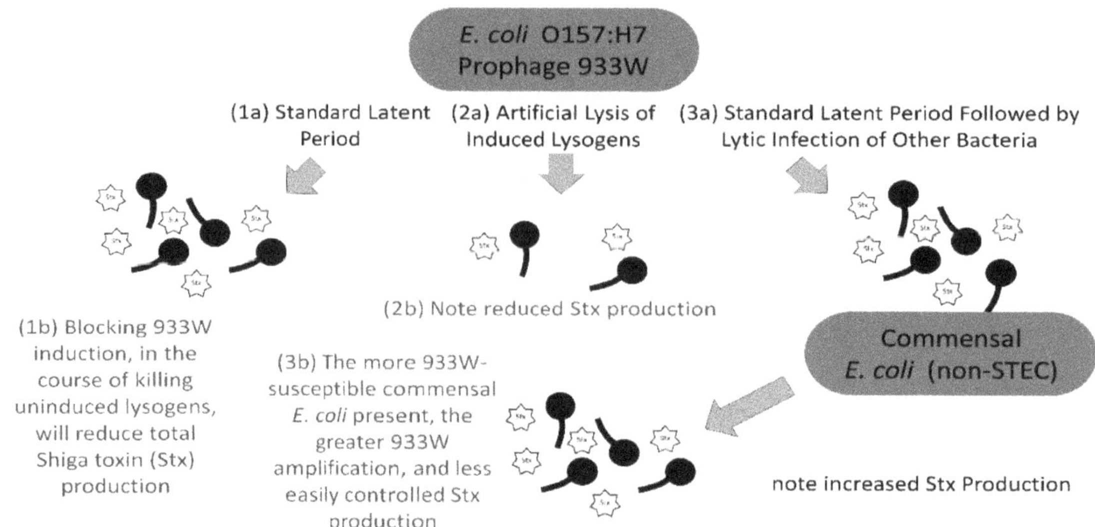

Figure 4. Different routes towards Shiga toxin (Stx) release: (1) 933W prophage induction followed by normal lytic cycles; (2) artificial lysis, for example by exogenous phage, of induced lysogens, resulting in truncated lytic cycles; and (3) subsequent lytic infection of non-Shiga toxigenic *E. coli* strains giving rise to more lytic cycles. Greater Stx production (stars in the figure) can occur given artificial induction of *E. coli* O157:H7 lysogens, but this both is not explicitly illustrated in the figure and is distinct from artificial lysis of already induced lysogens (2). Given the linkage between 933W induction and Shiga toxin production, the killing of *E. coli* O157:H7 lysogens without inducing the 933W prophage should result in reductions in future 933W induction events (Figure 3 and Table 2) along with subsequent reductions in Shiga toxin production.

Here we have confirmed that an exogenously supplied obligately lytic phage "treatment" can interfere with the spontaneous production of Shiga-toxigenic prophages encoded by an *E. coli* O157:H7 strain. The mechanism of reduction in prophage induction presumably is due to the killing of prophage-containing lysogens, apparently prior to natural or artificially triggered induction. It remains unconfirmed, however, how such phage treatment will impact Shiga toxin production or release. It is likely, though, as Shiga-toxogenic prophage induction is tightly coupled to Shiga toxin production [20,38], that phage treatment of *E. coli* O157:H7-exposed patients at the very least should mitigate Shiga toxin production by killing prophage-carrying Shiga-toxigenic lysogens.

To most effectively treat such Shiga-toxigenic pathogens, future research will need to explore several areas. First, it is not known to what extent, or with what variability, different treatment phages can impact the lytic cycles of already-induced lysogens (Figure 4, 2a). Additionally, recent research with environmental phage–host systems depicts the importance of also considering the host's response, given that they are often the ones driving the infection outcomes instead of the phages [43–45]. Second, it needs to be determined whether rapid treatment-phage-mediated *E. coli* O157:H7 killing is achievable in situ. It is likely, however, that achieving relatively high in-situ phage titers, e.g., 10^8 per ml or higher [46], would be required to attain such rapid treatment-phage impact, while substantial reductions in overall Stx production will require early initiation of treatment, such as in response to suspected rather than confirmed pathogen exposure (i.e., so-called "inundative" and prophylactic phage treatment, respectively). Third, while phage therapy is generally considered as a safe treatment, given the relative lack of toxicities and side effects, especially during oral delivery [47], further verification is needed prior to generalizing clinical implementation. Generally, these issues point to a broader "pharmacologically aware" approach to the development of any phage-based *E. coli* O157:H7 infection treatment, involving iteration between continued in vitro and in vivo as well as in silico studies. In this vein, the observations reported here are consistent with *E. coli* O157:H7 phage treatment likely not giving rise to negative outcomes, as can stem from the exacerbation of 933W prophage induction.

4. Materials and Methods

Raw data is provided in the Dataset, and additional methods can be found in the Supplementary Materials.

4.1. Bacterial Strain and Phages Used in This Study

The Shiga-toxigenic *E. coli* serotype O157:H7 (STEC) used in this study was obtained from the American Type Culture Collection (ATCC) under identifier 43895, which is published as EDL933 under GenBank accession numbers CP008957 and CP008958 [11,12]. The T4-like Myoviridae phages p000v and p000y are described elsewhere [32], and can be found in the Cyverse data repository [48] under DOI 10.7946/P2HP89 (https://www.doi.org/10.7946/P2HP89), and in GenBank under accession numbers MK047717 and MK047718, respectively.

4.2. Cell Growth

Bacteria were streaked onto TSA (Tryptic Soy Agar, 40 g/L, Ward's Cat. 38-1010) plates from glycerol stocks, grown overnight at room temperature (RT), and held at 4 °C. Single colonies were then inoculated in TSB (Tryptic Soy Broth, 30 g/L, Ward's Cat. 38-1012) and grown shaking at ~200 rpm at 37 °C overnight.

4.3. Lysates for Phage Amplification

An overnight bacterial culture was diluted 1:50 in fresh TSB and grown shaking at ~200 rpm at 37 °C until the optical density (OD) reached ~0.3 (2.94×10^8 CFUs/mL). Phages were added to 10–50 mL of the host culture at a low MOI (10^{-6}–0.1), and incubated shaking at ~200 rpm at 37 °C for ~5 h. Chloroform was added to the infection at 1% (*v/v*) and incubated shaking at ~70 rpm at RT for 2 h. The chloroform was allowed to settle for 30 min, and the aqueous phase was 0.2 μm-filtered to remove any remaining cells. Some lysates were also concentrated via polyethylene glycol (PEG)-precipitation. For those, both NaCl (6.5 g) and PEG-8000 (10 g) were added per 100 mL lysate. This was incubated overnight at 4 °C, then centrifuged at 10,000 *g* in a Beckman J2-MC centrifuge (Beckman Coulter, Brea, CA, USA) for 10 min. The supernatant was removed, and the pellet resuspended in phage buffer (4 g NaCl, 0.1 g gelatin, 10 mL 1 M Tris Base (pH 7.6), and 1 mL 1 M $MgSO_4$ per L).

4.4. DNA Extraction

The STEC strain obtained from ATCC (ATCC43895) was sequenced. For that, its genomic DNA was extracted using the ZymoBIOMICS DNA mini kit (Zymo Research, Irvine, CA, USA) following the manufacturer's protocol. Similarly, sequenced phage infections and phage-free cultures from which prophage induction was assessed were also sequenced. The DNA of these samples was extracted using the Phage DNA Isolation Kit (Norgen Biotek Corp., Thorold, ON, Canada) following the manufacturer's protocol. Any remaining host DNA was degraded by adding 10 μL (20 U) of DNase I from the RNase-free DNase I kit (Norgen Biotek Corp., Thorold, ON, Canada) prior to proteinase K treatment. Bacterial host DNA concentrations were quantified using the Qubit 3.0 Fluorometer and the Qubit dsDNA High Sensitivity Kit (Thermo Fisher Scientific, Waltham, MA, USA).

4.5. Library Preparation and Illumina Miseq Sequencing of Phage and Host Genomes

Extracts from the previous step were prepared for sequencing on the Illumina MiSeq platform (Illumina, San Diego, CA, USA) using the Nextera XT Library Preparation Kit (Illumina, San Diego, CA, USA) according to the manufacturer's protocol (Part # 15031942, revision D). The magnetic bead normalization step was replaced with a manual normalization step, based on library concentration and average size as measured by the Qubit 3.0 Fluorometer and Qubit dsDNA High Sensitivity Kit (Thermo Fisher Scientific, Waltham, MA, USA) and the Fragment Analyzer (AATI, Ankeny, IA,

USA), respectively. Paired-end sequencing was performed using the MiSeq Reagent v3 (600 cycle) kit (Illumina, San Diego, CA, USA).

4.6. Whole-Genome Sequencing and Read-Mapping to Assess Prophage Induction

Two sample types were obtained for sequencing whole bacterial and phage genomes, mapping reads to such genomes, and assessing prophage induction: phage-free and phage-infected bacterial cultures. The phage-infected samples were lysates grown as described in the "Lysates for Phage Amplification" section. The phage-free samples were mock lysates prepared as the infection samples, but without phages and in 30 mL containing 3.5 mL of phage buffer. After DNA extraction and library preparation procedures as described, samples were sequenced via the MiSeq technology described.

4.7. Read Mapping and Visualization of Prophage Induction

Reads from each of the lysates were mapped to the STEC and respective phage genome using the Burrows–Wheeler Aligner (BWA) [49] version 0.7.13, with default parameters. The resulting SAM files were converted to BAM files using samtools [50] version 1.3.1. Coverage across either phage or host genome was calculated using the Bayesian Analysis of Macroevolutionary Mixtures (BaMM) [51], software version 1.4.1, with the parse tool and the "tpmean" setting. Coverage values were then normalized by the number of reads that mapped to the virulent phages or STEC (i.e., the sequencing depth), as inferred by the samtools version 1.3.1 flagstat tool, and by the genome length of either prophage 933W, the virulent phages, or STEC without the prophage 933W. All depth- and length-normalized coverage values were then multiplied by 10^{11} to derive more comprehensible whole-genome coverage values. Coverage values per base were visualized by creating bedgraph files, using the bedtools [52] version 2.27.1 package and the genomecov -bg option. These bedgraph files were then uploaded to the Integrative Genomics Viewer (IGV) version 2.4.6 package [53] and Circos [54] version 0.69.

4.8. qPCR of Phage Lysates' DNA

The OD of an overnight bacterial culture was read to determine the volume containing 10^{10} cells, which was then added to 100 mL of TSB. This was grown shaking at ~200 rpm at 37 °C; the OD was read after ~30 min and then every 10 min until the reading was 0.25–0.3. Phages were added to 2–5 mL of the host culture at MOIs lower than 0.1 or close to 6. A 0.3–1 mL sample was taken immediately and 0.2 µm-filtered to remove any cells, then stored at 4 °C. The infected culture was then incubated shaking at ~200 rpm at 37 °C for 5 h. Chloroform was added to the infection at 1% (*v*/*v*) and incubated shaking at ~70 rpm at RT for 2.5 h. The chloroform was allowed to settle for 20 min, and the aqueous phase was 0.2 µm-filtered to remove cells. Another 0.3–1 mL sample was taken and stored at 4 °C. DNA was extracted from the two filtered samples. First, the viral DNA was inactivated using DNase in a ratio of 1 µL of DNase to 9 µL of sample. Ethylenediamine tetraacetic acid (EDTA) and Ethylene glycol tetraacetic acid (EGTA) were added at 100 mM to inactivate the DNase. After the DNA was inactivated, extraction was continued using a Wizard DNA Clean-up Kit (Cat. #A7181, Promega Corporation, Madison, WI, USA). Then, 1 mL of DNA clean-up resin was added to each sample, and they were mixed by inversion. The samples were put into a syringe and pushed through a Wizzard minicolumn (Cat. #A7211, Promega Corporation, Madison, WI, USA), followed by the addition of 2 mL 80% isopropanol pushed through the column, 1 mL at a time. Samples were centrifuged for 2 min at 10,000 *g* to remove any excess isopropanol. Each sample was eluted in 50 µL of Tris EDTA (TE) that had been warmed to 80 °C. At the addition of TE, each sample was briefly vortexed and then centrifuged at 10,000 *g* for 30 s to elute the DNA. The samples were then analyzed for their prophage content via qPCR.

To run the qPCR, 2 µL of DNA extracted from a phage lysate was used as the template in the 15 µL qPCR reaction that contained 1× Perfecta SYBR Green FastMix (Quanta Biosciences, Gaithersburg, MD, USA) and 300 nM of each of the forward and reverse primers targeting prophage 933W (gene *stx2a* forward primer: 5′-ATGTGGCCGGGTTCGTTAAT-3′; reverse primer: 5′-TGCTGTCCGTTGTCATGGAA-3′). The qPCR reaction was carried out with the following thermocycler conditions: initial denaturation and enzyme activation at 95 °C for 5 min, 40 cycles of denaturation at 95 °C for 30 s, annealing at 57 °C for 30 s, and extension at 72 °C for 30 s, followed by one cycle of 95 °C for 15 s, 57 °C for 15 s, and 95 °C for 15 s for the dissociation curve. Fluorescence signal was collected at the end of the extension step and of the ramping period of dissociation curve. Serial dilution of the genomic DNA of strain STEC was used to generate the standard curve ($R^2 > 0.99$).

5. Conclusions

With the rise in antibiotic resistance in bacterial pathogens, phage therapy presents a promising alternative for treatment. Importantly, though, many of pathogens contain prophages that not only are commonly the source of pathogenesis [3,6], but have also been shown to impact cell-virus communication systems [55]. Thus, as phage therapy advances, it will be important to investigate the impacts of exogenous phages on prophage induction. Here we have provided a first step towards such investigation with whole-genome sequencing and PCR-based quantification approaches that enable a genome-wide view and quantification of what prophages are induced under both exogenous phage-free and phage-rich environments. Future work should investigate the levels of the Shiga toxin under such scenarios, as well as the impacts of phage treatment plus stressors that can induce lysogens, such as antibiotics. Additionally, research from environmental phage-host systems provides invaluable insight into 'phage-host biology' in nature by showing that even in prophage-free bacteria exogenous phages are not always efficient at infecting [44,45]; important when considering phage candidates for therapy. Altogether, advancing knowledge of phage-prophage-host interactions should provide a baseline for engineering phages [56–58] as well as inform what phages to choose to make phage cocktails that can eradicate bacterial pathogens.

Author Contributions: C.H.-V., N.E.S., L.C., M.C.G., Y.-F.L., J.K.S., A.E.J., P.A., and A.H.-V. contributed to designing and executing experiments. C.H.-V. and D.R.V. contributed to most data analysis and figure/table generation, and with S.T.A. and M.B.S. to the writing of the manuscript. A.A.K. contributed to methods writing and sequencing efforts, as well to providing partial funding, along with Ohio State University.

Acknowledgments: We thank Michelle Davison and Rebecca Lu at Epibiome for DNA extraction and sequencing, respectively, as well as Zachary Hobbs and Ryan Honaker from Epibiome for providing the phages. We also thank the following undergraduates for their help with initial phage–host optimizations: Alice L. Herneisen, Catherine E. Johnson, John M. Thomas, and Storm A. Mohn. We also thank OSU PhD rotation students Siavash Azari, Sravya Kovvali, and Yiwei Liu.

References

1. Penades, J.R.; Chen, J.; Quiles-Puchalt, N.; Carpena, N.; Novick, R.P. Bacteriophage-mediated spread of bacterial virulence genes. *Curr. Opin. Microbiol.* **2015**, *23*, 171–178. [CrossRef]
2. Feiner, R.; Argov, T.; Rabinovich, L.; Sigal, N.; Borovok, I.; Herskovits, A.A. A new perspective on lysogeny: Prophages as active regulatory switches of bacteria. *Nat. Rev. Microbiol.* **2015**, *13*, 641–650. [CrossRef]
3. Howard-Varona, C.; Hargreaves, K.R.; Abedon, S.T.; Sullivan, M.B. Lysogeny in nature: Mechanisms, impact and ecology of temperate phages. *ISME J.* **2017**, *11*, 1511–1520. [CrossRef]
4. Fortier, L.-C.; Sekulovic, O. Importance of prophages to evolution and virulence of bacterial pathogens. *Virulence* **2013**, *4*, 354–365. [CrossRef]
5. Davies, E.V.; Winstanley, C.; Fothergill, J.L.; James, C.E. The role of temperate bacteriophages in bacterial infection. *FEMS Microbiol. Lett.* **2016**, *363*, fnw015. [CrossRef]

6. Touchon, M.; Bernheim, A.; Rocha, E.P.C. Genetic and life-history traits associated with the distribution of prophages in bacteria. *ISME J.* **2016**, *10*, 2744–2754. [CrossRef]
7. Kaper, J.B.; O'Brien, A.D. Overview and Historical Perspectives. *Microbiol. Spectr.* **2014**, *2*. [CrossRef]
8. Brabban, A.D.; Hite, E.; Callaway, T.R. Evolution of foodborne pathogens via temperate bacteriophage-mediated gene transfer. *Foodborne Pathog. Dis.* **2005**, *2*, 287–303. [CrossRef]
9. Melton-Celsa, A.R. Shiga Toxin (Stx) Classification, Structure, and Function. *Microbiol. Spectr.* **2014**, *2*. [CrossRef]
10. Plunkett, G.; Rose, D.J.; Durfee, T.J.; Blattner, F.R. Sequence of Shiga Toxin 2 Phage 933W from *Escherichia coli* O157:H7: Shiga Toxin as a Phage Late-Gene Product. *J. Bacteriol.* **1999**, *181*, 1767–1778.
11. Perna, N.T.; Plunkett, G.; Burland, V.; Mau, B.; Glasner, J.D.; Rose, D.J.; Mayhew, G.F.; Evans, P.S.; Gregor, J.; Kirkpatrick, H.A.; et al. Genome sequence of enterohaemorrhagic *Escherichia coli* O157:H7. *Nature* **2001**, *409*, 529–533. [CrossRef]
12. Latif, H.; Li, H.J.; Charusanti, P.; Palsson, B.O.; Aziz, R.K. A gapless, unambiguous genome sequence of the enterohemorrhagic *Escherichia coli* O157:H7 strain EDL933. *Genome Announc.* **2014**, *2*. [CrossRef]
13. Colon, M.P.; Chakraborty, D.; Pevzner, Y.; Koudelka, G.B. Mechanisms that determine the differential stability of Stx(+) and Stx(−) lysogens. *Toxins (Basel)* **2016**, *8*, 96. [CrossRef]
14. Iversen, H.; L'Abee-Lund, T.M.; Aspholm, M.; Arnesen, L.P.S.; Lindback, T. Commensal *E. coli* Stx2 lysogens produce high levels of phages after spontaneous prophage induction. *Front. Cell. Infect. Microbiol.* **2015**, *5*, 5. [CrossRef]
15. Livny, J.; Friedman, D.I. Characterizing spontaneous induction of Stx encoding phages using a selectable reporter system. *Mol. Microbiol.* **2004**, *51*, 1691–1704. [CrossRef]
16. Herold, S.; Siebert, J.; Huber, A.; Schmidt, H. Global expression of prophage genes in *Escherichia coli* O157:H7 strain EDL933 in response to norfloxacin. *Antimicrob. Agents Chemother.* **2005**, *49*, 931–944. [CrossRef]
17. Asadulghani, M.; Ogura, Y.; Ooka, T.; Itoh, T.; Sawaguchi, A.; Iguchi, A.; Nakayama, K.; Hayashi, T. The defective prophage pool of *Escherichia coli* O157: Prophage–prophage interactions potentiate horizontal transfer of virulence determinants. *PLoS Pathog.* **2009**, *5*, e1000408. [CrossRef]
18. Herold, S.; Karch, H.; Schmidt, H. Shiga toxin-encoding bacteriophages–genomes in motion. *Int. J. Med. Microbiol.* **2004**, *294*, 115–121. [CrossRef]
19. Łoś, J.M.; Łoś, M.; Węgrzyn, G.; Węgrzyn, A. Differential efficiency of induction of various lambdoid prophages responsible for production of Shiga toxins in response to different induction agents. *Microb. Pathog.* **2009**, *47*, 289–298. [CrossRef]
20. Los, J.M.; Los, M.; Wegrzyn, G. Bacteriophages carrying Shiga toxin genes: Genomic variations, detection and potential treatment of pathogenic bacteria. *Future Microbiol.* **2011**, *6*, 909–924. [CrossRef]
21. Pacheco, A.R.; Sperandio, V. Shiga toxin in enterohemorrhagic *E. coli*: Regulation and novel anti-virulence strategies. *Front. Cell. Infect. Microbiol.* **2012**, *2*, 81. [CrossRef] [PubMed]
22. Obrig, T.G.; Karpman, D. Shiga toxin pathogenesis: Kidney complications and renal failure. *Curr. Top. Microbiol. Immunol.* **2012**, *357*, 105–136. [CrossRef] [PubMed]
23. Pruimboom-Brees, I.M.; Morgan, T.W.; Ackermann, M.R.; Nystrom, E.D.; Samuel, J.E.; Cornick, N.A.; Moon, H.W. Cattle lack vascular receptors for *Escherichia coli* O157:H7 Shiga toxins. *Proc. Natl. Acad. Sci. USA* **2000**, *97*, 10325–10329. [CrossRef] [PubMed]
24. Kruger, A.; Lucchesi, P.M.A. Shiga toxins and stx phages: Highly diverse entities. *Microbiology* **2015**, *161*, 451–462. [CrossRef] [PubMed]
25. Wagner, P.L.; Waldor, M.K. Bacteriophage control of bacterial virulence. *Infect. Immun.* **2002**, *70*, 3985–3993. [CrossRef] [PubMed]
26. Freedman, S.B.; Xie, J.; Neufeld, M.S.; Hamilton, W.L.; Hartling, L.; Tarr, P.I.; Nettel-Aguirre, A.; Chuck, A.; Lee, B.; Johnson, D.; et al. Shiga Toxin-Producing *Escherichia coli* Infection, Antibiotics, and Risk of Developing Hemolytic Uremic Syndrome: A Meta-analysis. *Clin. Infect. Dis.* **2016**, *62*, 1251–1258. [CrossRef] [PubMed]
27. Arndt, D.; Grant, J.R.; Marcu, A.; Sajed, T.; Pon, A.; Liang, Y.; Wishart, D.S. PHASTER: A better, faster version of the PHAST phage search tool. *Nucleic Acids Res.* **2016**, *44*, W16–W21. [CrossRef] [PubMed]
28. Hertel, R.; Rodríguez, D.P.; Hollensteiner, J.; Dietrich, S.; Leimbach, A.; Hoppert, M.; Liesegang, H.; Volland, S. Genome-based identification of active prophage regions by next generation sequencing in bacillus licheniformis DSM13. *PLoS ONE* **2015**, *10*, e0120759. [CrossRef] [PubMed]

29. Utter, B.; Deutsch, D.R.; Schuch, R.; Winer, B.Y.; Verratti, K.; Bishop-Lilly, K.; Sozhamannan, S.; Fischetti, V.A. Beyond the chromosome: The prevalence of unique extra-chromosomal bacteriophages with integrated virulence genes in pathogenic Staphylococcus aureus. *PLoS ONE* **2014**, *9*, e100502. [CrossRef] [PubMed]

30. Chen, F.; Wang, K.; Stewart, J.; Belas, R. Induction of multiple prophages from a marine bacterium: A genomic approach. *Appl. Environ. Microbiol.* **2006**, *72*, 4995–5001. [CrossRef] [PubMed]

31. Ogura, Y.; Mondal, S.I.; Islam, M.R.; Mako, T.; Arisawa, K.; Katsura, K.; Ooka, T.; Gotoh, Y.; Murase, K.; Ohnishi, M.; et al. The Shiga toxin 2 production level in enterohemorrhagic *Escherichia coli* O157:H7 is correlated with the subtypes of toxin-encoding phage. *Sci. Rep.* **2015**, *5*, 16663. [CrossRef] [PubMed]

32. Howard-Varona, C.; Vik, D.R.; Solonenko, N.E.; Gazitua, M.C.; Hobbs, Z.; Honaker, R.W.; Kinkhabwala, A.A.; Sullivan, M.B. Whole-genome sequence of phages p000v and p000y infecting the bacterial pathogen Shigatoxigenic *Escherichia coli*. *Press. Genome Announc.* **2018.**

33. Zhang, X.; McDaniel, A.D.; Wolf, L.E.; Keusch, G.T.; Waldor, M.K.; Acheson, D.W. Quinolone antibiotics induce Shiga toxin-encoding bacteriophages, toxin production, and death in mice. *J. Infect. Dis.* **2000**, *181*, 664–670. [CrossRef] [PubMed]

34. Los, J.M.; Los, M.; Wegrzyn, A.; Wegrzyn, G. Altruism of Shiga toxin-producing *Escherichia coli*: Recent hypothesis versus experimental results. *Front. Cell. Infect. Microbiol.* **2012**, *2*, 166. [CrossRef] [PubMed]

35. Tyler, J.S.; Beeri, K.; Reynolds, J.L.; Alteri, C.J.; Skinner, K.G.; Friedman, J.H.; Eaton, K.A.; Friedman, D.I. Prophage induction is enhanced and required for renal disease and lethality in an EHEC mouse model. *PLoS Pathog.* **2013**, *9*, e1003236. [CrossRef] [PubMed]

36. Tarr, P.I. *Escherichia coli* O157:H7: Clinical, diagnostic, and epidemiological aspects of human infection. *Clin. Infect. Dis.* **1995**, *20*, 1–10. [CrossRef] [PubMed]

37. Thorpe, C.M. Shiga toxin-producing *Escherichia coli* infection. *Clin. Infect. Dis.* **2004**, *38*, 1298–1303. [CrossRef] [PubMed]

38. Wagner, P.L.; Neely, M.N.; Zhang, X.; Acheson, D.W.; Waldor, M.K.; Friedman, D.I. Role for a phage promoter in Shiga toxin 2 expression from a pathogenic *Escherichia coli* strain. *J. Bacteriol.* **2001**, *183*, 2081–2085. [CrossRef] [PubMed]

39. Krysiak-Baltyn, K.; Martin, G.J.O.; Stickland, A.D.; Scales, P.J.; Gras, S.L. Computational models of populations of bacteria and lytic phage. *Crit. Rev. Microbiol.* **2016**, *42*, 942–968. [CrossRef] [PubMed]

40. Gamage, S.D.; Patton, A.K.; Strasser, J.E.; Chalk, C.L.; Weiss, A.A. Commensal bacteria influence *Escherichia coli* O157:H7 persistence and Shiga toxin production in the mouse intestine. *Infect. Immun.* **2006**, *74*, 1977–1983. [CrossRef] [PubMed]

41. Acheson, D.W.; Reidl, J.; Zhang, X.; Keusch, G.T.; Mekalanos, J.J.; Waldor, M.K. In vivo transduction with shiga toxin 1-encoding phage. *Infect. Immun.* **1998**, *66*, 4496–4498. [PubMed]

42. Schmidt, H.; Bielaszewska, M.; Karch, H. Transduction of enteric *Escherichia coli* isolates with a derivative of Shiga toxin 2-encoding bacteriophage phi3538 isolated from *Escherichia coli* O157:H7. *Appl. Environ. Microbiol.* **1999**, *65*, 3855–3861. [PubMed]

43. Doron, S.; Fedida, A.; Hernandez-Prieto, M.A.; Sabehi, G.; Karunker, I.; Stazic, D.; Feingersch, R.; Steglich, C.; Futschik, M.; Lindell, D.; et al. Transcriptome dynamics of a broad host-range cyanophage and its hosts. *ISME J.* **2016**, *10*, 1437–1455. [CrossRef] [PubMed]

44. Howard-Varona, C.; Roux, S.; Dore, H.; Solonenko, N.E.; Holmfeldt, K.; Markillie, L.M.; Orr, G.; Sullivan, M.B. Regulation of infection efficiency in a globally abundant marine Bacteriodetes virus. *ISME J.* **2017**, *11*, 284–295. [CrossRef] [PubMed]

45. Howard-Varona, C.; Hargreaves, K.R.; Solonenko, N.E.; Markillie, L.M.; White, R.A.; Brewer, H.M.; Ansong, C.; Orr, G.; Adkins, J.N.; Sullivan, M.B. Multiple mechanisms drive phage infection efficiency in nearly identical hosts. *ISME J.* **2018**, *12*, 1605–1618. [CrossRef] [PubMed]

46. Abedon, S.T. Phage therapy: Eco-physiological pharmacology. *Scientifica (Cairo)* **2014**, *2014*, 581639. [CrossRef] [PubMed]

47. Sarker, S.A.; Berger, B.; Deng, Y.; Kieser, S.; Foata, F.; Moine, D.; Descombes, P.; Sultana, S.; Huq, S.; Bardhan, P.K.; et al. Oral application of *Escherichia coli* bacteriophage: Safety tests in healthy and diarrheal children from Bangladesh. *Environ. Microbiol.* **2017**, *19*, 237–250. [CrossRef] [PubMed]

48. Merchant, N.; Lyons, E.; Goff, S.; Vaughn, M.; Ware, D.; Micklos, D.; Antin, P. The iPlant collaborative: Cyberinfrastructure for enabling data to discovery for the life sciences. *PLoS Biol.* **2016**, *14*, e1002342. [CrossRef] [PubMed]
49. Li, H.; Durbin, R. Fast and accurate short read alignment with Burrows-Wheeler transform. *Bioinformatics* **2009**, *25*, 1754–1760. [CrossRef] [PubMed]
50. Li, H.; Handsaker, B.; Wysoker, A.; Fennell, T.; Ruan, J.; Homer, N. The sequence alignment/map format and SAMtools. *Bioinformatics* **2009**, *25*, 2078–2079. [CrossRef] [PubMed]
51. Rabosky, D.L.; Grundler, M.; Anderson, C.; Title, P.; Shi, J.J.; Brown, J.W.; Huang, H.; Larson, J.G. BAMMtools: An R package for the analysis of evolutionary dynamics on phylogenetic trees. *Methods Ecol. Evol.* **2014**, *5*, 701–707. [CrossRef]
52. Quinlan, A.R.; Hall, I.M. BEDTools: A flexible suite of utilities for comparing genomic features. *Bioinformatics* **2010**, *26*, 841–842. [CrossRef] [PubMed]
53. Thorvaldsdottir, H.; Robinson, J.T.; Mesirov, J.P. Integrative genomics viewer (IGV): High-performance genomics data visualization and exploration. *Brief. Bioinform.* **2013**, *14*, 178–192. [CrossRef] [PubMed]
54. Krzywinski, M.I.; Schein, J.E.; Birol, I.; Connors, J.; Gascoyne, R.; Horsman, D.; Jones, S.J.; Marra, M.A. Circos: An information aesthetic for comparative genomics. *Genome Res.* **2009**. [CrossRef] [PubMed]
55. Erez, Z.; Steinberger-Levy, I.; Shamir, M.; Doron, S.; Stokar-Avihail, A.; Peleg, Y.; Melamed, S.; Leavitt, A.; Savidor, A.; Albeck, S.; et al. Communication between viruses guides lysis–lysogeny decisions. *Nature* **2017**, *541*, 488–493. [CrossRef] [PubMed]
56. Yoichi, M.; Abe, M.; Miyanaga, K.; Unno, H.; Tanji, Y. Alteration of tail fiber protein gp38 enables T2 phage to infect *Escherichia coli* O157:H7. *J. Biotechnol.* **2005**, *115*, 101–107. [CrossRef] [PubMed]
57. Yosef, I.; Goren, M.G.; Globus, R.; Molshanski-Mor, S.; Qimron, U. Extending the host range of bacteriophage particles for DNA transduction. *Mol. Cell* **2017**, *66*, 721.e3–728.e3. [CrossRef] [PubMed]
58. Roach, D.R.; Debarbieux, L. Phage therapy: Awakening a sleeping giant. *Emerg. Top. Life Sci.* **2017**, *1*, 93–103. [CrossRef]

9

Use of a Regression Model to Study Host-Genomic Determinants of Phage Susceptibility in MRSA

Henrike Zschach [1,*], Mette V. Larsen [2], Henrik Hasman [3], Henrik Westh [4,5], Morten Nielsen [1,6,*], Ryszard Międzybrodzki [7,8], Ewa Jończyk-Matysiak [7], Beata Weber-Dąbrowska [7] and Andrzej Górski [7,8]

1 Department of Bio and Health Informatics, Technical University of Denmark, 2800 Kgs. Lyngby, Denmark
2 GoSeqIt ApS, Ved Klaedebo 9, 2970 Hoersholm, Denmark; MVL@goseqit.com
3 Department of Bacteria, Fungi and Parasites, Statens Serum Institut, 2300 Copenhagen S, Denmark, henh@ssi.dk
4 Department of Clinical Microbiology, MRSA Knowledge Center, Hvidovre Hospital, 2650 Hvidovre, Denmark; Henrik.torkil.westh@regionh.dk
5 Faculty of Health and Medical Sciences, Institute of Clinical Medicine, University of Copenhagen, 2200 Copenhagen, Denmark
6 Instituto de Investigaciones Biotecnológicas, Universidad Nacional de San Martín, San Martín, B 1650 HMP, Buenos Aires, Argentina
7 Bacteriophage Laboratory, Hirszfeld Institute of Immunology and Experimental Therapy, Polish Academy of Sciences, 53-114 Wroclaw, Poland; mbrodzki@iitd.pan.wroc.pl (R.M.); ewa.jonczyk@iitd.pan.wroc.pl (E.J.-M.); weber@iitd.pan.wroc.pl (B.W.-D.); agorski@ikp.pl (A.G.)
8 Department of Clinical Immunology, Transplantation Institute, Medical University of Warsaw, 02-006 Warsaw, Poland
* Correspondence: henrike@bioinformatics.dtu.dk (H.Z.); mniel@bioinformatics.dtu.dk (M.N.)

Abstract: *Staphylococcus aureus* is a major agent of nosocomial infections. Especially in methicillin-resistant strains, conventional treatment options are limited and expensive, which has fueled a growing interest in phage therapy approaches. We have tested the susceptibility of 207 clinical *S. aureus* strains to 12 (nine monovalent) different therapeutic phage preparations and subsequently employed linear regression models to estimate the influence of individual host gene families on resistance to phages. Specifically, we used a two-step regression model setup with a preselection step based on gene family enrichment. We show that our models are robust and capture the data's underlying signal by comparing their performance to that of models build on randomized data. In doing so, we have identified 167 gene families that govern phage resistance in our strain set and performed functional analysis on them. This revealed genes of possible prophage or mobile genetic element origin, along with genes involved in restriction-modification and transcription regulators, though the majority were genes of unknown function. This study is a step in the direction of understanding the intricate host-phage relationship in this important pathogen with the outlook to targeted phage therapy applications.

Keywords: phage therapy; bacterial phage resistance; regression modeling; MRSA

---

1. Introduction

Methicillin-resistant *Staphylococcus aureus* (MRSA) is a growing health concern. It is the agent of many chronic bacterial infections in hospitals as well as in the community. Its resistance to beta-lactamases severely limits treatment options, drives up the price for therapy, increases unwanted side effects, and leads in many cases to worse clinical outcomes [1]. MRSA has been classified as a high-priority pathogen on the 2017 list of antibiotic-resistant priority pathogens published by the World Health Organization [2]. Pathogens on this list are considered to pose the greatest threat to human health and to require urgently discovery and development of new antibiotics.

Phage therapy has been proposed as a promising substitute for conventional antibiotics or a co-treatment in the treatment of multi-resistant bacterial pathogens [3–7]. Of the *S. aureus* phage known to date, most are temperate phages and belong to the Siphoviridae family [8]. Strictly lytic staphylococcal phages, as are typically required for therapy, are almost exclusively found in the Podoviridae and Myoviridae families [8].

The Hirszfeld Institute of Immunology and Experimental Therapy of the Polish Academy of Science in Wroclaw (HI) has been producing staphylococcal phages for therapeutic purposes since the 1970s [9]. At present, its collection consists of nine monovalent staphylococcal phages (see Materials and Methods) [10]. Those phages are used at the Phage Therapy Unit in Wrocław under the rules of a therapeutic experiment to conduct treatment of patients with chronic bacterial infections resistant to antibiotic therapy. The result have been encouraging, as a good response has been observed in one third of patients [6].

However, in order for phage therapy to be efficient, it is necessary to have a good understanding of the specific interaction between phage and host. There are many strategies by which bacteria aim to evade predation by phages, which is a significant fitness factor and therefore under high evolutionary pressure. *S. aureus* is known to be deficient in CRISPR, one of the major phage defense mechanisms [11]. Instead, its principle defense against invading DNAs are extensive restriction-modification (RM) systems [12]. RM systems are two-part system composed of a methylase and a nuclease. The methylase introduces specific modifications on the organism's DNA, thereby marking it is as self. DNA lacking those modifications, i.e., DNA of foreign origin, will be cleaved by the nuclease. All four types of RM systems known to date are present in *S. aureus* [12]. Another, highly specialized phage defense mechanism is present in the form of staphylococcal pathogenicity islands (SaPIs) [13]. These mobile genetic elements interfere with the packaging of phage DNA in the late phase of infection, instead packaging and thereby disseminating copies of themselves. However, a small percentage of phage particles are still produced normally, leading to a reduced load of phage progeny instead of a total block. It has been implied that this may be an advantage to *S. aureus* as a species as it facilitates gene transfer [14]. Akin to abortive infection mechanisms, phage resistance by SaPI includes the lysis of the infected cell [13].

S. aureus is known to have a rather large accessory genome that can make up as much as 25% of total genome size [8]. We therefore hypothesize in this study that *S. aureus* may be carrying accessory genes that encode various mechanisms that are geared toward phage resistance. The presence of such mechanisms may hamper the efficacy of phage therapy, and it is therefore important to study these in order to perform optimization of phages used for treatment. With the advent of affordable high-throughput sequencing methods, it is now becoming possible to determine the whole genome sequences of the infecting strain in a clinical setting, making them accessible to this kind of investigation.

The relationship between *S. aureus* and its phages is intricate. A large proportion of *S. aureus* virulence factors are phage-encoded [8], and phages are the major agents of horizontal gene transfer in this species [11]. Furthermore, *S. aureus* is known to harbor prophages with a very high frequency, as detailed in a review by Lindsay in 2010 that states that all *S. aureus* sequenced up to that point contained at least one prophage [15]. In accordance with that, there is a sizeable body of research into staphylococcal phages, their genomes, their influence on their host's evolution, and their contribution to *S. aureus*' virulence (see for example [8,14,16]). Furthermore, phage susceptibility patterns have been used to classify *S. aureus* before the advent of molecular typing methods [17]. Despite that, there is a distinct lack of studies investigating the genetic basis for phage susceptibility and resistance in *S. aureus* from the host perspective, in particular with regard to whole genome approaches as opposed to studies focusing on single loci.

In this study, we seek to elucidate the interplay between *S. aureus* and therapeutic phage preparations. To do so, we have tested the susceptibility of a collection of clinical MRSA isolates towards a collection of staphylococcal phage preparations from HI. Both the bacterial and phage collections we used are of great relevance to the phage therapy efforts, since the phages are either already in use or under consideration for experimental therapy in accordance with European Union (EU) rules concerning compassionate use. Furthermore, the bacterial isolates were provided by Hvidovre Hospital in Hvidovre, Denmark and were obtained from patients showing complicated nosocomial MRSA infections. This strain set represents the most prevalent clonal complexes observed in Denmark. MRSA is predominantly imported, making the collection very diverse [18]. However, it is not representative of MRSA in all localities. The genomes of the bacterial strains were determined by whole genome sequencing and through employing a number of bioinformatics tools and machine-learning methods. We attempted to shed light on the genes of MRSA that play a role in determining the susceptibility or resistance towards phages. A similar approach but with different methodology was proposed by Allen et al., who tested for associations between phage and antibiotic resistance profiles with phylogenetic similarity in *E. coli* [19].

In this way, we aim to contribute to the development of predictive tools of phage susceptibility in the phage therapy–targeted bacteria and ultimately to devising strategies for the prevention, delay, or circumvention of phage resistance in a phage therapy setting.

2. Results

2.1. General Results of the Susceptibility Testing

A total of 207 MRSA strains were successfully tested for susceptibility to 12 phage preparations. The ratio of susceptible to resistant strains differed between the preparations. Note that phage preparations were standardized to routine test dilution (RTD). The percentage of susceptible strains ranged from 19% to 68%, as can be seen in Table 1. We have chosen to regard both weakly susceptible and resistant reactions as negatives for the modelling. We did not observe a large difference in efficacy between single phage preparations and mixtures.

Table 1. Wet lab results of susceptibility testing. All phage preparations were tested at RTD, see Methods. MS-1, OP_MS-1 and OP_MS-1_TOP are mixtures of P4/6409, A5/80 and 676/Z.

Phage Preparation	Percent Sensitive	Percent Resistant
1N/80	31.9%	68.1%
676/F	50.7%	49.3%
676/T	68.1%	31.9%
676/Z	40.6%	59.4%
A3/R	18.8%	81.2%
A5/L	47.3%	52.7%
A5/80	55.1%	44.9%
P4/6409	37.7%	62.3%
phi200/6409	44.0%	56.0%
MS-1	33.8%	66.2%
OP_MS-1	38.6%	61.4%
OP_MS-1 TOP	39.6%	60.4%

2.2. Genetic Diversity of the Strain Collection

Genetic distance between the MRSA strains was measured as 1-orthoANI (see Methods), and the result is depicted in form of a heatmap in Figure 1. This figure reveals a clear clustering of strains into groups with high identity, which follows the established clonal complexes and sequence types of *S. aureus* [20]. Based on this clustering, the strains were split into five partitions by visual inspection.

Partition 1 is substantially larger than the other four. This is due to the fact that the strains belonging to clonal complexes CC1, CC5, CC8, and CC80 have a high degree of identity to each other, compare large blue area in the upper left corner. Partitions 2 and 3 are well defined, encompassing CC22 and CC30, respectively. Partition 4 is made up of CC45 and CC398. CC398 is known for its prevalence in swine and cattle. Those strains are genetically distant from the rest of the strains, though there is some degree of similarity to CC30. Partition 5 is composed of two clusters of related strains, as indicated in Figure 1. It contains a number of rarer CCs that also show a comparatively high distance in terms of orthoANI to the rest of the data set.

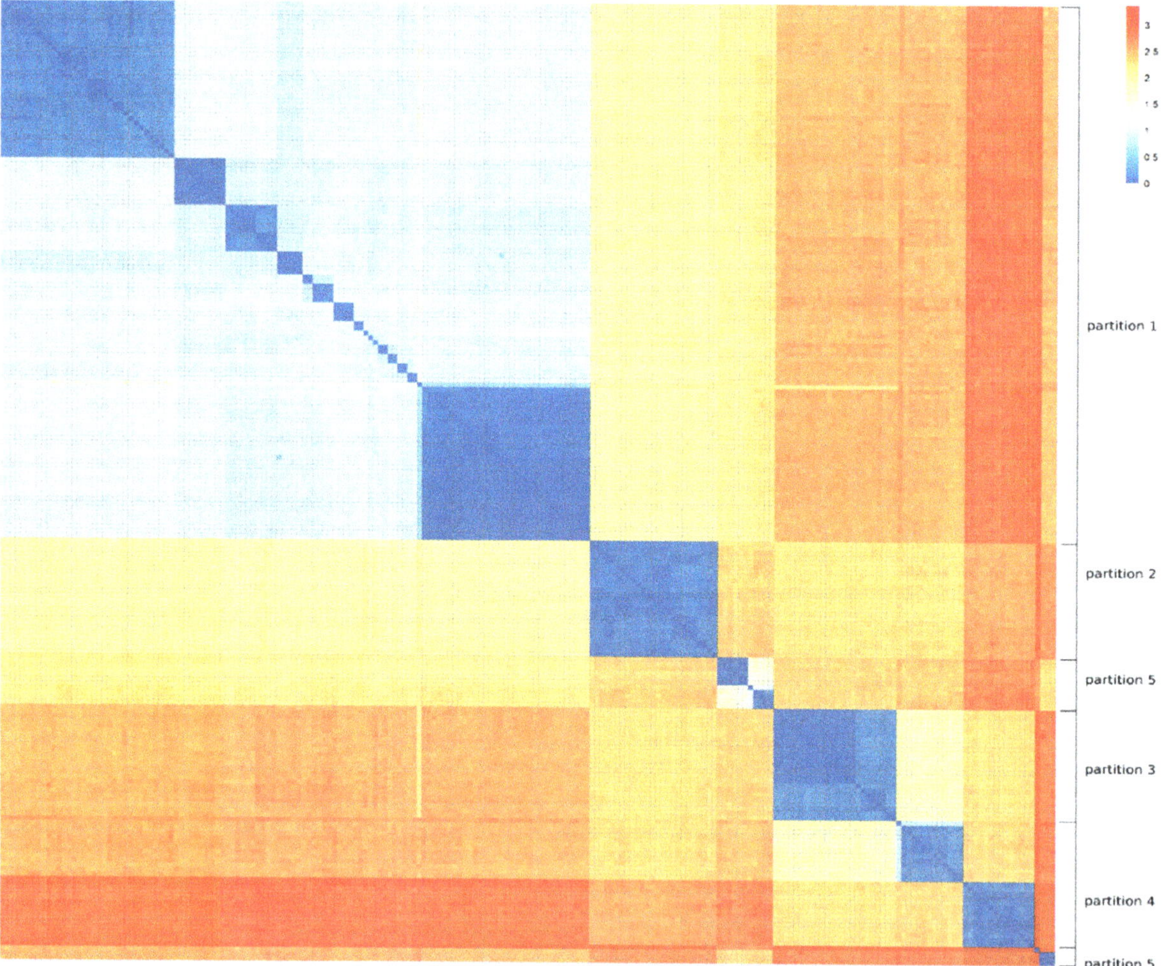

Figure 1. All-against-all matrix of the genetic distance between the 207 methicillin-resistant *Staphylococcus aureus* (MRSA) strains used for this study. Distance is calculated as 1-orthoANI and represented as color, where blue corresponds to lower and red corresponds to greater distance. The assignment of strains to partitions is marked on the right margin.

2.3. *Identification of Gene Families*

When predicting and clustering genes, we identified a total of 6419 gene families in the MRSA strain dataset. The distribution of these gene families across the 207 MRSA strains can be seen in Figure 2, which shows a histogram of abundances of the gene families. Here, 1777 gene families were identified in all 207 strains. These are the housekeeping genes. Furthermore, there is a heavy tail of gene families that were only observed in few strains (left side of the histogram).

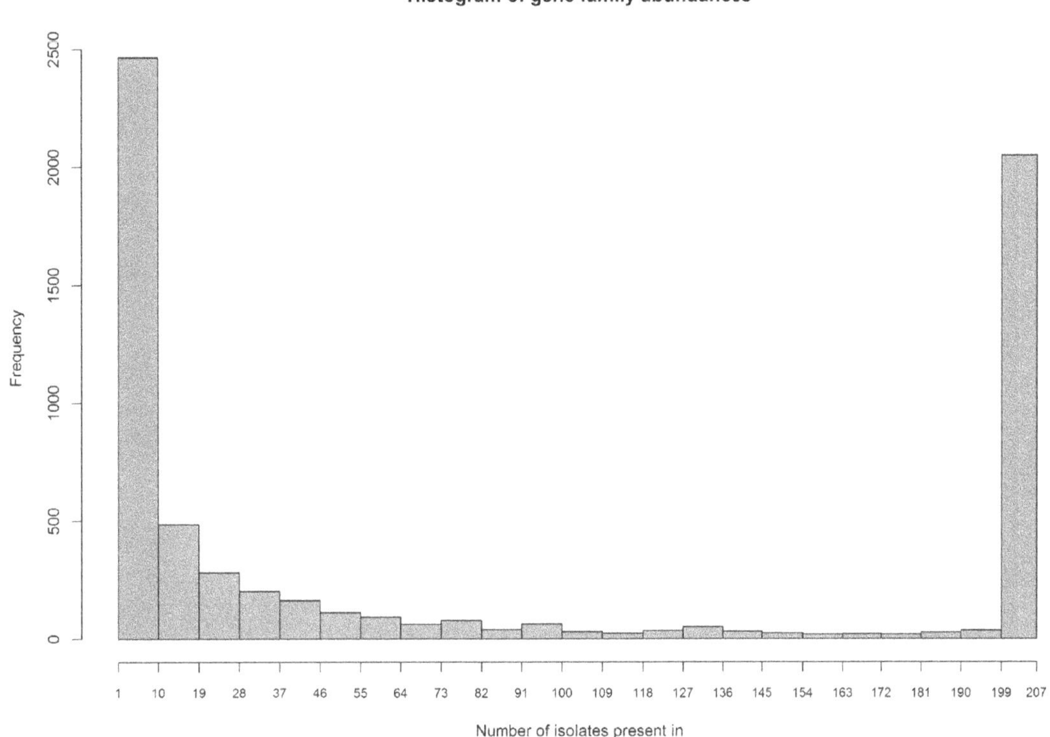

Figure 2. Abundance of gene families in the 207 strains. The peak depicted in the histogram is slightly higher than the number of housekeeping genes, 1.777, since the bin is wider than 1.

2.3.1. p-Value Distribution from Association Tests

Models are set up in five-fold cross validation frameworks (see Methods Section 4.5). For each cross validation fold, each gene family was assigned a p-value calculated from its corresponding contingency table estimated once from the original data and once from permuted data. We chose here to illustrate results for phage P4/6409 as it was representative of the other phage preparations.

When plotting the distributions of these p-values, see Figure 3, we can make several observations.

(a) In most phage interactions, there is a small tail of gene families with very low p-values, while the majority of gene families have non-significant p-values.

(b) In the permuted data, this tail vanishes, as was to be expected. We also observed that the p-value distributions of phages 1N/80, A3/R and cocktail MS-1 resemble those of the permuted data much more than those of the real data (see Supplementary Figure S1). This indicates there were not enough positive examples of lysed strains to produce a signal that is distinguishable from random.

Based on these observations, a p-value threshold of 0.01 or lower was implemented to admit gene families to the first step model. As seen in Table 2, the number of gene families picked by enrichment varied both by fold as well as by phage. In preparations 1N/80, A3/R, and mix MS-1, the number of gene families picked was very low. Further, as expected, we find that no or only very few gene families are selected when analyzing the permuted data.

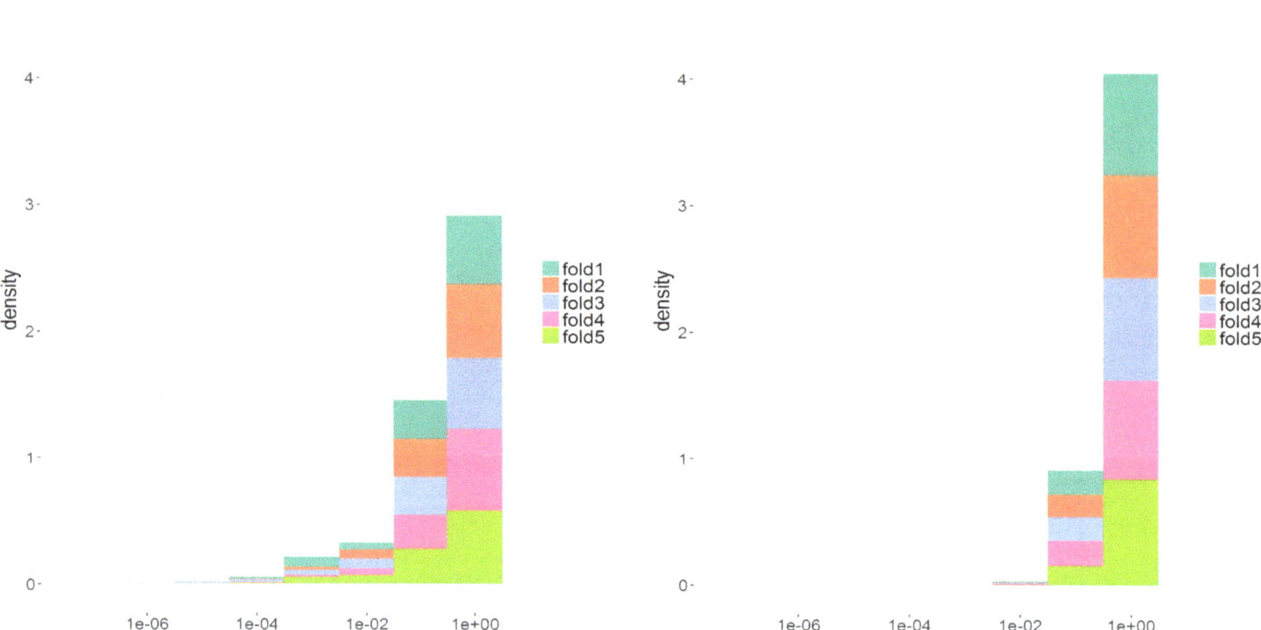

Figure 3. Stacked histogram of *p*-value distributions across the five folds for the interaction with phage P4/6409. The density is shown instead of counts to account for fold 1 having a 100 times less *p*-values compared to the other folds, since it does not include partition 1 and therefore did not need to be subsampled. **Left**: Real data. **Right**: Permuted data.

2.3.2. Refinement Based on Regression Models

In the second step of feature selection, we employed linear regression models fitted using Ridge regression. An internal cross validation was used to identify the optimal parameter for the Ridge penalty lambda. The optimal lambda penalty value across the different folds in the cross validation were comparable, indicating that the models are robust, though the size of the feature space varies (see Supplementary Figure S2).

We next required that a gene family should have absolute regression weights greater than 0.01 in at least three of the five partitions to have passed a second selection step. The number of gene families selected in this manner is listed per phage on the right side of Table 2. We term this the set of significant gene families for a certain phage. The number of significant gene families in interaction with phages 1N/80, A3/R, and mix MS-1 was too small to train a final model. For the remaining phages, the amount of significant gene families varied between the different phages, though the sets were comparable in size, with the smallest comprising 13 and the largest 80 gene families (see Table 2). In total, there were 167 significant gene families. When performing the same procedure on permuted data, significant gene families could only be identified in four phages, and a final model could only be trained for two.

Table 2. Summary of the modelling results for real and permuted data. The "First Model" section reports the results of the first filtering procedure based of association analyses. The "Final Model" section gives the result of the second filtering procedure based on regression model fitting combined with consistency constraints. The area under the curve (AUC) is used as performance measure of the final model. The number of gene families selected given in the left part of the table is calculated as the average ± standard deviation across the five folds. If less than two gene families were selected based on regression weights, a final model could not be trained and the associated AUC is reported as NA (not applicable).

	First Model		Final Model			
	Real Data	Permuted Data	Real Data		Permuted Data	
Phage Preparation	No. of Gene Families Selected by Enrichment	No. of Gene Families Selected by Enrichment	No. of Gene Families Selected on Regression Weights	AUC	No. of Gene Families Selected on Regression Weights	AUC
1N/80	10 ± 16	0	2	NA	0	NA
676/F	222 ± 144	0	45	0.78	0	NA
676/T	361 ± 243	12 ± 11	79	0.87	3	0.63
676/Z	112 ± 87	11 ± 14	31	0.72	4	0.61
A3/R	13 ± 26	0	1	NA	0	NA
A5/L	184 ± 124	0	37	0.8	0	NA
A5/80	265 ± 148	0	80	0.78	0	NA
P4/6409	200 ± 137	2 ± 4	61	0.79	0	NA
phi200/6409	160 ± 138	0	56	0.79	0	NA
MS-1	6 ± 10	0	0	NA	0	NA
OP_MS-1	86 ± 78	0	29	0.65	0	NA
OP_MS-1_TOP	54 ± 52	1 ± 1	13	0.67	0	NA

2.3.3. Final Model

Final models were next retrained including only the significant gene families passing both steps of feature selection (low association p-values and high regression weights) as input features. Plots of the regression weights assigned by those final models showed the direction of weights to be consistent across folds, i.e., gene families are consistently found to have either positive or negative weights across all of the five partitions. This is depicted for the example of phage P4/6409 in Figure 4. Results for other phage preparations were comparable.

Out of all the 167 gene families, a total of 97 increased phage resistance, 62 increased phage susceptibility, and eight were ambiguous, meaning that they increased resistance to some phages but susceptibility to others. This further shows that the vast majority of significant gene families identified were consistent in their direction of influence across all 12 tested phage preparations.

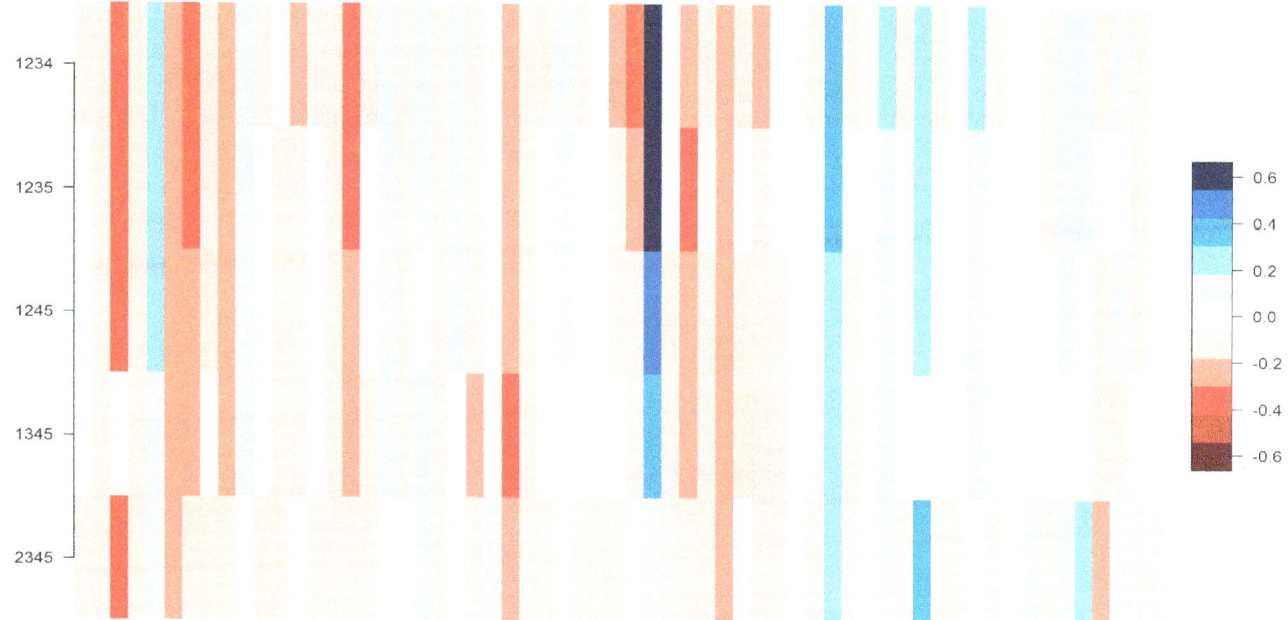

Figure 4. Heat map of the regression weights for the final model of phage P4/6409. Columns are gene families, rows are cross validation folds. The color indicates the value and direction of each weight, with blue being strongly positive and red being strongly negative. Weights with low values are white. Results were comparable for other phages with the exception of 1N/80, A3/R, and mix MS-1 (see Table 2).

2.4. Functional Annotation of the Significant Genes

We further sought to characterize the function of the identified significant gene families by comparing them to the eggNOG database. The distribution of functional annotation terms identified for the full set of significant genes is shown in Figure 5 and shows that it was possible to identify a match in eggNOG for only 60% of gene families. Most genes had either no hit in the eggNOG database or a hit to a NOG of unknown function.

Case-by-case inspection of the functional annotation terms retrieved from both RAST and eggNOG for the 167 significant gene families identified 13 gene families that have terms directly related to phages, while another 18 were related either to other mobile genetic elements such as genomic islands and transposons or to processes associated to them such as transposase activity. Of these, three gene families have homologs found in SaPIs, which are a phage defense system of *S. aureus* [13]. Four additional gene families appeared to be part of restriction-modification systems and six had hits to transcriptional regulators.

Out of these groups, the gene families related to restriction-modification systems and SaPIs were found to consistently be associated with resistance to phage infection (as measured by the sign of the weights in the final model described earlier), as can be seen in Supplementary Table S1. Of the gene families associated with transcriptional regulators, five were found to increase phage resistance, while one was found to increase susceptibility. The gene families related to phages and mobile elements encompass both gene families promoting resistance and families promoting susceptibility, further pointing to the complexity of the host–phage interaction. The full list of annotation terms for all significant gene families can be found in the Supplementary Table S1, together with the gene family's average regression weight across the five cross validation folds per phage.

We have estimated cumulative density functions (CDF) for each eggNOG category from the full gene set and next evaluated which functional categories in the significant gene set were enriched or depleted. With a threshold of $p = 0.05$, we found that categories "No hit" and "Replication, recombination, and repair" were enriched, while "Post-translational modification, protein turnover, and chaperones" and "Inorganic ion transport and metabolism" were depleted (see Supplementary Table S2).

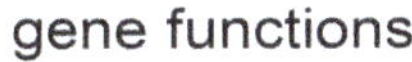

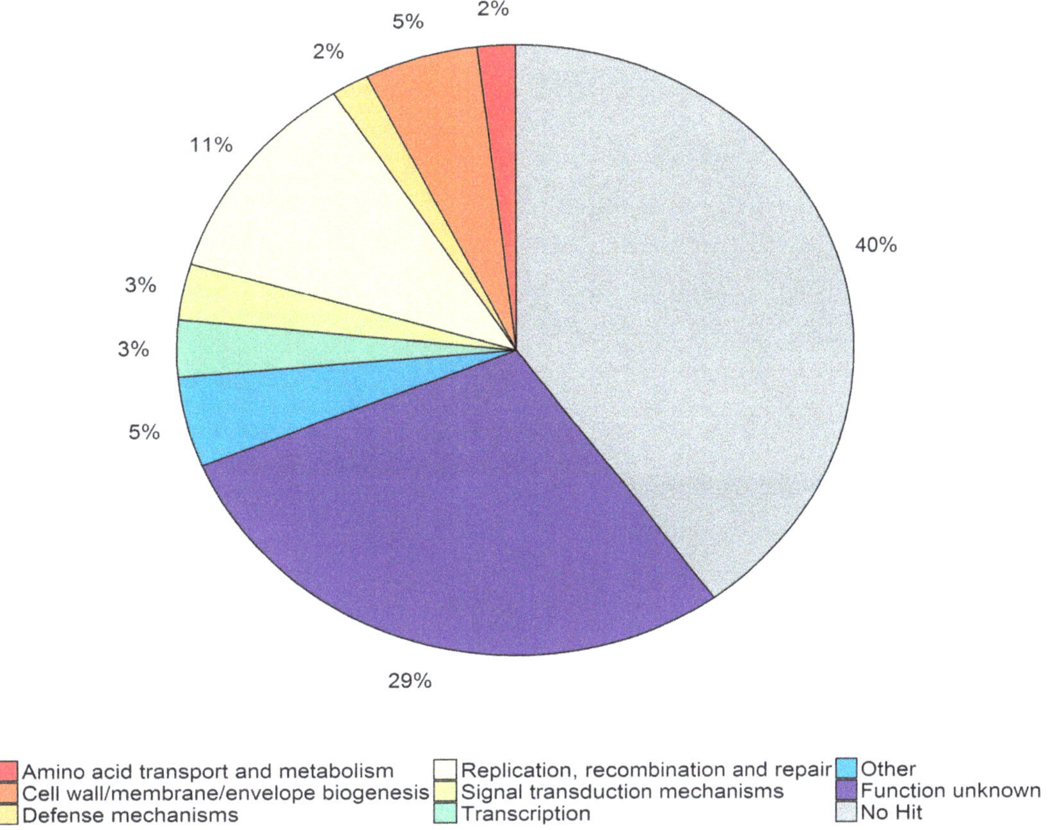

Figure 5. Functional annotation categories of the eggNOGs matching to the set of significant genes across all nine phages.

2.5. Overlap of Significant Gene Family Sets

We further analyzed the overlap between the significant gene family sets found for each phage model. Figure 6 shows a histogram of the number of phage models where a given gene family was identified as significant. It clearly presents that very few significant gene families are shared by many phage models, and only one is shared by all nine. The majority of significant gene families have been observed in interaction with only one or two different phages. This in turn means that each of the phages we tested has a distinct and specific interaction with our bacterial strain set, since different genes in the bacterial host dictate whether infection will be successful.

Further, the significant gene families of the three cocktails are not a linear combination of the sets identified for their component phages, though there is a sizeable overlap (data not shown).

There were four gene families found significant in at least eight phage models. They are listed in Table 3, along with their direction of influence and the annotation and category of their matching eggNOG, if any. Out of the four, three increase resistance to phage, while one was ambiguous in its direction of influence. Two gene families had no hit in the eggNOG database and one was categorized as being of "unknown function". We were therefore unable to deduce a possible function for them though they appear to be of great importance for phage susceptibility. One, cluster 3112, appears to be involved in regulation of transcription and signal transduction that may play a role in host takeover. There were no direct indications for how exactly those gene families effect their influence biologically, but it is evident from the models that they do.

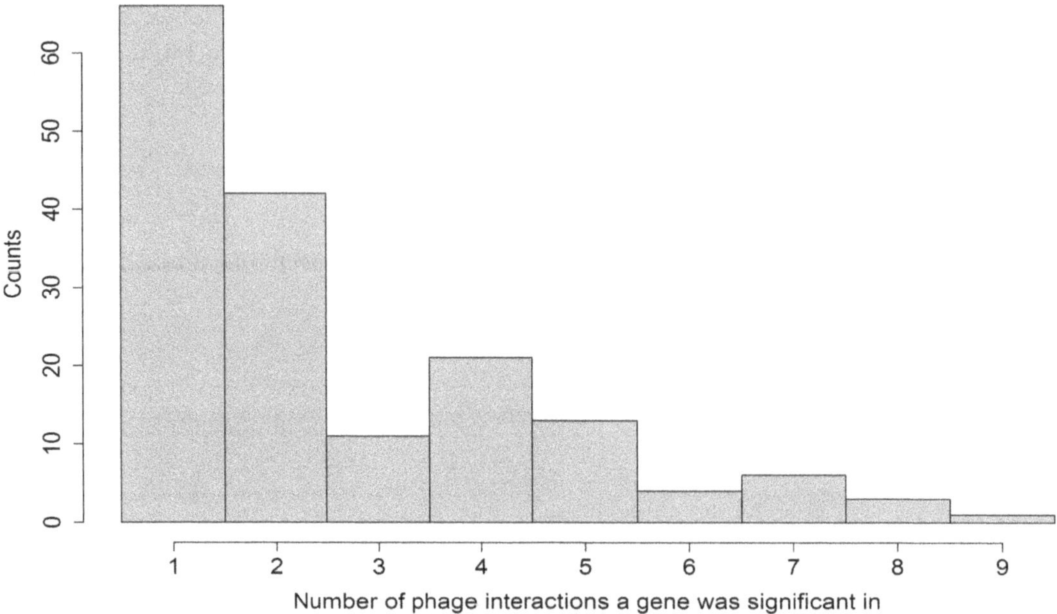

Figure 6. Histogram depicting the number of phage models where a given gene family was identified significant.

Table 3. Predicted functions of the gene families found significant in interaction with eight or more phages.

Gene Family ID	Times Observed	Increases	eggNOG Annotation	eggNOG Category
cluster_1791	9	Resistance	-	No Hit
cluster_389	8	Resistance	-	Function unknown
cluster_3112	8	Resistance	Transcriptional regulator	Transcription
cluster_3992	8	Ambiguous *	-	No Hit

* This gene family always confers phage resistance except in one interaction in which it confers susceptibility.

3. Discussion

In this study, we sought to model the host-genetic determinants of MRSA phage susceptibility with a two-step logistic regression model fitted via ridge regression. We succeeded in building models of acceptable performance for nine of the 12 tested phage preparations with AUCs ranging from 0.65 to 0.87. By doing so, we identified 167 host gene families that influence *S. aureus*' interaction with those nine phages.

Our dataset is, with 207 observations, rather small for this type of analysis, since there are many more covariates—i.e., gene families—than observations. We have addressed this by building a two-step model and including a filtering step based on *p*-values, thereby greatly reducing the number of covariates going into the analysis. As biological entities are shaped by evolution, the strains share some degree of relatedness, and the testing results are not completely independent observations. We have partitioned the data according to phylogeny in a way that ensures highly similar strains are located to the same partition. Doing that ensures that the observations we are aiming to predict are more independent from the ones we feed into the model during training. The partitioning was maintained at all steps, ensuring that data from highly similar strains was never used to predict the outcome. Furthermore, there was an uneven partitioning of the data due to a high percentage of strains from two very related sequence types, which may lead to bias. The challenge of uneven partitions was addressed by subsampling the oversized partition 1 so we could obtain a realistic distribution of *p*-values for the association of all genes to the observed phenotype. Finally, our set of strains with its composition of clonal complexes is specific to Denmark [18]. It is not necessarily representative of *S. aureus* populations observed in different settings.

It should further be noted that our approach can only identify gene families that are part of the accessory genome, since the first selection step is based on differential abundance of those gene families in susceptible vs. resistant strains. Furthermore, this analysis does not consider point mutations as far wild type and mutant version of a gene are more than 90% identical, since we have clustered genes into families with that threshold.

Regarding the electronic gene family annotation, we were able to identify four gene families related to restriction-modification systems and three related the genes found in SaPIs, all of which increased the resistance to phage as expected. Further, six of the significant gene families were related to transcriptional regulation, which fits well with the fact that phages try to shut down host transcription during takeover.

A multitude of gene families found appear to be mobile elements of some kind. Interestingly, Ram et al. have stated that "Most genes involved in phage resistance are carried by plasmids and other mobile genetic elements, including bacteriophages and their relatives" [14], though this statement is quite possibly related to SaPIs and phage-inducible chromosomal islands (PICIs) in general. Those mobile element related gene families had varying direction of influence. They may be related to the interplay of integrated prophages and external phages, which can either complement each other or oppose each other. An integrated prophage may for example protect from further infection via a principle known as superinfection-exclusion [21]. For a large proportion of the significant gene families, however, no hit could be found in the eggNOG database, and of those that had a hit, the most common category was "Function unknown". This may be due to the fact *S. aureus* has a large accessory genome that is made up mostly of different types of mobile genetic elements, among them prophages, that are highly diverse and not well characterized [8]. We have not determined whether either the gene families with hits to phage related proteins or those without hits or with hits to proteins of unknown functions are parts of integrated prophages. Identification of the prophages present in our strain set could add to the interpretation of the analysis; however, it is out of the scope of this study.

We also found that there is only a minor overlap between the sets of significant gene families identified for different phages. This means that each phage had a different and specific interaction with the set of bacterial strains.

Further, we found that generally more gene families promoted resistance than susceptibility. Among the four gene families that were found significant in interaction with at least eight different phages, three promote resistance, and one was ambiguous (see Table 3). This overrepresentation of gene families promoting resistance was expected, since in our set-up resistance to phage can more easily be explained by a gain of function model, meaning the gaining of a defense mechanism of which there are plenty found in nature. We were unfortunately unable to identify the nature of the defense mechanism in most resistance promoting gene families from electronic annotation alone.

Conversely, a gain in susceptibility linked to the presence of a certain gene family is more difficult to explain. The most ready interpretation is that these gene families somehow improve conditions for the phage. The observation can also be explained by integrated prophages that may become activated upon infection or stress caused by the adsorption of an external phage and then lyse their host after completing the lytic cycle. Since the products of the bacterial lysis by the phages were not sequenced, we cannot say whether the external, therapeutic phage or an integrated prophage is the agent of the lysis. Intriguingly, evidence of an interplay between virulence and phage resistance has also been shown. Laanto et al. report that after co-cultivation with lytic phage, strains of the fish pathogen *Flavobacterium columnare* that have acquired phage-resistance have also lost their virulence compared to phage-sensitive paternal strains [22]. Similar observations have been made for *S. aureus* by Capparelli et al. [23], who show that phage-resistance is associated with reduced fitness. Accordingly, the opposite correlation may hold as well, meaning that genes associated with higher virulence and host fitness may at the same time effect higher susceptibility to phages. As our strain set was isolated from patients displaying severe *S. aureus* infections, it is conceivable that these strains are both very virulent and of high fitness.

In conclusion, we have shown that while our methodology does not have predictive power, it allows for the association of the observed phenotype with the genetic background, thereby producing interpretable results that can be used for gene function discovery. This type of analysis, which combines phenotypic and whole genome sequencing (WGS) data, can be used to identify genetic determinants of observed bacterial phenotypes in other settings as well and is expected to be a useful tool in future analyses of phage-host relationships

4. Materials and Methods

4.1. Collection of Clinical MRSA Strains Used for Susceptibility Testing

The collection of 207 MRSA strains tested in this project as well as their whole genome sequences (WGS) were obtained from the Clinical Microbiology Department of Hvidovre Hospital, Hvidovre, Denmark. The strains originate from patient samples. They were selected to represent a broad genetic diversity of the more than 5000 WGS MRSA from Hvidovre Hospital. The fasta sequences of the 207 selected strains have been submitted to the European Nucleotide Archive (Hinxton, Cambridgeshire, UK) [24] with the accession numbers ERZ485118–ERZ485325. They can be viewed under the link: http://www.ebi.ac.uk/ena/data/view/<AccessionNumbers>.

Although no methicillin-sensitive (MSSA) strains were included in the study, we nonetheless chose MRSA strains of the spa-types that are common in MSSA infections [25]. Spa-typing is a single-locus classification scheme for *S. aureus* based on the polymorphic region in protein A [26]. We included MRSA strains positive for PVL and containing *mecC*. All inclusion criteria are listed Supplementary Section 1 'List of inclusion criteria for MRSA strains' and the properties of selected isolates can be found in the Supplementary Table S3.

4.2. Collection of Phages Used for Susceptibility Testing

A total of 12 therapeutic staphylococcal phage preparations were used for susceptibility testing. They contain phages which are part of the proprietary collection of therapeutic phages used by the phage therapy unit of the Hirszfeld Institute of Immunology and Experimental Therapy of the Polish Academy of Science in Wroclaw (HI) [27]. Nine of the preparations are monovalent phage lysates: 1N/80, 676/F, 676/T, 676/Z, A3/R, A5/L, A5/80, P4/6409, and phi200/6409. Crude phage lysates were prepared according to the modified method of Ślopek et al. [9]. Six of those phages (1N/80, 676/Z, A3/R, A5/80, P4/6409, and phi200/6409) were sequenced and confirmed to be obligatory lytic and belonging to a Twortlikevirus genus of a Spounavirinae subfamily of Myoviruses. A detailed report on characteristics of these six phages can be found in Łobocka et al. [28]. All monovalent phage preparations were standardized to routine test dilution (RTD) and had a titer between 10^6 and 10^8. RTD is the highest dilution that still gives confluent lysis on the designated propagating strain of *S. aureus* [17] and the standardization method of choice at HI.

MS.1, OP_MS.1, and OP_MS.1_TOP were equal mixtures of A5/80, P4/6409, and 676/Z phages prepared at the Institute of Biotechnology, Sera and Vaccines BIOMED S.A. in Cracow, Poland. MS-1 phage cocktail lysate contained each component phage in a titer no less than 5×10^5 pfu/mL, OP_MS-1_TOP cocktail of purified phages was suspended in phosphate buffered saline containing each phage at no less than 10^9 pfu/mL [29], and OP_MS-1 phage cocktail had similar characteristics as OP_MS-1_TOP but contained up to 10% of saccharose as a phage stabilizer.

4.3. Susceptibility Testing Procedure

Testing for phage susceptibility was performed as described by Ślopek et al. [30]. In short, 50 μL of phage preparation was applied onto a fresh bacterial lawn from day culture and the results were assessed the next day following 6 h incubation at 37 °C.

Results were assessed according to a 7-point scale as described by Ślopek et al. [30] and shortly summarized in the supplement Section 9 'Details on susceptibility testing as described by Ślopek et al.'

Results were further discretized into two levels: "susceptible" and "resistant". The "susceptible" label was applied to the two strongest reactions, resulting in confluent or semi confluent lysis. According to standards applied at the Bacteriophage Laboratory of the HI, those two levels enable the phage procurement for therapeutic phage preparation. All other weak reactions as well as a negative reaction and opaque lysis were regarded as "resistant". Susceptibility testing results in these two levels, as used for the modelling, can be found in Table 1, while Supplementary Table S4 details results in three levels: resistant, weakly susceptible and strongly susceptible.

The full set of 207 strains was challenged with each of the 12 phage preparations. We call the result of susceptibility testing to a preparation the "interaction" of our strain set with said phage.

4.4. Data Partitioning

For the purpose of modelling the phage response from the genomic composition of the bacterial strains, the 207 MRSA strains were divided into five partitions. This division was based on the orthogonal average nucleotide identity (orthoANI) as described by Lee et al. [31]. OrthoANI is suitable for creating a distance matrix, because it is a symmetric measure of distance, unlike the traditional ANI. Calculations were performed on all pairs of strains with the standalone tool OAT by Lee et al. Distances were subsequently calculated as 1-orthoANI, and a heat map was generated that can be found in Figure 1.

The resulting heat map showed very clear clusters of closely related sequences. Partitioning was therefore done by visual inspection.

The partitions thus obtained were then used in a five-fold cross validation framework, i.e., four of them were combined into the training set, and one was left out for testing. This process was repeated five times so that each partition was in turn the testing set.

4.5. Model Framework

We sought to model a binary outcome (resistant/susceptible) based on weighted binary features (absence/presence of gene families). Logistic regression models were chosen for this task and set-up inside a five-fold cross validation. Each cross validation fold was trained using a Ridge regression to avoid overfitting. A nested cross validation was used to identify the optimal parameter for the Ridge penalty lambda.

Due to challenges posed by the large feature space, the modelling was further split into a two-step process: a first-step model in which we performed feature selection by association testing, and a second-step model whose features were selected based on the regression weights obtained from the first model. The following sections describe details of each modelling step.

4.6. Feature Selection by Association Testing

The genetic background of the MRSA strains was established by first predicting genes and performing functional annotation through the RAST service [32] for all 207 strains. The predicted genes were then clustered with cd-hit [33] using a cutoff of 90% on global sequence identity, word size 5 and the -g 1 option to cluster with the best match instead of the first match. This resulted in a total of 6.419 gene families in the 207 MRSA strains.

Next, the feature space, i.e., the number of gene families included in the model, was reduced by removing gene families with limited power for distinguishing susceptible from non-susceptible bacterial strains. This was done by constructing 2×2 contingency tables as illustrated in Supplementary Table S5, and from these tables calculating a p-value to each gene family in each phage interaction using Fischer-Boschloo's exact unconditional test. We then imposed a threshold of 0.01 on the p-value for the gene family to be admitted to the second step of modelling.

As can be seen in Figure 1, one of the partitions was significantly larger than the other four. This obliged us to employ bootstrapping in every fold that included partition 1 so as to not bias the feature selection on partition size. Details to this can be found in the Supplementary Section 10 'Details on Feature selection by association testing'.

4.7. Feature Selection by Regression Weights

Due to the five-fold cross validation setup, each gene family was assigned five regression weights for interaction with each phage preparation. These may be NA (not applicable) if the gene family was not chosen by association testing for that fold. Weights can be either positive or negative. As we chose to model susceptibility as the positive outcome and resistance as the negative outcome, this means that positive weights point towards increased susceptibility, while negative weights point towards increased resistance.

We hypothesized that gene families with a high weight across many folds drive the response to this particular phage. Therefore, we next trained and tested a second five-fold cross validated regression model with only the genes that (1) were significant according to the Fischer-Boschloo's test ($p \leq 0.01$) and (2) had absolute regression weights greater or equal to 0.01 in at least three folds in the first regression model. We term the gene families selected in this fashion the set of significant gene families. They are the main focus of this study as they are thought to be driving the response to the tested phage preparations.

In order to verify that the set of gene families we identified were indeed descriptive of the phage susceptibility and not an artifact of overfitting, we repeated the model construction and feature selection with shuffled target values. That is, we randomly associated susceptibility outcomes and bacterial genomes while keeping the ratio between susceptible and resistant as in the original data. We then re-ran the modelling and evaluated the predictive performance and the number of predictive gene-families identified.

4.8. Assignment of eggNOGs

We compared each selected gene family to the eggNOG database [34] by using the eggNog-mapper available on their webpage. eggNOG is a database of non-supervised orthologous groups (NOG) of proteins based on the clustering of the 9.6 million proteins from 2031 genomes. Each NOG has only one annotation term compiled from the integrated and summarized functional annotation of its group members, as well as being part of a broader functional category. EggNOG was chosen primarily because of this functional category assignment that allows a broad overview of the functions present in a set of genes.

To estimate whether the observed distribution of functional categories in the set of significant gene families was different from what could be expected by chance, we employed the cumulative density function (CDF). We first drew 10,000 random subsamples of the same size as the full set of significant genes families from the total set of 6419 gene families. From these data, we established an estimated cumulative density function (eCDF) for each functional category. We could then calculate likelihoods for each category of obtaining the actual observed frequency or lower or, conversely, the actual observed frequency or higher.

Supplementary Materials: Figure S1:
p-Value distributions of gene enrichment analysis on phage preparations 1N_80, A3_R and cocktail MS-1. Figure S2: Plot of the cumulative mean square error of the inner cross validation vs. strength of the ridge penalty. Table S1: List of all significant gene families along with their functional annotation terms. Table S2: Probabilities of observing a given prevalence per functional category based on the cumulative density function. Table S3: List of MRSA strains included in the test set and their properties. Table S4: Detailed phage typing results. Table S5: Layout of the contingency tables. The supplement further contains sections one the following: Details of inclusion criteria for MRSA strains. Details on susceptibility testing as described by Ślopek et al. Details on Feature selection by association testing.

Acknowledgments: This work was supported financially by a full PhD scholarship granted by the Technical University of Denmark (DTU).

Author Contributions: Mette V. Larsen and Ryszard Międzybrodzki conceived and designed the overall project idea. Morten Nielsen coordinated the modeling part. Mette V. Larsen and Morten Nielsen coordinated the gene functional analysis. Ryszard Międzybrodzki and Ewa Jończyk-Matysiak coordinated the experimental part. Ewa Jończyk-Matysiak and Henrike Zschach conducted the laboratory work. Beata Weber-Dąbrowska supplied the phage preparations. Henrik Westh supplied the bacterial strains and advised on the strain selection criteria. Henrik Hasman, Henrik Westh, and Andrzej Górski provided feedback on the biological relevance of the findings. Henrike Zschach and Ryszard Międzybrodzki wrote the paper. Mette V. Larsen, Morten Nielsen, and Andrzej Górski advised the paper writing and performed edits. All authors contributed to the final proof read.

References

1. World Health Organization (WHO). Antimicrobial Resistance Fact Sheet. 2016. Available online: http://www.who.int/mediacentre/factsheets/fs194/en/ (accessed on 5 September 2017).
2. World Health Organization (WHO). WHO Global Priority List of Antibiotic-Resistant Bacteria. 2017. Available online: http://www.who.int/medicines/publications/WHO-PPL-Short_Summary_25Feb-ET_NM_WHO.pdf (accessed on 27 February 2017).
3. Chhibber, S.; Kaur, T.; Kaur, S.S.; Wilson, B.; Cheung, A. Co-Therapy Using Lytic Bacteriophage and Linezolid: Effective Treatment in Eliminating Methicillin Resistant *Staphylococcus aureus* (MRSA) from Diabetic Foot Infections. *PLoS ONE* **2013**, *8*, e56022. [CrossRef] [PubMed]
4. Abedon, S.T.; Kuhl, S.J.; Blasdel, B.G.; Kutter, E.M. Phage treatment of human infections. *Bacteriophage* **2011**, *1*, 66–85. [CrossRef] [PubMed]
5. Pincus, N.B.; Reckhow, J.D.; Saleem, D.; Jammeh, M.L.; Datta, S.K.; Myles, I.A. Strain specific phage treatment for *Staphylococcus aureus* infection is influenced by host immunity and site of infection. *PLoS ONE* **2015**, *10*, e0124280. [CrossRef] [PubMed]
6. Miedzybrodzki, R.; Borysowski, J.; Weber-Dabrowska, B.; Fortuna, W.; Letkiewicz, S.; Szufnarowski, K.; Pawelczyk, Z.; Rogóz, P.; Klak, M.; Wojtasik, E.; et al. Clinical aspects of phage therapy. *Adv. Virus Res.* **2012**, *83*, 73–121. [PubMed]
7. Borysowski, J.; Łobocka, M.; Międzybrodzki, R.; Weber-Dabrowska, B.; Górski, A. Potential of Bacteriophages and Their Lysins in the Treatment of MRSA. *BioDrugs* **2011**, *25*, 347–355. [CrossRef] [PubMed]
8. Deghorain, M.; van Melderen, L. The Staphylococci Phages Family: An Overview. *Viruses* **2012**, *4*, 3316–3335. [CrossRef] [PubMed]
9. Ślopek, S.; Durlakowa, I.; Weber-Dąbrowska, B.; Kucharewicz-Krukowska, A.; Dąbrowski, M.; Bisikiewicz, R. Results of bacteriophage treatment of suppurative bacterial infections. I. General evaluation of the results. *Arch. Immunol. Ther. Exp.* **1983**, *31*, 267–291.
10. Weber-Dąbrowska, B.; Jończyk-Matysiak, E.; Żaczek, M.; Łobocka, M.; Łusiak-Szelachowska, M.; Górski, A. Bacteriophage Procurement for Therapeutic Purposes. *Front. Microbiol.* **2016**, *7*, 1177. [CrossRef] [PubMed]
11. Sadykov, M.R. Restriction-Modification Systems as a Barrier for Genetic Manipulation of *Staphylococcus aureus*. In *The Genetic Manipulation of Staphylococci. Methods in Molecular Biology*; Bose, J., Ed.; Humana Press: New York, NY, USA, 2016; Volume 1373, pp. 9–23.
12. Seed, K.D. Battling Phages: How Bacteria Defend against Viral Attack. *PLoS Pathog.* **2015**, *11*, e1004847. [CrossRef] [PubMed]
13. Ram, G.; Chen, J.; Ross, H.F.; Novick, R.P. Precisely modulated pathogenicity island interference with late phage gene transcription. *Proc. Natl. Acad. Sci. USA* **2014**, *111*, 14536–14541. [CrossRef] [PubMed]
14. Xia, G.; Wolz, C. Phages of *Staphylococcus aureus* and their impact on host evolution. *Infect. Genet. Evol.* **2014**, *21*, 593–601. [CrossRef] [PubMed]
15. Lindsay, J.A. Genomic variation and evolution of *Staphylococcus aureus*. *Int. J. Med. Microbiol.* **2010**, *300*, 98–103. [CrossRef] [PubMed]
16. Goerke, C.; Pantucek, R.; Holtfreter, S.; Schulte, B.; Zink, M.; Grumann, D.; Bröker, B.M.; Doskar, J.; Wolz, C. Diversity of prophages in dominant *Staphylococcus aureus* clonal lineages. *J. Bacteriol.* **2009**, *191*, 3462–3468. [CrossRef] [PubMed]
17. Blair, J.E.; Williams, R.E.O. Phage typing of staphylococci. *Bull World Heal. Organ.* **1961**, *24*, 771–784.
18. Bartels, M.D.; Larner-Svensson, H.; Meiniche, H.; Kristoffersen, K.; Schonning, K.; Nielsen, J.B.; Rohde, S.M.; Christensen, L.B.; Skibsted, A.W.; Jarlov, J.O.; et al. Monitoring meticillin resistant *Staphylococcus aureus* and

its spread in Copenhagen, Denmark, 2013, through routine whole genome sequencing. *Eurosurveillance* **2015**, *20*, 21112. [CrossRef] [PubMed]
19. Allen, R.C.; Pfrunder-Cardozo, K.R.; Meinel, D.; Egli, A.; Hall, A.R. Associations among Antibiotic and Phage Resistance Phenotypes in Natural and Clinical *Escherichia coli* Isolates. *MBio* **2017**, *8*, e01341-17. [CrossRef] [PubMed]
20. Monecke, S.; Coombs, G.; Shore, A.C.; Coleman, D.C.; Akpaka, P.; Borg, M.; Chow, H.; Ip, M.; Jatzwauk, L.; Jonas, D.; et al. A field guide to pandemic, epidemic and sporadic clones of methicillin-resistant *Staphylococcus aureus*. *PLoS ONE* **2011**, *6*, e17936. [CrossRef] [PubMed]
21. Hofer, B.; Ruge, M.; Dreiseikelmann, B. The superinfection exclusion gene (sieA) of bacteriophage P22: Identification and overexpression of the gene and localization of the gene product. *J. Bacteriol.* **1995**, *177*, 3080–3086. [CrossRef] [PubMed]
22. Laanto, E.; Bamford, J.K.H.; Laakso, J.; Sundberg, L.R. Phage-Driven Loss of Virulence in a Fish Pathogenic Bacterium. *PLoS ONE* **2012**, *7*, e53157. [CrossRef] [PubMed]
23. Capparelli, R.; Nocerino, N.; Lanzetta, R.; Silipo, A.; Amoresano, A.; Giangrande, C.; Becker, K.; Blaiotta, G.; Evidente, A.; Cimmino, A.; et al. Bacteriophage-resistant *Staphylococcus aureus* mutant confers broad immunity against staphylococcal infection in mice. *PLoS ONE* **2010**, *5*, e11720. [CrossRef] [PubMed]
24. Leinonen, R.; Akhtar, R.; Birney, E.; Bower, L.; Cerdeno-Tárraga, A.; Cheng, Y.; Cleland, I.; Faruque, N.; Goodgame, N.; Gibson, R.; et al. The European Nucleotide Archive. *Nucleic Acids Res.* **2011**, *39*, D28–D31. [CrossRef] [PubMed]
25. Aanensen, D.M.; Feil, E.J.; Holden, M.T.; Dordel, J.; Yeats, C.A.; Fedosejev, A.; Goater, R.; Castillo-Ramírez, S.; Corander, J.; Colijn, C.; et al. Whole-Genome Sequencing for Routine Pathogen Surveillance in Public Health: A Population Snapshot of Invasive *Staphylococcus aureus* in Europe. *MBio* **2016**, *7*, e00444-16. [CrossRef] [PubMed]
26. Shopsin, B.; Gomez, M.; Montgomery, S.O.; Smith, D.H.; Waddington, M.; Dodge, D.E.; Bost, D.A.; Riehman, M.; Naidich, S.; Kreiswirth, B.N. Evaluation of protein A gene polymorphic region DNA sequencing for typing of *Staphylococcus aureus* strains. *J. Clin. Microbiol.* **1999**, *37*, 3556–3563. [PubMed]
27. Weber-Dąbrowska, B.; Mulczyk, M.; Górski, A.; Boratyński, J.; Łusiak-Szelachowska, M.; Syper, D. Methods of Polyvalent Bacteriophage Preparation for the Treatment of Bacterial Infections. U.S. Patent US7232564 B2, 2002.
28. Łobocka, M.; Hejnowicz, M.S.; Dąbrowski, K.; Gozdek, A.; Kosakowski, J.; Witkowska, M.; Ulatowska, M.I.; Weber-Dąbrowska, B.; Kwiatek, M.; Parasion, S.; et al. Genomics of Staphylococcal Twort-like Phages—Potential Therapeutics of the Post-Antibiotic Era. *Adv. Virus Res.* **2012**, *83*, 143–216. [PubMed]
29. Górski, A.; Weber-Dąbrowska, B.; Miedzybrodzki, R.; Stefański, G.; Dechnik, K.; Olchawa, E. A Method for Obtaining Bacteriophage Purified Preparations. Polish Patent No. PL 212811 B1, 2012.
30. Slopek, S.; Durlakowa, I.; Kucharewicz-Krukowska, A.; Krzywy, T.; Slopek, A.; Weber, B. Phage typing of Shigella flexneri. *Arch. Immunol. Ther. Exp.* **1972**, *20*, 1–60.
31. Lee, I.; Kim, Y.O.; Park, S.C.; Chun, J. OrthoANI: An improved algorithm and software for calculating average nucleotide identity. *Int. J. Syst. Evol. Microbiol.* **2016**, *66*, 1100–1103. [CrossRef] [PubMed]
32. Overbeek, R.; Olson, R.; Pusch, G.D.; Olsen, G.J.; Davis, J.J.; Disz, T.; Edwards, R.A.; Gerdes, S.; Parrello, B.; Shukla, M.; et al. The SEED and the Rapid Annotation of microbial genomes using Subsystems Technology (RAST). *Nucleic Acids Res.* **2014**, *42*, D206–D214. [CrossRef] [PubMed]
33. Fu, L.; Niu, B.; Zhu, Z.; Wu, S.; Li, W. CD-HIT: Accelerated for clustering the next-generation sequencing data. *Bioinformatics* **2012**, *28*, 3150–3152. [CrossRef] [PubMed]
34. Huerta-Cepas, J.; Szklarczyk, D.; Forslund, K.; Cook, H.; Heller, D.; Walter, M.C.; Rattei, T.; Mende, D.R.; Sunagawa, S.; Kuhn, M.; et al. eggNOG 4.5: A hierarchical orthology framework with improved functional annotations for eukaryotic, prokaryotic and viral sequences. *Nucleic Acids Res.* **2016**, *44*, D286–D293. [PubMed]

10

Bacteriophages in the Dairy Environment: From Enemies to Allies

Lucía Fernández *, Susana Escobedo, Diana Gutiérrez, Silvia Portilla, Beatriz Martínez , Pilar García and Ana Rodríguez

Instituto de Productos Lácteos de Asturias (IPLA-CSIC), Paseo Río Linares s/n, Villaviciosa, 33300 Asturias, Spain; s.escobedo@ipla.csic.es (S.E.); dianagufer@ipla.csic.es (D.G.); silvia.portilla@ipla.csic.es (S.P.); bmf1@ipla.csic.es (B.M.); pgarcia@ipla.csic.es (P.G.); anarguez@ipla.csic.es (A.R.)

* Correspondence: lucia.fernandez@ipla.csic.es

Academic Editor: Christopher C. Butler

Abstract: The history of dairy farming goes back thousands of years, evolving from a traditional small-scale production to the industrialized manufacturing of fermented dairy products. Commercialization of milk and its derived products has been very important not only as a source of nourishment but also as an economic resource. However, the dairy industry has encountered several problems that have to be overcome to ensure the quality and safety of the final products, as well as to avoid economic losses. Within this context, it is interesting to highlight the role played by bacteriophages, or phages, viruses that infect bacteria. Indeed, bacteriophages were originally regarded as a nuisance, being responsible for fermentation failure and economic losses when infecting lactic acid bacteria, but are now considered promising antimicrobials to fight milk-borne pathogens without contributing to the increase in antibiotic resistance.

Keywords: bacteriophages; dairy industry; pathogens; lactic acid bacteria; fermentation failure; biofilms; antimicrobial resistance

---

1. Introduction

1.1. Origins and Industrialization of Dairy Production

Archaeological evidence indicates that already in ancient times, the people of Mesopotamia learned to domesticate milk-producing animals, using and preserving milk for nourishment [1]. Thousands of years later, milk is still the most consumed dairy product worldwide, playing a fundamental role in the diet of all populations [2,3]. It is precisely from the exercise of milk extraction by man that the dairy industry was developed [1,4]. Indeed, cheese and yogurt, the first dairy derivatives, were accidentally discovered as a result of the difficulties encountered to transport and preserve milk. From that time to the present, there has been a continuous development of new and improved dairy products. One of the most striking features of the traditional dairy industry is the manner in which chemical, microbiological, physical, and engineering principles were integrated to allow the manufacture of high quality and safe products. This multidisciplinary strategy has led to the wide variety of products available today. Nowadays, aspects like the availability and presentation of products are very important for the consumer. An example of this is the diversification of dairy products by the inclusion of fruits and cereals [3,5,6]. Moreover, the creation of new and sophisticated products that contribute to improving the health of final users, the so-called functional foods, is on high demand [2,5]. Some examples include products with added vitamins and minerals or those supplemented with living beneficial microorganisms (probiotics). Besides dairy products, the technological development of the dairy industry has made it possible to separate solids from milk, and subsequently transform these components into raw material for other food industry sectors [4,7]. It is also worth noting that the diversity of dairy products varies considerably from region to region depending on dietary habits, available milk-making technologies, market demand, and sociocultural circumstances [8].

1.2. Economic Importance of the Dairy Industry in Different Countries

The dairy sector is a dynamic global industry that plays an important economic role in the agricultural sector of most industrialized and developing countries [8,9]. Currently, in the face of rising global demand and imminent industrial globalization, there has been an increase in both the scope and the intensity of world trade of dairy products [8]. Based on data estimates by the Food and Agricultural Organization (FAO), world milk production for 2016 was 817 million tons. In addition, the expected increase in global demand and production of dairy products until 2025 is estimated to be around 6–20 percent [9]. The most important milk producers are Europe, Asia and the Americas. More specifically, the European Union (EU) is the largest producing economic region worldwide, while India is the largest producer as a country [10]. According to the International Dairy Federation [9], milk production has increased by 50 percent in the last three decades, with a total of 150 million smallholders around the world participating in this activity. On the other hand, developed countries account for one-third of the world milk production, while the remaining two-thirds correspond to developing countries. In developing countries, however, growth in the dairy sector is limited by refrigeration, marketing and transportation problems as well as nutritional and zootechnical issues [8]. Thus, smallholders often lack the necessary skills to manage their farms as companies because they have limited access to animal health services, genetic improvement and training of personnel, which results in low yields and poor quality milk. In addition, the economic importance of dairy production both nationally and internationally is directly related to the sustainability of pasture production areas and the size of herds [11]. Other important factors that influence the success of the dairy sector are the degree of government intervention through subsidies and the demand in the export markets. Furthermore, the success of dairy development programs in different countries also depends to a large extent on traditional habits of consumption of dairy products [7,10]. Nonetheless, food safety remains a key global challenge in the dairy industry of any country to prevent economic losses and health concerns. Within this context, bacteriophages (or phages) have consistently played a significant role in the success of the dairy industry. Indeed, bacterial fermentation processes are threatened by contamination of raw milk with phages that infect lactic acid bacteria. This makes necessary the development of techniques to ensure control of the phage load in starting materials and equipment. In contrast, more recently, phages have been proposed as biocontrol agents to eliminate pathogenic or spoilage bacteria in dairy products. This review aims to summarize and discuss both the negative and positive impact of phages in dairy settings, depending on their specific bacterial hosts.

2. Bacteriophages as Unwanted Guests

Phage infection of dairy starter cultures remains the main cause of fermentation failures in the dairy industry. Phage outbreaks can lead to substantial economic losses due to manufacturing delays, waste of ingredients, lower quality product, growth of spoilage and pathogenic microorganisms or even total production loss [12]. Close monitoring of entry routes, quick and effective phage detection methods and control measurements are currently applied to reduce the risk of phage propagation within dairy settings (Figure 1).

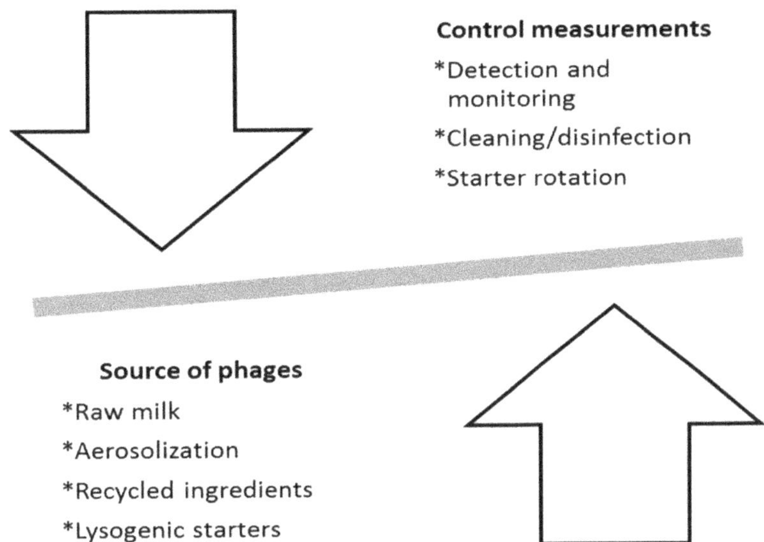

Figure 1. Factors that contribute to the presence of phages in dairy settings.

2.1. *Sources of Contamination*

The sources of phage entry into dairy plant facilities and dissemination routes must be identified in order to implement corrective actions to limit their propagation. Due to the wide diversity of phages present in raw milk, either as free virions or as prophages in wild lactic acid bacteria (LAB) strains, milk is considered to be the primary entry route for phages into the dairy environment [13]. As much as 10% of milk samples obtained from different dairies in Spain yielded viable *Lactococcus lactis* phages, while lactococcal and streptococcal phages were detected in 37% of raw milk samples used for yogurt production [14,15].

Personnel and equipment movement, raw materials handling, air displacements around contaminated surfaces and liquid splashes can aerosolize viruses and cause dissemination of phage particles in the air to the entire factory environment [16]. Concentrations ranging from 10^2 PFU/m^3 to 10^8 PFU/m^3 in air have been detected in different areas of a cheese manufacturing plant during the fermentation process [17]. A variety of samplers are now available for viral detection in the air; however, there is no standard sampling procedure [18]. In many cases, these devices may have damaging effects on the virus structure that can lead to false-negative results; that is why analytical methods that are independent of viral infectivity, such as quantitative PCR (qPCR), are more suitable for the analysis of air samples [19]. Other reservoirs of phages include materials and equipment used in the manufacturing process as well as surfaces in dairy facilities. Phages can be found in places where conditions for development of their host are favorable and where cleaning and disinfection are difficult.

A common practice in the manufacturing of yogurt and other fermented products consists in the utilization of reconstituted milk from powder and whey proteins obtained from cheese production to increase the product yield and improve the texture and nutritional value of the final products [20]. However, whey proteins may protect phages during heat; there is a correlation between thermal stability of molecular structures and their ability to protect lactococcal virulent phage P1532 from thermal treatments [21]. In addition, whey protein concentrate often contains high temperature-resistant phages, which are able to survive pasteurization and contaminate starters during the manufacturing process [14]. Furthermore, separation and concentration steps of the whey products, consisting in ultrafiltration and microfiltration, may also increase significantly phage titers in these ingredients [22].

LAB strains used as starter cultures can also be a source of phages since they may contain temperate phages integrated into the bacterial chromosome. Lysogeny is widely distributed among dairy lactococci, lactobacilli and with lower incidence in *Streptococcus thermophilus* strains [23,24]. Prophages may be induced and enter into the lytic life cycle under stress conditions such as heat, salts, bacteriocins, starvation, ultraviolet light or may also occur naturally with a frequency of even up to 9% [25–27].

2.2. Detection and Elimination

Great research efforts have focused on early detection of infective phages in dairy manufacturing. Phage monitoring methods include microbiological and molecular assays designed for rapid, low cost and high sensitive evaluation [28].

One of the most common methods for the detection of phages from industrial dairy plants is the activity test based on the acidification rate of milk that provides a reliable indication of their presence when acid production slows down. Acidification can be evaluated by pH measurements, color change of an indicator compound or variations in the electrical conductance of milk [29]. Another method is the double layer plaque assay, which allows a quantitative analysis of infective phage levels, but requires availability of a sensitive strain [30,31]. Flow cytometry can also be used for detection lysed bacterial cells that are found late in the lytic cycle, allowing an accurate and rapid monitoring of phage contamination [32].

Because microbiological tests are time consuming and mostly rely on the availability of single indicator strains, a number of alternative molecular methods focused on detecting the presence of phage particles or their components (DNA, proteins) have been developed. Immunological assays are based on the use of specific antibodies against principal structural proteins of the virion, while viral DNA can be detected with specific DNA-hybridization probes or by polymerase chain reaction [28]. PCR methods have been successfully adapted to detect and identify phages in different stages of dairy product manufacture. In a single reaction, multiplex PCR test allows the detection of several of the most common phages infecting LAB, such as *L. lactis* phage species P335, 936, and c2 and phages infecting *S. thermophilus* and *Lactobacillus delbrueckii* [15,33]. More sensitive than conventional PCR, real-time qPCR can be used to estimate the copy number of a target gene, allowing quantitative viral contamination diagnosis. By using different fluorogenic reporters in the same reaction it is possible to develop multiplex qPCR to detect different targets [34]. qPCR suppliers constantly offer new solutions to get automated systems adapted to industrial needs. Recently, phage metagenomics studies have been conducted to assess the biodiversity and dynamics of phage populations in dairy settings, providing a rational basis for suitable control strategies [35].

2.3. Control Methods

Significant progress in the control of phage populations within the dairy sector has been made in order to keep these bacterial viruses at bay. Although cleaning of equipment and facilities can remove a large proportion of microorganisms, the presence of residual LAB may increase the risk of phage contamination. The role of disinfection is to kill microorganisms that survived the cleaning procedures, reducing the spread of phages within the facility. Disinfectants active against bacteria are not always efficient to inactivate phages [36]. Several biocides used in the dairy industry as well as cleaning procedures have been tested for viral effectiveness on different phages infecting LAB strains. Peracetic acid and sodium hypochlorite containing products are shown to be the most efficient biocides for inactivation of phage particles, while ethanol and isopropanol were usually not effective [37]. The majority of disinfectants consist of several biocides and they must ensure the lack of negative impact on the final product and be able to degrade into harmless final compounds. Combining biocides and heat or using them at extreme pH conditions have shown to give the best results [38]. Photocatalysis intended to destroy fungi, bacteria and spores in the air has been recently explored for inactivating viruses infecting *Lactobacillus casei*, *Lb. delbrueckii* and *Lactobacillus plantarum* [39]. Photocatalytic reaction has shown to completely eliminate two 936-type phages, CHD and QF9 within 120 and 60 min of exposure; respectively [39]. Of note, UV-A radiation assayed by the authors has the advantage of safe use, thus allowing their application for long periods even in the presence of personnel.

The viral load of the ingredients used in dairy production should be reduced as much as possible. Although heating can reduce the activity of phage particles, many LAB phages are not inactivated by classical pasteurization procedures (63 °C for 30 min or 72 °C for 15 s). Therefore, emerging non-thermal technologies such as pulsed electric field, high hydrostatic pressure and high pressure homogenization as well as the combination with heat are currently being explored for inactivating phages [40]. It is important to take into consideration that phages also react differently to heat depending on the medium. Moreover, protective effects due to the presence of proteins, salt or fat have been reported [21,22].

Phage inhibitory media have been developed for starter propagation in dairy plants. The addition of components that inhibit or delay phage propagation such as chelating agents, sodium tripolyphosphate or purified phage peptides can help protect from further phage infection [41–43].

Rotation of defined phage-free cultures is an efficient phage control method to avoid recontamination by the same phage and the build-up of specific phages. A follow up is necessary in order to detect the emergence of new virulent phages to adjust the strain rotation protocol. Recently, a multiplex PCR method based on the genetic locus of the cell wall polysaccharide that acts as phage receptor for many lactococcal phages has been developed to predict phage susceptibility and aid to design suitable starter rotation schemes [44].

The availability of alternative phage resistant starters is of paramount importance and many efforts are being made to search for potential new starter bacteria with different phage sensitivity profiles or to engineer phage-resistant starters. Bacteria have developed natural defense mechanisms against phage infection based on adsorption inhibition, blockage of phage DNA injection, restriction-modification, abortive infection and CRISPR-Cas systems [45]. Many of these systems are plasmid encoded and can be moved from one strain to another for genetically improving dairy starters. Isolation of spontaneous bacteriophage insensitive mutants (BIMs) is a feasible alternative for bacteria without conjugative plasmids, and involves no genetic manipulation. On the other hand, construction of genetically engineered strains has been intensively studied. Several genetic tools, based in the LAB native phage defense mechanisms as well as phage elements have been designed. Examples of these engineered antiphage approaches include cloning of replication origin, antisense RNA technology, phage triggered suicide systems, overproduction of phage proteins, DARPins and neutralizing antibody fragments [12]. Nevertheless, legislation and consumers' concerns regarding genetically modified organisms (GMOs) makes its application to dairy industry difficult.

3. Problems Associated with Bacterial Contamination

3.1. Foodborne Infectious Diseases in Dairy Products

Ensuring access to safe food products remains one of the major global health challenges. Indeed, foodborne diseases constitute a sanitary and economic burden in countries all over the world. To be effective, food safety measures require the participation of all the different actors along the food supply chain, "from farm to fork", including farmers, manufacturers, vendors and consumers. This has become particularly difficult in our global market economy, as these different actors are often far away from each other, frequently across national borders. In this context, adequate regulatory frameworks need to be in place to ensure that the required safety standards are met throughout the process. Nonetheless, foodborne infections are still a major health care concern, with a total of 600 million people falling ill and 420,000 dying every year from eating contaminated food [46].

Dairy products can get contaminated at different points along the production chain (Figure 2). For instance, raw milk can carry microorganisms from the udder or teat canal, the milking equipment, storage containers, the animal's or handler's skin, etc. [47]. Since some of these microbes can be human pathogens, milk can be a potential source of infections if consumed unpasteurized. These pathogens may even persist in aged products made from raw milk, like some traditionally-manufactured cheeses [48]. Pasteurization, on the other hand, can kill most potentially dangerous microorganisms present in milk [47]. However, outbreaks may still occur due to improper pasteurization or post-pasteurization contamination of the milk. Indeed, proper cleaning and hygiene procedures are essential to prevent milk-borne infections.

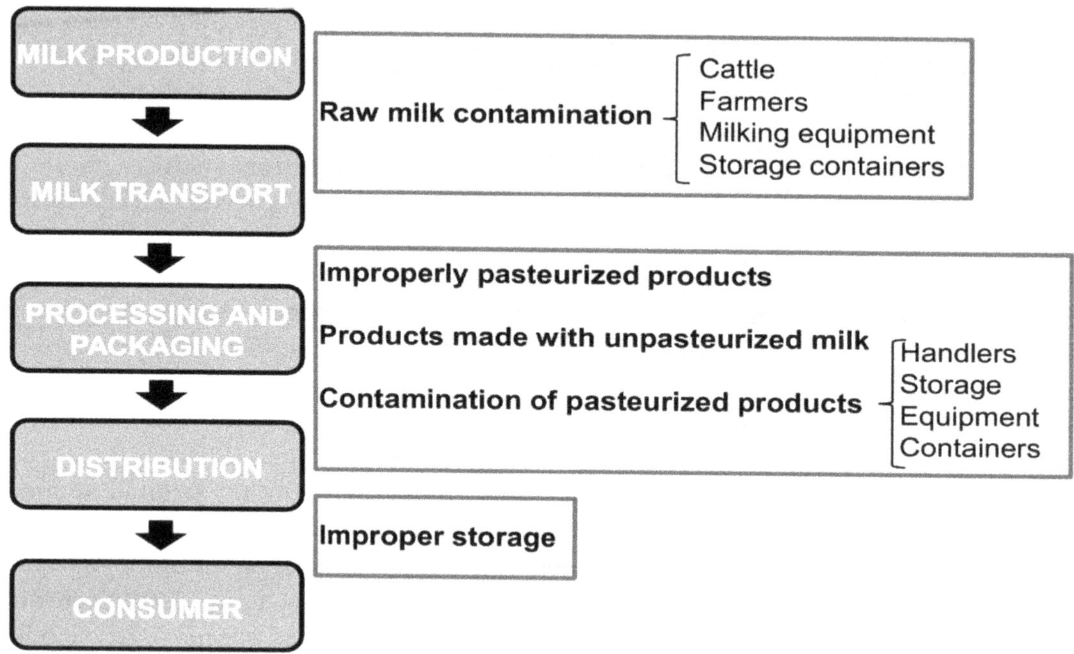

Figure 2. Schematic representation of different points of the dairy supply chain susceptible to microbial contamination.

The pathogens commonly found in the dairy environment include viruses, parasites, fungi and bacteria [49]. Some of the most notorious bacterial pathogens are *Brucella* spp., *Campylobacter jejuni*, *Bacillus cereus*, Shiga toxin-producing *Escherichia coli* (*E. coli* O157:H7), *Staphylococcus aureus*, *Listeria monocytogenes*, *Coxiella burnietti*, *Mycobacterium tuberculosis*, *Mycobacterium bovis*, *Salmonella* spp. and *Yersinia enterocolitica*. Consumption of unpasteurized milk and its derived products is the main source of contamination for most of these pathogens [50–62]. Although unpasteurized milk is not easily available to consumers, it is still consumed by dairy farmers and raw-milk health advocates [51,63]. The human pathogenic bacterium *S. aureus* is one of the microorganisms responsible for mastitis in dairy cows and can also be a source of raw milk contamination [64]. However, this microbe can frequently contaminate food after pasteurization as a result of improper handling during production. *S. aureus* is also problematic due to the production by some strains of heat stable enterotoxins that cannot be easily destroyed by cooking the product [65]. As a result, contaminated products will remain dangerous even after the bacterium has been killed, potentially leading to intoxications.

Taking all of this into account, it is evident that proper hygiene and disinfection measures are essential along the dairy production chain, from the handling of dairy cows to the final product before it reaches the consumer. On top of that, consumers need to be aware that following the instructions for preservation of dairy products and obeying expiry dates are important to ensure their safety.

3.2. *Antimicrobial Resistance in the Dairy Environment*

Antimicrobials have been overused and misused in human and veterinary medicine ever since their introduction in the clinic. One of the main consequences of this has been the spread of antibiotic resistance determinants amongst microorganisms, including human pathogens, even in environments where antimicrobials themselves were not present [66]. This increase in antibiotic resistance has ultimately led to a decrease in the efficacy of routine disinfection regimes. Indeed, strains belonging to some species have acquired resistance to almost all antibiotics available in the market. The so-called "superbugs" have raised the alarms within the medical and scientific community at large as an indicator that the antibiotic era might be coming to an end. From a less dramatic perspective, perhaps superbugs remind us of the need to understand resistance mechanisms and develop new antimicrobials.

The use of antibiotics in the context of the dairy industry is subject to strict regulations, which are in place to avoid the presence of antibiotic residues in milk aimed for human consumption. For instance, in the US, safety standards for milk are specified in the Grade "A" Pasteurized Milk Ordinance and the Regulation EC 853/2004 defines food safety standards for foodstuffs in the EU [67,68]. In the dairy environment, antimicrobials are used for the treatment of infections in cattle, as growth promoters and as prophylactic agents. The most prevalent infectious illness affecting dairy cattle is mastitis, followed by respiratory infections, lameness, infections of the reproductive system and diarrhea/gastrointestinal tract infections [69]. In many cases, cows require antibiotic treatment with cephalosporins and tetracycline being the most frequently used for mastitis and lameness, respectively [69]. Also, farmers often administer antibiotics to prevent infections, usually penicillin G or dihydrostreptomycin, following the end of the lactation period, the so-called dry cow therapy [69]. The most common routes of antibiotic administration in cows are intramammary and intramuscular [70].

Generalized used of antimicrobials in agriculture and animal farming is considered a potential risk factor for the increased prevalence of antimicrobial resistance in bacteria from food-producing animals [71,72]. Thus, antibiotic pressure would favor the selection and spread of resistance markers by horizontal transfer [73–75]. It must be pointed out, however, that there is no definitive scientific evidence of a direct link between the two. Nevertheless, there have been numerous studies that tried to determine whether antibiotic resistance increased in microorganisms from dairy environments as a result of antimicrobial exposure. However, the results obtained have shown contradictory information. Thus, some studies point that there is an increase in antibiotic resistance over time under antibiotic pressure, while others show no change whatsoever, with differences observed for certain species or antimicrobials [76,77]. Also, some studies have assessed whether there are differences in the amount of antimicrobial resistant organisms in conventional versus organic (antibiotic-free) dairies. For instance, Pol and Ruegg [78] observed that some microorganism-antibiotic combinations were indeed dependent on the farm type while others showed no difference.

Due to the concern regarding antibiotic resistance in pathogenic bacteria, there has been a boom in research regarding the development of novel antimicrobials and new disinfection regimes. Amongst these therapeutic alternatives, phages have been gaining particular attention, as we will discuss below.

4. Bacteriophages as Unexpected Allies

4.1. Phages as Disinfectants and Preservatives in the Dairy Industry

As we mentioned previously, foodborne diseases continue to be a hurdle for human health and those associated to dairy industries are not an exception. Thus, many pathogenic bacteria can spread along the food chain from "farm to fork". In this regard, phages can be used as antimicrobials and biocontrol agents in food industries to prevent and control step by step the pathogenic bacterial contamination during food production (Figure 3). The use of phages has some advantages over conventional disinfectants such as their narrow host range, targeting specifically bacteria from one species or genus, being also effective against bacteria resistant to antibiotics. Moreover, phages have been described as safe for humans, animals, plants and the environment [79]. Besides, they do not cause equipment or surface damage or alter the organoleptic properties of food.

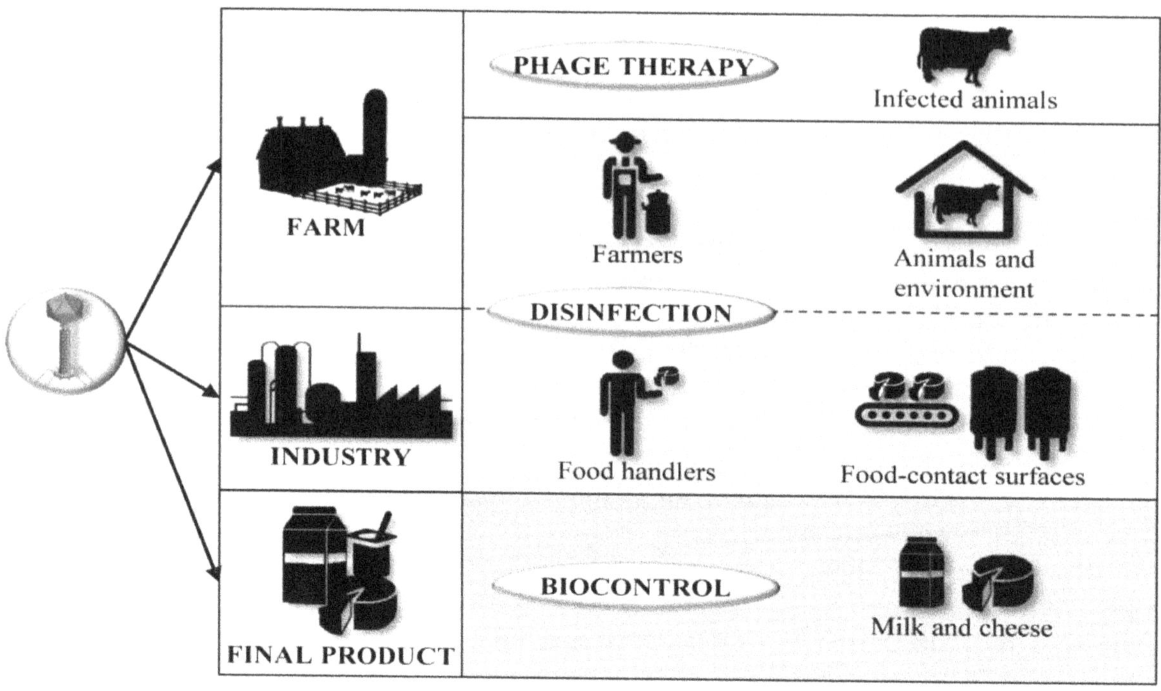

Figure 3. Principal points of disinfection and biocontrol along the dairy chain (from "farm to fork"), where phages can be applied to ensure dairy safety.

The efficacy of phages as an intervention strategy in primary production to reduce bacterial infections in food-producing animals has been widely demonstrated [80]. Nevertheless, data regarding the use of phages in the dairy industry are still scarce. The treatment of subclinical *S. aureus* mastitis in lactating dairy cattle with phage K resulted in a cure rate of 16.7%, although the difference between the treated and non-treated groups was not statistically significant. This can be the consequence of phage inactivation in the udder due to milk proteins and fats [81]. However, utilization of phages as biocontrol agents in milk seems to be a better approach, since the combination of two temperate phages ΦH5 and ΦA72 inhibited the growth of *S. aureus* at 37 °C in ultra-high-temperature (UHT) and traditionally pasteurized whole-fat milk [82]. Moreover, lytic derivatives of these phages, Φ88 and Φ35 were successfully used to completely remove *S. aureus* during curd manufacturing and also during the maturation of fresh and hard-type cheeses [83,84]. Similarly, the application of listeriaphages in combination with a bacteriocin (coagulin C23) to extended shelf life (ESL) milk contaminated with *L. monocytogenes* prevented bacterial growth at 4 °C after 10 days [85].

In the dairy industry, recurrent contamination comes from inadequate cleaning of the equipment and the growth of pathogenic bacteria forming biofilms. Biofilms are structures where bacterial cells are protected by a surrounding matrix, thus becoming difficult to clean and remove. Several studies using biofilms preformed in laboratory conditions (onto polystyrene) have confirmed the potential of phages for staphylococcal biofilm removal. Phage K and a mixture of derivative phages removed biofilms in a time-dependent manner, with the highest reduction occurring after 72 h at 37 °C [86]. The combination of phage K with another staphylococcal phage (DRA88), completely removed biofilms after 48 h at 37 °C [87]. In a similar way, phages phiIPLA-RODI, phiIPLA-C1C, and a mixture of both phages, achieved a reduction of 2 log units after 8 h of treatment at 37 °C [88]. On the other hand, *E. coli* biofilms formed onto materials typically used in food processing surfaces (stainless steel, ceramic tile and high density polyethylene) were removed below the detection level after treatment with a phage mixture named BEC8 [89]. Biofilms formed by *L. monocytogenes* onto stainless steel were reduced up to 5.4 log-units/cm^2 by phage P100 [90]. In this regard, a commercial phage-based product ListShield^{TM}, developed by Intralytix Inc. (Baltimore, MD, USA), has been proposed as a disinfectant for food facilities and also on cheese surfaces [91].

The potential of phages in the food industry is so extensive that several companies have developed phage-based products against important foodborne pathogens that could be used as disinfectants and as food-processing aids. But only Intralytix Inc. (Baltimore, MD, USA) and Micreos BV (Wageningen, The Netherlands) commercialize phage-based products (ListShield^{TM} and PhageGuard Listex, respectively) that can be applied in dairy settings. PhageGuard Listex can be applied as a surface intervention against *Listeria* contamination on cheese by spraying or by immersion, without affecting the color, texture or taste of the product [92]. These phage-based products provide a basis for the future approval of phages as disinfectants and preservatives, overcoming the specific regulatory shortcomings of each country.

4.2. Regulatory Framework for the Application of Phage-Derived Products in the Food Industry

One of the major difficulties for the use of phages as antimicrobial agents is the lack of a proper regulatory framework for their authorization. Moreover, the European Food Safety Authority (EFSA) expressed concerns regarding the efficacy of phages and the danger of recontamination of the food products [93]. In the case of the dairy industry, and food industry at large, phages have great potential for the control of foodborne pathogens. As mentioned previously, phages can be used as food preservatives or for the disinfection of food-contact surfaces, especially against biofilms. However, depending on their intended use and label claims, the procedure for their approval may vary and, in some cases, be time-consuming and costly. Moreover, legislation can differ considerably from country to country.

Probably the easiest route for placing a phage-based product on the market is for application as a food-processing aid. Indeed, several products have been granted clean label processing in the USA, Canada, Israel, Australia, New Zealand, Switzerland, Norway and the EU (The Netherlands). The first product to be approved by the Food and Drug Administration (FDA) and the US Department of Agriculture (USDA) was LISTEX^{TM} P100, now named PhageGuard Listex, in 2007 (EBI Food Safety, Wageningen, The Netherlands). More recently, three phage-based products manufactured by Intralytix Inc. (Baltimore, MD, USA), have also been approved by the FDA for application in food-processing facilities against *L. monocytogenes*, *E. coli* O157:H7, and several *Salmonella* species.

Another potential application of phage-based products is as food additives. So far, only Intralytics has achieved FDA approval for commercializing the phage product ListShield^{TM} as a food additive.

The approval of phage-based products as surface disinfectants for the food industry is proving to be more complicated than the previously discussed applications. Indeed, only one product, ListShield^{TM}, produced by Intralytix Inc., has been granted approval by the FDA and the Environmental Protection Agency (EPA) in the United States to be used for disinfection of non-food contact surfaces and equipment in food-processing facilities and food establishments. In the EU, use of these products as disinfectants in food environments requires authorization under the current Biocidal Products Regulation 528/12 [94]. Preparation of a dossier for this purpose can be somewhat complicated and, most especially, very expensive as it requires a number of studies demonstrating the safety for humans and the environment as well as the efficacy of the active substance, in this case phages, and the product itself. Analysis of potential resistance development is also quite frequently requested by the authorities.

Overall, despite the obvious difficulties encountered for marketing phage-based products, the need for alternatives to conventional antimicrobials and disinfectants seems to be encouraging progress in this field. Hopefully, this will only be the first step towards the development of a proper legal framework that allows an easier path to authorization and commercialization of phage-based products.

5. Concluding Remarks

One century after phages were first described, there is no doubt regarding their importance in diverse fields including ecology, biotechnology, medicine and industrial activities. The dairy industry provides a perfect example of the diverse ways in which bacterial viruses can affect human activities.

This review intends to compile these different aspects, both positive and negative, and gives an overview of how phages have in some ways shaped the development of a whole industrial sector. Thus, achieving a good understanding of phages that infect lactic acid bacteria has enabled the development and implementation of strategies to limit the economic losses associated to fermentation failures. On the other hand, phages appear as a viable alternative to conventional disinfectants for application in food industrial surfaces and dairy products themselves. In the midst of a crisis of rising resistance rates to antimicrobials, phages are giving new hope in the fight against bacterial pathogens. Nevertheless, it is still necessary to conduct further research and develop the appropriate regulatory framework in order to ensure that phage disinfection procedures are effective, safe and easily available.

Acknowledgments: Our research was funded by grants AGL2015-65673-R (Ministry of Science and Innovation, Spain), BIO2013-46266-R (MINECO, Spain), EU ANIWHA ERA-NET BLAAT, GRUPIN14-139 (Program of Science, Technology and Innovation 2013–2017 and FEDER EU funds, Principado de Asturias, Spain). L.F. and S.P. were respectively awarded a "Marie Curie Clarin-Cofund" grant and a CONCACYT (Mexico) postdoctoral fellowship. P.G., B.M. and A.R. are members of the bacteriophage network FAGOMA II and the FWO Vlaanderen funded "Phagebiotics" research community (WO.016.14).

Author Contributions: Lucía Fernández, Susana Escobedo, Diana Gutiérrez, Silvia Portilla, Beatriz Martínez, Ana Rodríguez and Pilar García wrote the paper.

References

1. Rodríguez González, A.; Roces Rodríguez, C.; Martínez Fernández, B. Chapter 9: Cultivos Iniciadores en Quesería: Tradición y Modernidad. In *Biocontrol en la Industria Láctea*; Roa, I., Pacheco, M., Tabla, R., Rebollo, J.E., Eds.; Bubok Publishing, S.L.: Madrid, Spain, 2014; pp. 110–125, ISBN 978-84-686-5316-7. (In Spanish)
2. Dugdill, B.; Bennett, A.; Phelan, J.; Scholten, B.A. Chapter 8: Dairy-industry development programmes: Their role in food and nutrition security and poverty reduction. In *Milk and Dairy Products in Human Nutrition*; Muehlhoff, E., Bennett, A., McMahon, D., Eds.; FAO: Rome, Italy, 2013; pp. 313–348, ISBN 978-92-5-107863-1.
3. Kongerslev Thorning, T.; Raben, A.; Tholstrup, T.; Soedamah-Muthu, S.S.; Givens, I.; Astrup, A. Milk and dairy products: Good or bad for human health? An assessment of the totality of scientific evidence. *Food Nutr. Res.* **2016**, *60*. [CrossRef]
4. Chandan, R.C. Dairy Industry: Chapter 2: Production and Consumption Trends. In *Dairy Processing & Quality Assurance*; Chandan, R.C., Kilara, A., Schah, N.P., Eds.; Wiley-Blackwell: Ames, IA, USA, 2008; pp. 41–58, ISBN 978-0813827568.
5. Moncada Jiménez, A.; Pelayo Consuegra, B.H. Chapter 4: El Proceso Industrial de los Productos Lácteos. In *El libro blanco de la Leche y los Productos Lácteos*; Cámara Nacional de Industriales de la Leche: Mexico City, Mexico, 2011; pp. 52–65.
6. Visioli, F.; Strata, A. Milk, dairy products, and their functional effects in humans: A narrative review of recent evidence. *Adv. Nutr.* **2014**, *5*, 131–143. [CrossRef] [PubMed]
7. Chandan, R.C. Chapter 1: Dairy Processing and Quality Assurance: An Overview. In *Dairy Processing & Quality Assurance*; Chandan, R.C., Kilara, A., Schah, N.P., Eds.; Wiley-Blackwell: Ames, IA, USA, 2008; pp. 1–38, ISBN 978-0813827568.
8. OECD/FAO. *OECD-FAO Agricultural Outlook 2016–2025*; OECD Publishing: Paris, France, 2016; ISBN 9789264253223.
9. International Dairy Federation. *The IDF Guide on Biodiversity for the Dairy Sector*; Bulletin of the International Dairy Federation; International Dairy Federation: Schaerbeek, Belgium, 2017; Volume 488.
10. FAO. *Food Outlook Biannual Report on Global Food Markets*; FAO: Rome, Italy, 2016; ISSN 0251-1959.
11. Hemme, T.; Uddin, M.M.; Oghaiki Asaah Ndambi, O.A. Benchmarking cost of milk production in 46 countries. *J. Rev. Glob. Econ.* **2014**, *3*, 254–270.
12. Samson, J.E.; Moineau, S. Bacteriophages in food fermentations: New frontiers in a continuous arms race. *Annu. Rev. Food Sci. Technol.* **2013**, *4*, 347–368. [CrossRef] [PubMed]
13. Kleppen, H.P.; Bang, T.; Nes, I.F.; Holo, H. Bacteriophages in milk fermentations: Diversity fluctuations of normal and failed fermentations. *Int. Dairy J.* **2011**, *21*, 592–600. [CrossRef]

14. Madera, C.; Monjardin, C.; Suarez, J.E. Milk contamination and resistance to processing conditions determine the fate of *Lactococcus lactis* bacteriophages in dairies. *Appl. Environ. Microbiol.* **2004**, *70*, 7365–7371. [CrossRef] [PubMed]
15. Del Rio, B.; Binetti, A.G.; Martin, M.C.; Fernandez, M.; Magadan, A.H.; Alvarez, M.A. Multiplex PCR for the detection and identification of dairy bacteriophages in milk. *Food Microbiol.* **2007**, *24*, 75–81. [CrossRef] [PubMed]
16. Verreault, D.; Moineau, S.; Duchaine, C. Methods for sampling of airborne viruses. *Microbiol. Mol. Biol. Rev.* **2008**, *72*, 413–444. [CrossRef] [PubMed]
17. Neve, H.; Berger, A.; Heller, K.J. A method for detecting and enumerating airborne virulent bacteriophage of dairy starter cultures. *Kieler Milchwirtschaftliche Forschungsberichte* **1995**, *47*, 193–207.
18. Verreault, D.; Gendron, L.; Rousseau, G.M.; Veillette, M.; Masse, D.; Lindsley, W.G.; Moineau, S.; Duchaine, C. Detection of airborne lactococcal bacteriophages in cheese manufacturing plants. *Appl. Environ. Microbiol.* **2011**, *77*, 491–497. [CrossRef] [PubMed]
19. Verreault, D.; Rousseau, G.M.; Gendron, L.; Massé, D.; Moineau, S.; Duchaine, C. Comparison of polycarbonate and polytetrafluoroethylene filters for sampling of airborne bacteriophages. *Aerosol Sci. Technol.* **2010**, *44*, 197–201. [CrossRef]
20. Ipsen, R. Microparticulated whey proteins for improving dairy product texture. *Int. Dairy J.* **2017**, *67*, 73–79. [CrossRef]
21. Geagea, H.; Gomaa, A.I.; Remondetto, G.; Moineau, S.; Subirade, M. Investigation of the protective effect of whey proteins on lactococcal phages during heat treatment at various pH. *Int. J. Food Microbiol.* **2015**, *210*, 33–41. [CrossRef] [PubMed]
22. Atamer, Z.; Samtlebe, M.; Neve, H.; Heller, K.; Hinrichs, J. Review: Elimination of bacteriophages in whey and whey products. *Front. Microbiol.* **2013**, *4*. [CrossRef] [PubMed]
23. Sun, X.; Van Sinderen, D.; Moineau, S.; Heller, K.J. Impact of lysogeny on bacteria with a focus on Lactic Acid Bacteria. In *Contemporary Trends in Bacteriophage Research*; Adams, H.T., Ed.; Nova Science Publishers, Inc.: New York, NY, USA, 2009; pp. 309–336, ISBN 978-1-60692-181-4.
24. Brüssow, H.; Frémont, M.; Bruttin, A.; Sidoti, J.; Constable, A.; Fryder, V. Detection and classification of *Streptococcus thermophilus* bacteriophages isolated from industrial milk fermentation. *Appl. Environ. Microbiol.* **1994**, *60*, 4537–4543. [PubMed]
25. Lunde, M.; Aastveit, A.H.; Blatny, J.M.; Nes, I.F. Effects of diverse environmental conditions on ϕLC3 prophage stability in *Lactococcus lactis*. *Appl. Environ. Microbiol.* **2005**, *71*, 721–727. [CrossRef] [PubMed]
26. Madera, C.; Garcia, P.; Rodriguez, A.; Suarez, J.E.; Martinez, B. Prophage induction in *Lactococcus lactis* by the bacteriocin Lactococcin 972. *Int. J. Food Microbiol.* **2009**, *129*, 99–102. [CrossRef] [PubMed]
27. Lunde, M.; Blatny, J.M.; Lillehaug, D.; Aastveit, A.H.; Nes, I.F. Use of real-time quantitative PCR for the analysis of ϕLC3 prophage stability in lactococci. *Appl. Environ. Microbiol.* **2003**, *69*, 41–48. [CrossRef] [PubMed]
28. Magadán, A.H.; Ladero, V.; Martínez, N.; del Río, B.; Martín, M.C.; Alvarez, M.A. Detection of bacteriophages in milk. In *Handbook of Dairy Foods Analysis*; Nollet, L.M.L., Toldrá, F., Eds.; CRC Press, Taylor & Francis Group: Boca Raton, FL, USA, 2009; pp. 469–482, ISBN 978-1-4200-4631-1.
29. Marcó, M.B.; Moineau, S.; Quiberoni, A. Bacteriophages and dairy fermentations. *Bacteriophage* **2012**, *2*, 149–158. [CrossRef] [PubMed]
30. Lillehaug, D. An improved plaque assay for poor plaque-producing temperate lactococcal bacteriophages. *J. Appl. Microbiol.* **1997**, *83*, 85–90. [CrossRef] [PubMed]
31. Cormier, J.; Janes, M. A double layer plaque assay using spread plate technique for enumeration of bacteriophage MS2. *J. Virol. Methods* **2014**, *196*, 86–92. [CrossRef] [PubMed]
32. Michelsen, O.; Cuesta-Dominguez, A.; Albrechtsen, B.; Jensen, P.R. Detection of bacteriophage-infected cells of *Lactococcus lactis* by using flow cytometry. *Appl. Environ. Microbiol.* **2007**, *73*, 7575–7581. [CrossRef] [PubMed]
33. Labrie, S.; Moineau, S. Multiplex PCR for detection and identification of lactococcal bacteriophages. *Appl. Environ. Microbiol.* **2000**, *66*, 987–994. [CrossRef] [PubMed]
34. Del Río, B.; Martín, M.C.; Martínez, N.; Magadán, A.H.; Alvarez, M.A. Multiplex fast real-time polymerase chain reaction for quantitative detection and identification of cos and pac *Streptococcus thermophiles* bacteriophages. *Appl. Environ. Microbiol.* **2008**, *74*, 4779–4781. [CrossRef] [PubMed]

35. Muhammed, M.K.; Kot, W.; Neve, H.; Mahony, J.; Castro-Mejía, J.L.; Krych, L.; Hansen, L.H.; Nielsen, D.S.; Sørensen, S.J.; Heller, K.J.; et al. Metagenomic analysis of dairy bacteriophages: Extraction method and pilot study on whey samples derived from using undefined and defined mesophilic starter cultures. *Appl. Environ. Microbiol.* **2017**, *83*. [CrossRef] [PubMed]
36. Campagna, C.; Villion, M.; Labrie, S.J.; Duchaine, C.; Moineau, S. Inactivation of dairy bacteriophages by commercial sanitizers and disinfectants. *Int. J. Food Microbiol.* **2014**, *171*, 41–47. [CrossRef] [PubMed]
37. Guglielmotti, D.M.; Mercanti, D.J.; Reinheimer, J.A.; Quiberoni, A.L. Review: Efficiency of physical and chemical treatments on the inactivation of dairy bacteriophages. *Front. Microbiol.* **2011**, *2*, 282–297. [CrossRef] [PubMed]
38. Murphy, J.; Mahony, J.; Bonestroo, M.; Nauta, A.; van Sinderen, D. Impact of thermal and biocidal treatments on lactococcal 936-type phages. *Int. Dairy J.* **2014**, *34*, 56–61. [CrossRef]
39. Marcó, M.B.; Quiberoni, A.; Negro, A.C.; Reinheimer, J.A.; Alfano, O.M. Evaluation of the photocatalytic inactivation efficiency of dairy bacteriophages. *Chem. Eng. J.* **2011**, *172*, 987–993. [CrossRef]
40. Capra, M.J.; Patrignani, F.; Guerzoni, M.E.; Laciotti, R. Non-thermal technologies: Pulsed electric field, high hydrostatic pressure and high pressure homogenization. Application on virus inactivation. In *Bacteriophages in Dairy Processing*; Nova Science Publishers, Inc.: New York, NY, USA, 2012; pp. 215–238, ISBN 978-1-61324-517-0.
41. Mahony, J.; Tremblay, D.M.; Labrie, S.J.; Moineau, S.; van Sinderen, D. Investigating the requirement for calcium during lactococcal phage infection. *Int. J. Food Microbiol.* **2015**, *201*, 47–51. [CrossRef] [PubMed]
42. Carminati, D.; Giraffa, G.; Quiberoni, A.; Binetti, A.; Suárez, V.; Reinheimer, J. Advances and trends in starter cultures for dairy fermentations. In *Biotechnology of Lactic Acid Bacteria: Novel Applications*; Mozzi, F., Raya, R., Vignolo, G., Eds.; Wiley-Blackwell: Ames, IA, USA, 2010; pp. 177–192, ISBN 9781118868409.
43. Hicks, C.L.; Clark-Safko, P.A.; Surjawan, I.; O'Leary, J. Use of bacteriophage derived peptides to delay phage infections. *Food Res. Int.* **2004**, *37*, 115–122. [CrossRef]
44. Mahony, J.; Kot, W.; Murphy, J.; Ainsworth, S.; Neve, H.; Hansen, L.H.; Heller, K.J.; Sørensen, S.J.; Hammer, K.; Cambillau, C.; et al. Investigation of the relationship between lactococcal host cell wall polysaccharide genotype and 936 phage receptor binding protein phylogeny. *Appl. Environ. Microbiol.* **2013**, *79*, 4385–4392. [CrossRef] [PubMed]
45. Labrie, S.J.; Samson, J.E.; Moineau, S. Bacteriophage resistance mechanisms. *Nat. Rev. Microbiol.* **2010**, *8*, 317–327. [CrossRef] [PubMed]
46. World Health Organization. *WHO Estimates of the Global Burden of Foodborne Diseases*; World Health Organization: Geneva, Switzerland, 2015; ISBN 978 92 4 156516 5.
47. Rampling, A. The microbiology of milk and milk products. In *Topley and Wilson's Principles of Bacteriology, Virology, and Immunity*, 8th ed.; Parker, M.T., Collier, L.H., Eds.; B.C. Decker: Philadelphia, PA, USA, 1990; pp. 265–287.
48. Altekruse, S.F.; Timbo, B.B.; Mowbray, J.C.; Bean, N.H.; Potter, M.E. Cheese associated outbreaks of human illness in the United States, 1973 to 1992: Sanitary manufacturing processes protect consumers. *J. Food Prot.* **1998**, *61*, 1405–1407. [CrossRef] [PubMed]
49. Dhanashekar, R.; Akkinepalli, S.; Nellutla, A. Milk-borne infections. An analysis of their potential effect on the milk industry. *Germs* **2012**, *2*, 101–109. [CrossRef] [PubMed]
50. Costard, S.; Espejo, L.; Groenendaal, H.; Zagmutt, F.J. Outbreak-related disease burden associated with consumption of unpasteurized cow's milk and cheese, United States, 2009–2014. *Emerg. Infect. Dis.* **2017**, *23*, 957–964. [CrossRef] [PubMed]
51. Claeys, W.L.; Cardoen, S.; Daube, G.; De Block, J.; Dewettinck, K.; Dierick, K.; De Zutter, L.; Huyghebaert, A.; Imberechts, H.; Thiange, P.; et al. Raw or heated cow milk consumption: Review of risks and benefits. *Food Control* **2013**, *31*, 251–262. [CrossRef]
52. Christidis, T.; Pintar, K.D.; Butler, A.J.; Nesbitt, A.; Thomas, M.K.; Marshall, B.; Pollari, F. *Campylobacter* spp. prevalence and levels in raw milk: A systematic review and meta-analysis. *J. Food Prot.* **2016**, *79*, 1775–1783. [CrossRef] [PubMed]
53. Jamali, H.; Paydar, M.; Radmehr, B.; Ismail, S. Prevalence, characterization, and antimicrobial resistance of *Yersinia* species and *Yersinia enterocolitica* isolated from raw milk in farm bulk tanks. *J. Dairy Sci.* **2015**, *98*, 798–803. [CrossRef] [PubMed]

54. Bernardino-Varo, L.; Quiñones-Ramírez, E.I.; Fernández, F.J.; Vázquez-Salinas, C. Prevalence of *Yersinia enterocolitica* in raw cow's milk collected from stables of Mexico City. *J. Food Prot.* **2013**, *76*, 694–698. [CrossRef] [PubMed]
55. Chmielewski, T.; Tylewska-Wierzbanowska, S. Q fever at the turn of the century. *Pol. J. Microbiol.* **2012**, *61*, 81–93. [PubMed]
56. Mailles, A.; Rautureau, S.; Le Horgne, J.M.; Poignet-Leroux, B.; d'Arnoux, C.; Dennetière, G.; Faure, M.; Lavigne, J.P.; Bru, J.P.; Garin-Bastuji, B. Re-emergence of brucellosis in cattle in France and risk for human health. *Euro Surveill.* **2012**, *17*. [CrossRef]
57. Ning, P.; Guo, M.; Guo, K.; Xu, L.; Ren, M.; Cheng, Y.; Zhang, Y. Identification and effect decomposition of risk factors for *Brucella* contamination of raw whole milk in China. *PLoS ONE* **2013**, *8*. [CrossRef] [PubMed]
58. Pearson, L.J.; Marth, E.H. *Listeria monocytogenes*—Threat to a safe food supply: A review. *J. Dairy Sci.* **1990**, *73*, 912–928. [CrossRef]
59. Swaminathan, B.; Gerner-Smidt, P. The epidemiology of human listeriosis. *Microbes Infect.* **2007**, *9*, 1236–1243. [CrossRef] [PubMed]
60. Bolaños, C.A.D.; Paula, C.L.; Guerra, S.T.; Franco, M.M.J.; Ribeiro, M.G. Diagnosis of mycobacteria in bovine milk: An overview. *Rev. Inst. Med. Trop. Sao Paulo* **2017**, *59*. [CrossRef] [PubMed]
61. Doyle, M.P. *Escherichia coli* O157:H7 and its significance in foods. *Int. J. Food Microbiol.* **1991**, *12*, 289–301. [CrossRef]
62. Honish, L.; Predy, G.; Hislop, N.; Chui, L.; Kowalewska-Grochowska, K.; Trottier, L.; Kreplin, C.; Zazulak, I. An outbreak of *E. coli* O157:H7 hemorrhagic colitis associated with unpasteurized gouda cheese. *Can. J. Public Health* **2005**, *96*, 182–184. [PubMed]
63. Buzby, J.C.; Gould, L.H.; Kendall, M.E.; Jones, T.F.; Robinson, T.; Blayney, D.P. Characteristics of consumers of unpasteurized milk in the United States. *J. Consum. Aff.* **2013**, *47*, 153–166. [CrossRef]
64. Zecconi, A. *Staphylococcus aureus* mastitis: What we need to control them. *Israel J. Vet. Med.* **2010**, *65*, 93–99.
65. Schelin, J.; Wallin-Carlquist, N.; Cohn, M.T.; Lindqvist, R.; Barker, G.C.; Radstrom, P. The formation of *Staphylococcus aureus* enterotoxin in food environments and advances in risk assessment. *Virulence* **2011**, *2*, 580–592. [CrossRef] [PubMed]
66. Martínez, J.L. Natural antibiotic resistance and contamination by antibiotic resistance determinants: The two ages in the evolution of resistance to antimicrobials. *Front. Microbiol.* **2012**, *3*. [CrossRef] [PubMed]
67. United States Food and Drug Administration, Department of Health and Human Services. Grade "A" Pasteurized Milk Ordinance. 2015 Revision. Available online: https://www.fda.gov/downloads/food/guidanceregulation/guidancedocumentsregulatoryinformation/milk/ucm513508.pdf (accessed on 1 October 2017).
68. European Parliament and Council. Regulation EU No 853/2004 laying down specific hygiene rules for on the hygiene of foodstuffs. *Off. J. Eur. Union* **2004**, *139*, 55–205.
69. United States Department of Agriculture, Animal Plant Health Inspection Service National Animal Health Monitoring System. Antibiotic Use on U.S. Dairy Operations, 2002 and 2007. 2008. Available online: https://www.aphis.usda.gov/animal_health/nahms/dairy/downloads/dairy07/Dairy07_is_AntibioticUse.pdf (accessed on 1 October 2017).
70. United States Department of Agriculture, Animal Plant Health Inspection Service National Animal Health Monitoring System. Injection Practices on U.S. Dairy Operations, 2007. 2009. Available online: https://www.aphis.usda.gov/animal_health/nahms/dairy/downloads/dairy07/Dairy07_is_InjectionPrac.pdf (accessed on 1 October 2017).
71. World Health Organization. *WHO Global Principles for the Containment of Antimicrobial Resistance in Animals Intended for Food*; Report of a WHO Consultation, 5–9 June 2000; World Health Organization: Geneva, Switzerland, 2000.
72. World Health Organization. *Monitoring Antimicrobial Usage in Food Animals for the Protection of Human Health*; Report of a WHO Consultation, Oslo, Norway, 10–13 September 2001; World Health Organization: Geneva, Switzerland, 2002.
73. Witte, W. Medical consequences of antimicrobial use in agriculture. *Science* **1998**, *279*, 996–997. [CrossRef] [PubMed]

74. O'Brien, T.F. Emergence, spread, and environmental effect of antimicrobial resistance: How use of an antimicrobial anywhere can increase resistance to any antimicrobial anywhere else. *Clin. Infect. Dis.* **2002**, *34*, S78–S84. [CrossRef] [PubMed]
75. Molbak, K. Spread of resistant bacteria and resistance genes from animals to humans—The public health consequences. *J. Vet. Med. B Infect. Dis. Vet. Public Health* **2004**, *51*, 364–369. [CrossRef] [PubMed]
76. Erskine, R.J.; Walker, R.D.; Bolin, C.A.; Bartlett, P.C.; White, D.G. Trends in antibacterial susceptibility of mastitis pathogens during a seven-year period. *J. Dairy Sci.* **2002**, *85*, 1111–1118. [CrossRef]
77. Rajala-Schultz, P.J.; Smith, K.L.; Hogan, J.S.; Love, B.C. Antimicrobial susceptibility of mastitis pathogens from first lactation and older cows. *Vet. Microbiol.* **2004**, *102*, 33–42. [CrossRef] [PubMed]
78. Pol, M.; Ruegg, P.L. Treatment practices and quantification of antimicrobial drug usage in conventional and organic dairy farms in Wisconsin. *J. Dairy Sci.* **2007**, *90*, 249–261. [CrossRef]
79. Bruttin, A.; Brussow, H. Human volunteers receiving *Escherichia coli* phage T4 orally: A safety test of phage therapy. *Antimicrob. Agents Chemother.* **2005**, *49*, 2874–2878. [CrossRef] [PubMed]
80. Carvalho, C.; Costa, A.R.; Silva, F.; Oliveira, A. Bacteriophages and their derivatives for the treatment and control of food-producing animal infections. *Crit. Rev. Microbiol.* **2017**, *43*, 583–601. [CrossRef] [PubMed]
81. Gill, J.J.; Pacan, J.C.; Carson, M.E.; Leslie, K.E.; Griffiths, M.W.; Sabour, P.M. Efficacy and pharmacokinetics of bacteriophage therapy in treatment of subclinical *Staphylococcus aureus* mastitis in lactating dairy cattle. *Antimicrob. Agents Chemother.* **2006**, *50*, 2912–2918. [CrossRef] [PubMed]
82. García, P.; Madera, C.; Martínez, B.; Rodríguez, A.; Suárez, J.E. Prevalence of bacteriophages infecting *Staphylococcus aureus* in dairy samples and their potential as biocontrol agents. *J. Dairy Sci.* **2009**, *92*, 3019–3026. [CrossRef] [PubMed]
83. García, P.; Madera, C.; Martínez, B.; Rodríguez, A. Biocontrol of *Staphylococcus aureus* in curd manufacturing processes using bacteriophages. *Int. Dairy J.* **2007**, *17*. [CrossRef]
84. Bueno, E.; García, P.; Martínez, B.; Rodríguez, A. Phage inactivation of *Staphylococcus aureus* in fresh and hard-type cheeses. *Int. J. Food Microbiol.* **2012**, *158*, 23–27. [CrossRef] [PubMed]
85. Rodríguez-Rubio, L.; García, P.; Rodríguez, A.; Billington, C.; Hudson, J.A.; Martínez, B. Listeriaphages and coagulin C23 act synergistically to kill *Listeria monocytogenes* in milk under refrigeration conditions. *Int. J. Food Microbiol.* **2015**, *205*, 68–72. [CrossRef] [PubMed]
86. Kelly, D.; McAuliffe, O.; Ross, R.P.; Coffey, A. Prevention of *Staphylococcus aureus* biofilm formation and reduction in established biofilm density using a combination of phage K and modified derivatives. *Lett. Appl. Microbiol.* **2012**, *54*, 286–291. [CrossRef] [PubMed]
87. Alves, D.R.; Gaudion, A.; Bean, J.E.; Perez Esteban, P.; Arnot, T.C.; Harper, D.R.; Kot, W.; Hansen, L.H.; Enright, M.C.; Jenkins, A.T. Combined use of bacteriophage K and a novel bacteriophage to reduce *Staphylococcus aureus* biofilm formation. *Appl. Environ. Microbiol.* **2014**, *80*, 6694–6703. [CrossRef] [PubMed]
88. Gutiérrez, D.; Vandenheuvel, D.; Martínez, B.; Rodríguez, A.; Lavigne, R.; García, P. Two phages, philPLA-RODI and philPLA-C1C, lyse mono- and dual-species staphylococcal biofilms. *Appl. Environ. Microbiol.* **2015**, *81*, 3336–3348. [CrossRef] [PubMed]
89. Viazis, S.; Akhtar, M.; Feirtag, J.; Diez-Gonzalez, F. Reduction of *Escherichia coli* O157:H7 viability on hard surfaces by treatment with a bacteriophage mixture. *Int. J. Food Microbiol.* **2011**, *145*, 37–42. [CrossRef] [PubMed]
90. Soni, K.A.; Nannapaneni, R. Removal of *Listeria monocytogenes* biofilms with bacteriophage P100. *J. Food Prot.* **2010**, *73*, 1519–1524. [CrossRef] [PubMed]
91. Intralytix Inc. Available online: http://www.intralytix.com (accessed on 1 October 2017).
92. PhageGuard. Available online: https://www.phageguard.com (accessed on 1 October 2017).
93. EFSA. Scientific opinion on the evaluation of the safety and efficacy of Listex™ P100 for the removal of surface contamination of raw fish. *EFSA J.* **2012**, *10*. [CrossRef]
94. European Parliament and Council. Regulation EU No 528/2012 concerning the making available on the market and use of biocidal products. *Off. J. Eur. Union* **2012**, *167*, 1–123.

11

Bystander Phage Therapy: Inducing Host-Associated Bacteria to Produce Antimicrobial Toxins against the Pathogen Using Phages

T. Scott Brady [1], Christopher P. Fajardo [1], Bryan D. Merrill [1], Jared A. Hilton [1], Kiel A. Graves [1], Dennis L. Eggett [2] and Sandra Hope [1,*]

[1] Department of Microbiology and Molecular Biology, Brigham Young University, Provo, UT 84602, USA; thomasscottbrady@gmail.com (T.S.B.); christopher.fajardo@gmail.com (C.P.F.); brymerr921@gmail.com (B.D.M.); thehumanjervis@gmail.com (J.A.H.); kielgraves@gmail.com (K.A.G.)

[2] Department of Statistics, Brigham Young University, Provo, UT 84602, USA; theegg@byu.edu

* Correspondence: sandrahope2016@gmail.com

Abstract: *Brevibacillus laterosporus* is often present in beehives, including presence in hives infected with the causative agent of American Foulbrood (AFB), *Paenibacillus larvae*. In this work, 12 *B. laterosporus* bacteriophages induced bactericidal products in their host. Results demonstrate that *P. larvae* is susceptible to antimicrobials induced from field isolates of the bystander, *B. laterosporus*. Bystander antimicrobial activity was specific against the pathogen and not other bacterial species, indicating that the production was likely due to natural competition between the two bacteria. Three *B. laterosporus* phages were combined in a cocktail to treat AFB. Healthy hives treated with *B. laterosporus* phages experienced no difference in brood generation compared to control hives over 8 weeks. Phage presence in bee larvae after treatment rose to 60.8 $\pm$ 3.6% and dropped to 0 $\pm$ 0.8% after 72 h. In infected hives the recovery rate was 75% when treated, however AFB spores were not susceptible to the antimicrobials as evidenced by recurrence of AFB. We posit that the effectiveness of this treatment is due to the production of the bactericidal products of *B. laterosporus* when infected with phages resulting in bystander-killing of *P. larvae*. Bystander phage therapy may provide a new avenue for antibacterial production and treatment of disease.

Keywords: American Foulbrood; bacteriophage; phage; phage therapy; *Paenibacillus larvae*; *Brevibacillus laterosporus*; treatment; safety; bystander phage therapy

---

1. Introduction

Brevibacillus laterosporus is a Gram-positive, spore-forming bacterium that can be found in myriad locations including the gut of honeybees [1–5]. While typically found at low levels in healthy honeybees, the population of *B. laterosporus* often increases as a secondary infection when a hive is infected with *Paenibacillus larvae* or *Melissococcus plutonius*, the causative agents of American Foulbrood and European foulbrood, respectively [6]. American Foulbrood (AFB) is the most devastating bacterial infection in honeybees, killing honeybee larvae and spreading easily from hive to hive within an apiary [7–9]. In the wake of antibiotic resistance in *P. larvae*, novel methods for controlling AFB outbreaks are needed, similar to the need for new approaches to treating antibiotic resistant bacterial infections in general.

Strains of *B. laterosporus* produce potent toxins that can kill a wide range of organisms [5,10,11]. *B. laterosporus* has been used as a bio control agent for decreasing the populations of unwanted bacteria and this method yielded modest results in attempts to control American Foulbrood [12,13]. While typically a symbiote to honeybees [14], *B. laterosporus* can produce toxins with insecticidal properties and certain strains of the bacterium are implicated in causing minor disease in honeybee hives after a primary infection [15–18]. The role of *B. laterosporus* as either a beneficial symbiote or as an opportunistic infector is yet to be fully understood.

Prior to this study, phages that specifically infect *B. laterosporus* were isolated from beehives and the genomes of most have been studied and published [19–21]. In this study, isolated phages were tested against strains of *B. laterosporus* to determine the most effective combination of phages to be included in a final cocktail. During isolation and experimentation, we discovered that when *B. laterosporus* was treated with phages, the bacteria began to produce antimicrobials that kill *P. larvae* when undiluted. These findings led us to believe that *B. laterosporus* phages could be used as a biocontrol for AFB by inducing antimicrobial production to kill *P. larvae*.

The studies presented here show: (1) The host range of identified phages; (2) the phages' presence and persistence in the larval gut after treatment; (3) the phages' ability to induce antimicrobial production compared to other forms of induction; (4) the phages' safety to healthy honeybee hives over time; and (5) the phages' ability to control an active AFB infection. We propose a new approach called "bystander phage therapy" as a method for treating pathogenic bacteria.

2. Results

2.1. Phage Characteristics and Host Range

The genome sequences for all of the phages used in these studies, except for Lauren and Fawkes, were previously sequenced and analyzed [19,21]. GenBank accession numbers for the phage genomes are as follows: Jimmer1-KC595515, Jimmer2-KC595514, Emery-KC595516, Abouo-KC595517, Davies-KC595518, Osiris-KT151956, Powder-KT151958, SecTim467-KT151957, Sundance-KT151959, Jenst-KT151955.

Electron microscopy images of Jimmer1, Jimmer2, Emery, Abouo, Davies, Osiris, and Powder were previously published [19,21]. Figure 1 includes electron microscopy images of the two previously unpublished images of phages used in this study, Lauren and Fawkes, from phage lysates. Figure 1C is an image of Fawkes attached to the side of BL2 *B. laterosporus* field isolate.

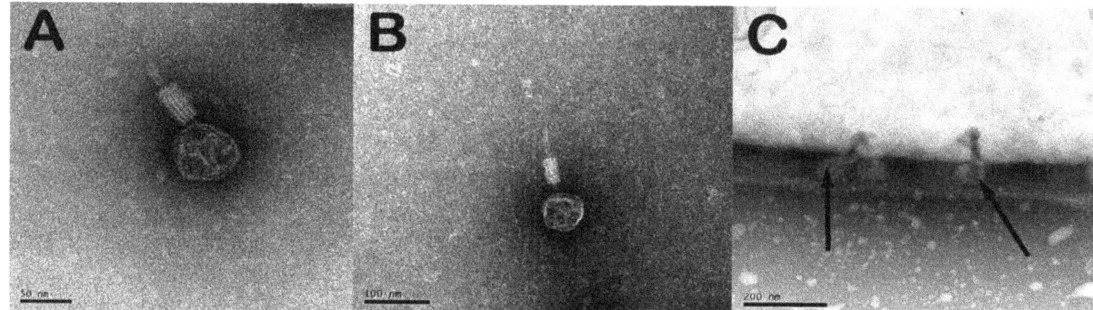

Figure 1. *Brevibacillus laterosporus* phages Lauren and Fawkes. (**A**) Single Lauren phage particle SEM image. (**B**) Single Fawkes phage particle SEM image. (**C**) Fawkes phage particles attached to BL2 bacterium SEM image, arrows point to attached phage particles. Images of the other phages mentioned were previously published by [19] and [21].

Upon isolation, *B. laterosporus* phages were challenged for their ability to infect three field isolates of *B. laterosporus* as well as nine type-strains of *B. laterosporus* from the Bacillus Genetic Stock Center (BGSC) by both spot tests and plaque formation assays. Table 1 indicates bacterial susceptibility to *B. laterosporus* phage infection using *P. larvae* bacteria as a negative control. Emery/Abouo had the largest host range against archived *B. laterosporus* strains, showing infectivity against eight of the 12 strains. Fawkes showed infectivity against seven strains of which three were not covered by Emery/Abouo. None of the tested *B. laterosporus* phages were capable of forming plaques on lawns of 40A4. Furthermore, no plaques formed on *P. larvae* ATCC 9545, a highly phage susceptible strain [22], indicating that the isolated phages are specific to *B. laterosporus* and do not have the ability to cross-infect into *P. larvae*.

Table 1. Host range of *B. laterosporus* phages. Twelve *B. laterosporus* strains and one *P. larvae* strain were challenged with 12 *B. laterosporus* phages. The number of plus signs indicate the level of clearing. A minus sign indicates that no bacterial clearing occurred. BL2–BL14 are our field isolates of *B. laterosporus*, 40A1–40A10 are type strains of *B. laterosporus* from BGSC, and PL ATCC is the type strain of *P. larvae ATCC 9545*.

Phage	BL2	BL6	BL14	40A1	40A2	40A3	40A4	40A5	40A6	40A8	40A9	40A10	PL ATCC
Jimmer1	++++	–	++++	+	–	–	–	–	–	–	–	–	–
Jimmer2	++++	–	++++	+	–	–	–	–	–	–	–	–	–
Osiris	++++	–	++	++	+	+	–	+	++	–	++	+	–
Fawkes	++++	–	++	+++	+	–	–	–	+	–	++++	++	–
Lauren	++++	–	++++	+	–	–	–	–	+	–	+	+	–
Powder/ Sundance	+++	–	+++	+++	–	+	–	–	–	–	+++	–	–
SecTim467	+++	++	+++	++	+	–	–	–	–	–	+++	–	–
Jenst	–	++++	–	+	–	–	–	–	+	–	+++	–	–
Davies	–	++++	–	++++	++	+	–	+++	+++	+++	–	–	–
Emery/ Abouo	–	++++	–	++++	++++	+	–	+++	+++	++	+++	–	–

Underlines designate the bacteria used for phage isolation.

2.2. *Phage Persistence in the Larval Honeybee*

This study aimed to determine whether phages would reach the larval gut and how long the phages would persist in a larval gut. Five hives were previously established in a single apiary and each hives' brood racks (with the worker bees covering the brood) were sprayed with *B. laterosporus* phage lysate suspended in sugar water. One hundred larval specimens were collected from each hive at spaced time points and were tested for the presence of viable phages, see Figure 2. The first samples were collected at time 0 immediately prior to treatment with the phage cocktail to establish a baseline for the presence of naturally occurring phages in honeybee larvae. Phage persistence studies showed that phage presence in bee larvae was 1.5 ± 0.8% before treatment and rose to 58.8 ± 3.2% 15 min after treatment, 60.8 ± 3.6% after 3 hours, 52.2 ± 1.8% after 24 h, 44.9 ± 1.8% after 48 h, and 0 ± 0.8% after 72 h. Phages were found in larvae within 15 min of the treatment and peaked at 3 hours where 60.8 ± 3.6% of larvae contained detectible, viable phages as determined by spot test. Phage presence in bee larvae remained well above the normal untreated control for 2 days after the treatment was administered. After 3 days, the phage presence returned to the normal nominal levels.

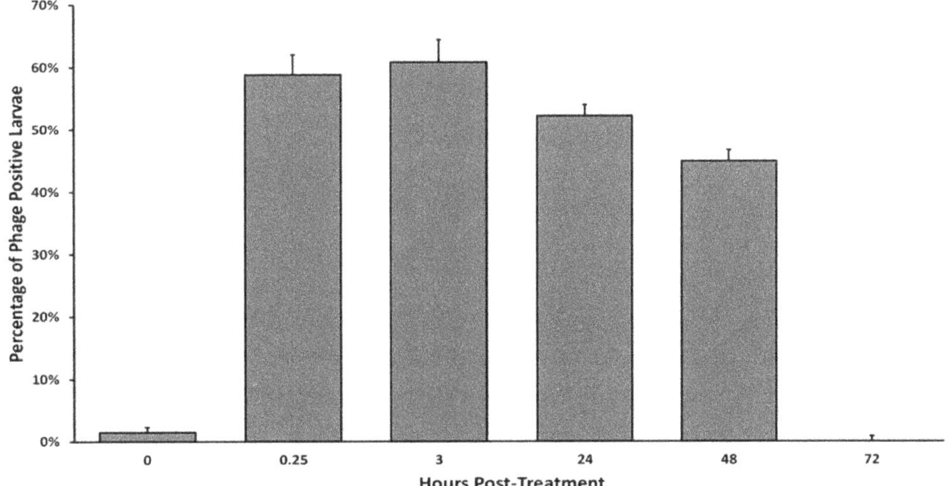

Figure 2. Average presence of phages in larvae samples after treatment. The time 0 sampling was taken just prior to initial treatment to serve as a baseline. Bees and racks were sprayed with phages and larvae were plucked from the racks at each timepoint and tested for the presence of phages.

2.3. Phage Infection Induces *B. laterosporus* to Produce Antimicrobials

During culture of *B. laterosporus* phages, we observed that bacterial lawns exhibited clearing from phage plaques as well as a diffusion of a bacterial component in the vicinity of a plaque. An experiment was designed to characterize the effects of *B. laterosporus* phage on the production/release of toxins from *B. laterosporus*. Strains BL-2 and BL-6 were infected with the phages Fawkes and Emery/Abouo, respectively in duplicate. The resulting lysates were filtered and three μLs spotted onto lawns of different bacteria. Antimicrobial activity was qualified by the creation of a hole in the bacteria on the plate indicating cell die off distinguished between plaques from phages by observing the shape and size of the clearing (Figure 3, Table 2). Lysates from Fawkes and Emery/Abouo both contained antimicrobial products that were lethal to BL-2, BL-6, *P. larvae* ATCC 9545, and *E. coli* MG1655. Neither lysate type was effective against *Agrobacterium tumefaciens* or *Sinorhizobium meliloti*.

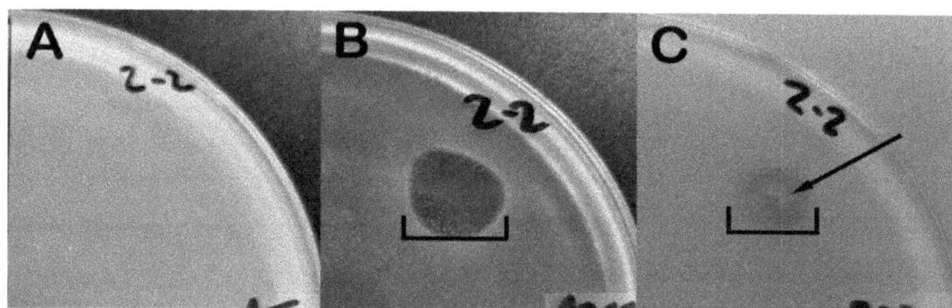

Figure 3. *B. laterosporus* antimicrobial product spot test. Drops of *B. laterosporus* phage lysate were placed and incubated for 24 h onto (**A**) a lawn of *A. tumefaciens* that did not respond to the antimicrobial product or generate plaque clearings, (**B**) a lawn of *P. larvae* that exhibited antimicrobial death, and (**C**) a lawn of *B. laterosporus* strain BL2 that showed antimicrobial death as well as phage infection formation. Brackets indicate antimicrobial clearing, arrow indicated phage plaque formation.

Table 2. Bacterial susceptibility to *B. laterosporus* antimicrobial products. *P. larvae, E. coli, A. tumefaciens, S. Meliloti,* and two strains of *B. laterosporus* were challenged with the supernatant from two phage lysates and the supernatant of live, dead, and mechanically lysed *B. laterosporus*. Antimicrobial-induced death is indicated by plus signs. A minus sign indicates no discernable antimicrobial clearing on the bacterial lawn.

Source Tested	B. Laterosporus (BL-2)	B. laterosporus (BL-6)	P. larvae	E. coli	A. tumefaciens	S. Meliloti
Emery/Abouo Phage lysate (BL-6)	+++	++ *	++++	+	–	–
Fawkes Phage lysate (BL-2)	++ *	+++	++++	+	–	–
Supernatant of live *B. Laterosporus*	–	–	–	–	–	–
Supernatant of UV killed *B. Laterosporus*	–	–	–	–	–	–
Supernatant of mechanically lysed *B. Laterosporus*	–	–	–	–	–	–

* Phage plaques were discernable on the bacterial lawns as well as death from antimicrobial products.

These data indicate the sensitivity of *P. larvae* to the antimicrobial product generated by *B. laterosporus*, and that it has limited killing against other bacteria.

Control samples recreated various stages of the phage life cycle to verify phage-induced antimicrobial production as opposed to products release from other mechanisms. Supernatant from UV killed bacteria was spotted onto lawns of bacteria to identify if bacterial death alone induces antimicrobial production. The supernatant from mechanically lysed bacteria was also tested to determine whether phage lysis releases antimicrobial products present in the bacterial cytoplasm. Supernatant from untreated vegetative *B. laterosporus* was also tested to identify whether unprovoked bacteria releases antimicrobial products. None of the control sample supernatants formed holes in bacterial lawns, indicating that these mechanisms did not result in any production or release as seen in Figure 3. The lack of antimicrobial production via UV killing and mechanical lysis indicates that the bactericidal produced by *B. laterosporus* is not a result of bacterial death or lysis. Phage-induced antimicrobial production may be the result of expression of genes encoded by the bacteria since no known antimicrobial genes reside in the sequenced phage genomes while several have been identified in *B. laterosporus* [5,10]. The fact that more than one genetically unique *B. laterosporus* phage can induce the bacteria to make an identically-acting antimicrobial (Table 3 and [19]), may further suggest that the product arises from the bacterial genome instead of the phage genome.

2.4. Phage-Induced B. laterosporus Antimicrobial Products Shows Inert Characteristics Against Honeybees

This study aimed to determine whether phage treatment for *B. laterosporus* would be problematic for honeybees. Since *B. laterosporus* has been suggested previously to be a commensal to honeybees, this study was conducted to observe if side effects of phage-induced toxin or phage killing of *B. laterosporus* in the bee gut would decrease the overall health of the hives. Twelve hives, six in a test group and six in a mock-treated group, were installed into new boxes with new frames in spring. New queens and approximately 1.1 kg of honeybees were installed into each box and weekly inspections were made to follow the bees' progress by observing the number of bees in the spaces between racks. Hives were allowed to become established for 9 weeks before receiving phage or mock treatments. Populations in all treated and untreated hives stayed below four full racks through early-summer. In mid-summer, the bees began to expand to fill the fourth rack, at which point the phage treatment commenced.

All 12 hives were treated three times at weeks nine and eleven, with 3 days between treatments for each regiment. Our data showed that all hives expanded at approximately the same rate during the study, see Figure 4. There was no statistical difference between the expansion of the bee populations in mock-treated controls versus the phage-treated group. The data was evaluated statistically using the repeated measures, mixed procedure, two-tailed analysis of the number of bee-filled spaces in the treated, and control hives over the 17-week period using an alpha level $\alpha = 0.05$ (p-value of 0.1104). These data indicate that antimicrobial products in the phage lysate treatment was sufficiently low or not active on honeybees. Further, it shows that the hives were either lacking *B. laterosporus* and thus this bacterium is not essential for honeybee health, and/or that any antimicrobials or killing from phage infection of *B. laterosporus* does not adversely affect honeybee expansion.

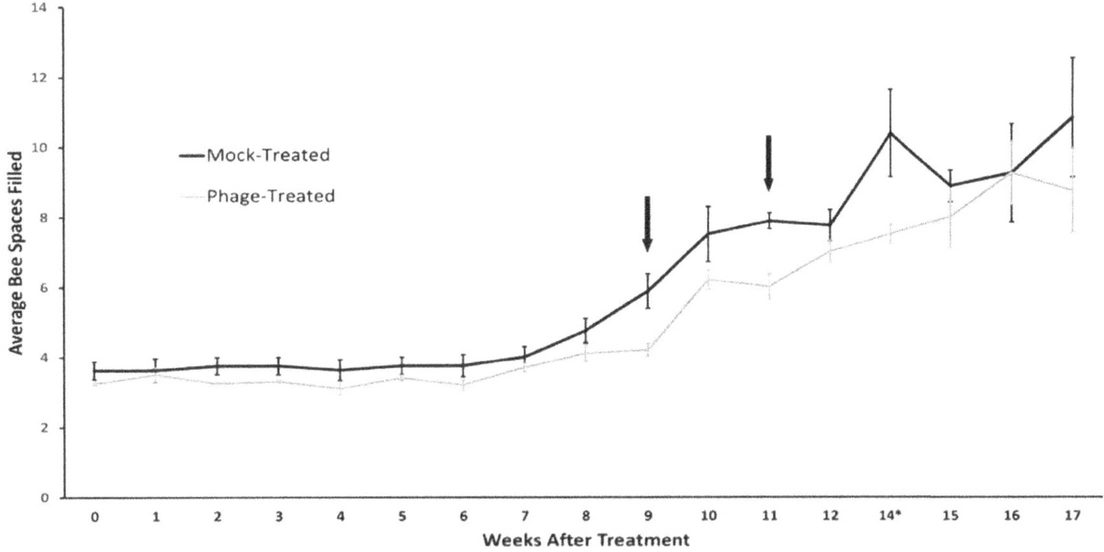

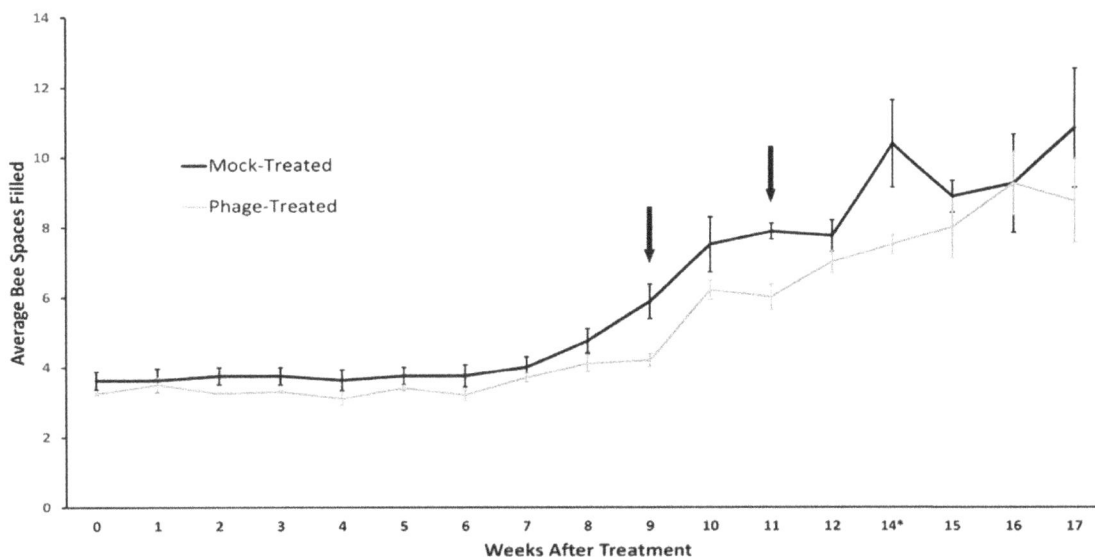

Figure 4. Colony expansion after phage treatment in beehives. New packets of bees with a fertilized queen were allowed to establish in new hives. Arrows indicate when phage treatments were administered to the bees and results demonstrate that healthy hives treated with *B. laterosporus* phage cocktail exhibited no difference in colony expansion when compared to healthy control hives. Bee spaces indicate honeybee population within the hive. Data not collected for week 13.

2.5. *B. laterosporus* Phages Can Effectively Treat an Active AFB Infection

The objective of this experiment was to determine the effectiveness *B. laterosporus* phages in curing honeybee hives of American Foulbrood caused by *P. larvae*. Forty hives of honeybees (*Apis mellifera*) were previously established in one apiary. Of the 40 colonies, 12 presented with American Foulbrood, the remaining 28 colonies were relocated to prevent the spread of the disease to the remaining healthy hives. Government regulation requires immediate treatment or destruction of known American Foulbrood-infected hives and any hives potentially exposed during an outbreak. Beekeepers are allowed to treat sick bees for 2 weeks at which point recovered hives can be kept and any hives with signs of the disease must be burned. Within these regulatory parameters, the 12 sick hives were all assigned to receive phage therapy and were followed for 2 weeks. All 12 sick hives were treated three times (each treatment was given 3 days apart) by spraying each rack on both sides with *B. laterosporus* phages in sugar water. The remaining 28 hives appeared healthy and were treated with antibiotics by the beekeeper. Treatment of the beehives occurred immediately before the onset of winter.

All 40 hives were inspected 2 weeks after the first treatment. Of the 12 infected hives treated with *B. laterosporus* phages, 9 recovered and showed no signs of AFB upon inspection at week two, which indicates a 75% cure rate (see Table 3). Of the 28 originally uninfected hives, two appeared healthy at the beginning of the study but were diagnosed with AFB at the two-week inspection. The two hives had received antibiotic treatments along with the other 26 healthy hives; however, both hives collapsed with severe signs of AFB. It is anticipated that the hives were in very early stages of infection at the time of the outbreak and were missed as infected during hive assessment at the beginning of the study. The complete AFB destruction of these two untreated hives within 2 weeks of the first inspection of the study indicates that the 12 diagnosed-infected hives which received bystander phage therapy from that apiary during that outbreak were infected with a strain of *P. larvae* that was both antibiotic resistant and lethal. Dead-out hives were burned. No further problems were reported with the other 26 hives healthy antibiotic treated hives. From the 12 sick beehives, dead larval samples were taken from the hives before the first phage treatment and healthy larvae were taken at 2 weeks post-phage treatment (healthy larvae were taken post-treatment because no dead larvae were observed). The larval samples were analyzed by PCR for the presence of bacteria as described in the Materials and Methods Section 4.1. Results of PCR confirmed the presence of *P. larvae* and *B. laterosporus* DNA at pre-treatment, and only *B. laterosporus* DNA with no amplification of *P. larvae* DNA at post-treatment from the larval samples. The nine hives that recovered from AFB were followed through winter. In spring, of the nine recovered hives, five survived, four died. No signs of AFB were found in the four dead hives; three of the hives appeared to have frozen to death, and one hive was destroyed by vandals.

Table 3. Survival rate of hives after treatment in fall and after winter. Infected hives received phage cocktail treatments and uninfected hives were prophylactically treated with antibiotics. Survival rates of the hives were evaluated after 2 and 16 weeks.

Hive Status	Total Hives	AFB-Free Post-Treatment	Hive Survival Over Winter
Uninfected hives	28	92.85% *	78.1% †
AFB infected hives	12	75%	62.5%

* Two hives of the 28 uninfected became infected when they were removed from the initial 12 infected hive. † Results excluding the two hives that became infected with AFB.

2.6. *B. Laterosporus* Phages Do not Prevent Reinfection by Latent *P. larvae* Spores

The five recovered, surviving hives were followed for 9 months to investigate the effectiveness of the *B. laterosporus* phage cocktail in the inactivation of latent *P. larvae* spores, see Table 4. Two weeks after phage treatment as well as in the following spring, 16 weeks after the first treatment, all five hives had no signs of AFB infection. At 18 weeks, one of the five surviving hives experienced an AFB infection and that hive recovered after another treatment of *B. laterosporus* phages. At each time of recurrence, all five hives in the apiary were preemptively treated with the phage cocktail. At week 22, the first hive and a second hive experienced symptoms of AFB, which were again treatable with *B. laterosporus*, signs of AFB disappearing within a week of the treatment. By week 26, all five hives presented with AFB symptoms and were treated with the phage cocktail, which again cleared all of the hives of AFB symptoms with 2 weeks. All hives were destroyed mid-summer due to the reoccurring infections. These data indicate that *B. laterosporus* phage treatment could kill active *P. larvae* infections, but could not kill *P. larvae* spores nor prevent future infection.

Table 4. Health of five hives after and AFB outbreak, *B. laterosporus* phage treatment, and overwintering. The surviving hives after *B. laterosporus* phage treatment were monitored for 28 weeks after initial treatment. When hives were seen to relapse, all hives were retreated with phage cocktail.

Hive Status	Week 16	Week 18 *	Week 20	Week 22 *	Week 24	Week 26 *	Week 28
Healthy	5	4	5	3	5	0	5
AFB+	0	1	0	2	0	5	0

* Weeks when phage cocktail was administered.

3. Discussion

The phage cocktail used in these studies was formulated to specifically infect a wide range of *B. laterosporus* field isolate strains. As seen in [23] and [24], phage cocktails designed in this manner (with phages in the cocktail selected according to the ability to kill as many field strains as possible) are effective at reducing the amount of their target bacteria. Here, we observed that the phages selected for a cocktail using laboratory-generated data of phage efficacy was predictive of the efficacy of phages in field tests, as observed by the reduction in the amount of *P. larvae* DNA present in hives and recovery of 75% of the hives with 2 weeks of bystander phage treatment. Furthermore, we studied the antimicrobial-inducing capabilities in the laboratory to observe whether or not the antimicrobials could be effective at reducing *P. larvae* bacteria, and then applied our results to safety and efficacy studies in the field.

Using *B. laterosporus* phages as a biocontrol comes with some inherent risk. We were concerned to know whether, by inducing antimicrobial synthesis and lysing *B. laterosporus*, the phage cocktail could release toxins with insecticidal properties or other adverse effects in honeybees. No such deleterious effects were seen in our studies. Firstly, we observed rapid loss of detectable phages in healthy larvae which indicates that a phage treatment has a relatively short exposure time to the bees. Secondly, we observed no short-term or long-term harm to healthy honeybees treated with multiple doses of phages. These studies add to the expanding literature that indicates that phage cocktails are a safe alternative to traditional antibiotic use [25–31].

The results of our studies further indicate that *B. laterosporus* is not a necessary symbiote for honeybee health, which conclusion is contrary to the postulations of several other researchers [11,12] but supports reports by others [5]. The current field of research surrounding *B. laterosporus* is tempestuous as to its merits and disadvantages. However, the research conducted in this article is uniquely equipped to demonstrate the effects of beehives with and without *B. laterosporus* in vivo and the results indicate that there are no significant differences between hives with or without the bacteria. This study also demonstrates advantages to having the bacteria naturally present and using phages to induce antimicrobials to kill pathogenic bacteria.

One aim of our studies was to determine whether a phage cocktail designed for a co-infecting of commensal bacteria (*B. laterosporus*), could reduce the presence of a pathogenic bacteria (*P. larvae*), during a disease state (AFB infection). Figure 5 depicts this new "bystander phage therapy" as a phage treatment approach compared to the current dogma of phage therapy. Such situations may be more common than just this *B. laterosporus/P. larvae* system because co-existing, non-pathogenic bacteria may evolve to secrete antimicrobials in order to out-compete a pathogenic bacteria. The "bystander" bacteria may be poised to produce antimicrobials under stress as we were able to do using phage infection. It is important to note that none of our *B. laterosporus* phages could infect *P. larvae*. Therefore, any activity of a cocktail of *B. laterosporus* phages against AFB must be either from antimicrobial release to induce bystander killing of AFB or that *B. laterosporus* is responsible for AFB. We do not believe the latter is true. It was already known that *B. laterosporus* can produce antimicrobial toxins [10,32] and results from our laboratory experimentation demonstrate that these compounds are effective against *P. larvae* as well as other unrelated bacteria. In addition, we demonstrated that the phage cocktail can clear an active AFB infection but is not curative as observed by the recurrent infections. We hypothesize that the antimicrobials released by the phage when infecting *B. laterosporus* are effective against the vegetative bacteria that infect the larval brood, but that the antimicrobials are not able to eradicate *P. larvae* spores. *P. larvae* spores resistant to the antimicrobial toxins, unfortunately indicate that in this system bystander phage therapy is not a preventative tool for AFB but a treatment for clearing active infection, which is true of current antibiotic treatments for AFB which also leave *P. larvae* spores intact and viable.

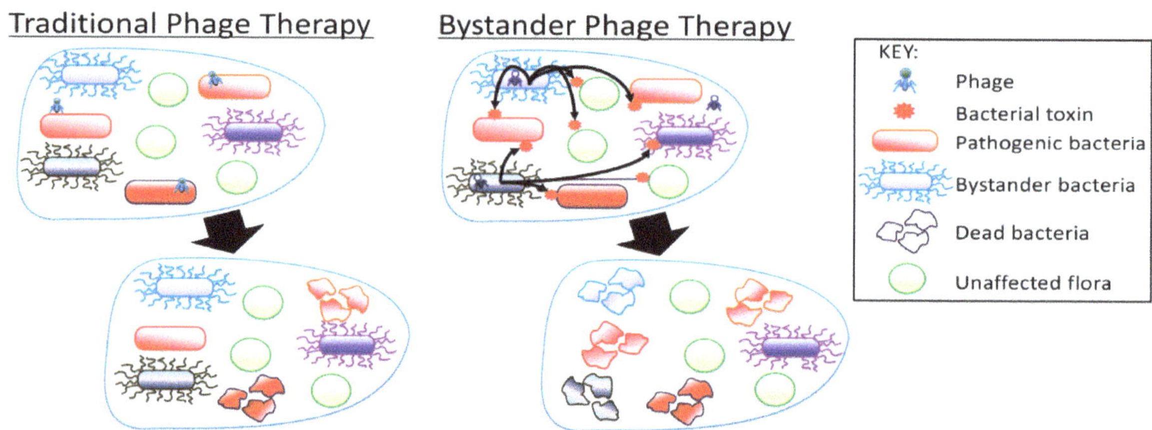

Figure 5. Mechanism of pathogen killing using phage therapy versus bystander phage therapy. In traditional phage therapy, phages against a pathogenic bacterium bind and lyse come bacterial strains, but may leave others unscathed (Left Panel). In Bystander Phage Therapy, phages against a bystander induce the bystander to make a toxin that kills all versions of the pathogenic bacteria while leaving an untouched population of itself that was not infected by phages (Right Panel).

Furthermore, our results show that the antimicrobial from *B. laterosporus* was capable of killing vegetative *B. laterosporus*, albeit at a much lower sensitivity than killing of *P. larvae*. Typically, bacteria are good at defending themselves against their own agents while having potency against others. In this instance, we do see preference of the toxin against the pathogen but still some potential loss of the bystander. This discrepancy may be due to the fact that the toxin does not affect spores. *B. laterosporus* is also a spore-former, so its survival strategy may have evolved to release an antimicrobial that is effective against other bacteria at the risk of killing a few self-bacteria with the confidence that the majority of its own will survive as well as self-survival of its spores. This approach would explain the lack of toxicity to *P. larvae* spores as well. In application of bystander phage therapy to other bacterial commensal/pathogen systems, the lack of complete killing of the pathogen may not be an issue if the commensal bystander is not a spore-former or if the pathogenic bacteria is not a spore former.

Bystander phage therapy has an advantage over typical phage therapy because the range of targets affected by the antimicrobials can be much greater than traditional phage therapy that has limited host range. For instance, bystander phage therapy does not rely on the phage killing all of its targets. Rather, the phages only need to infect and induce enough antimicrobials to kill the pathogen. By this method, a hive could be infected with several strains of *P. larvae* that could include phage resistant *P. larvae* because of the limited host range of the individual phages, but the bacteria could still be killed by the phage-induced *B. laterosporus* antimicrobial product. This bystander effect could occur regardless of whether or not all strains of the non-pathogenic bacteria (*B. laterosporus*) are killed.

An option not to kill all target bacterium is useful and desirable for a phage therapy approach because it means that the cocktail for bystander phage treatment would not need to include phages to kill every possible bacterial strain of its target. This simplifies the cocktail itself, and increases the chances of the treatment being functional since it is not dependent on killing all bystanders, but simply on activating the bystander to kill the pathogen. Bystander phage therapy may be a useful as an added component of phages in a traditional phage cocktail and/or in combination with antibiotics. Others have indicated the need for clinical phage treatments that include co-treatment of both phages and antibiotics at the time to restore antibiotic function as well as attempt complete elimination of all life-threatening bacteria [33]. Co-treatment of traditional phage and antibiotics may well indicate that bystander phages could step into the position of the antibiotic and a traditional/bystander cocktail of phages could be a highly effective therapeutic approach.

Due to the nature of the antimicrobial effects of products made by *B. laterosporus*, bystander phage therapy could function as treatment against other bacterial infections in beehives such as *Melissococcus plutonius*, the causative agent of European Foulbrood. If the phage-induced antimicrobial products are lethal to other pathogens such as *M. plutonius*, then it would be an attractive alternative to standard phage therapies because of its ability to treat various diseases. This approach is especially helpful in the case of misdiagnoses of the pathogen causing foulbrood in a hive. For instance, *B. laterosporus* is often found in the hive regardless of whether foulbrood disease is due to the European or American Foulbrood pathogens (*M. plutonius* or *P. larvae*, respectively). Therefore, a bystander treatment using phages against *B. laterosporus* could be effective in both instances. Furthermore, *M. plutonius* is difficult and expensive to culture due to anaerobic requirements, which presents a barrier to lab work that would otherwise lead to phage isolation for traditional phage therapy against European Foulbrood. This exemplifies a situation where bystander phage therapy is a sensible method to pursue as a phage treatment since the bystander is easy to grow in aerobic conditions and could be used to treat more than one bacterial pathogen whose pathogenic presentation is very similar. Such approaches can be applied to many infectious bacterial systems. By inducing bystander bacteria to produce an antimicrobial, phages can remain a treatment option even for difficult-to-culture bacteria.

4. Materials and Methods

4.1. Gathering B. laterosporus Field Isolates

Samples of honey and hive material were gathered from local apiaries and used for bacterial isolation. Samples were processed as described previously intended for *P. larvae* isolation [19,34] and isolated bacterial colonies were identified as *P. larvae* or *B. laterosporus* by PCR. Specifically, bacteria were initially streaked on *Paenibacillus larvae agar* PLA agar [35] and incubated at 37 °C. Catalase negative [36] and Gram-positive colonies were streaked on LB agar (Becton, Dickinson and Company, Sparks, MD, USA), gathered, archived in 20% glycerol, and stored at −80 °C. Bacteria were confirmed as *B. laterosporus* by PCR amplification of the *B. laterosporus rpo*B gene, see Table 5. Samples were also PCR tested with primers specific for *P. larvae* rpoB and *fts*A to confirm the presence of *P. larvae* [37]. Prior to PCR, bacterial samples were streaked out to single colonies. Template DNA for PCR was extracted by adding part of a colony to 50 μL of water in a PCR tube and incubating it at 100 °C for 10 min. The total PCR reaction volume was 25 μL composed of 22 μL standard PCR reagents (New England Biolabs, Ipswich, MA, USA) plus 3 μL of template DNA. After 30 cycles, PCR products were run in an agarose gel to confirm amplification. Amplicons from the reactions were sequenced using BigDye (Life Technologies, Carlsbad, CA, USA). MEGA6 was used to match sequence results with bacterial genomes.

Table 5. Primer List. Primers used for amplification and sequencing of *rpo*B, *fts*A, and 16S rRNA genes of *B. laterosporus* and *P. larvae*. Results were used to positively identify bacterial isolates from beehives.

Primer	Sequence	Direction	Purpose	Reference
27F 907R	5′-AGAGTTTGATCMTGGCTCAG-3′ 5′-CCGTCAATTCMTTTRAGTTT-3′	Forward Reverse	16S rRNA universal primer	[38]
BLrpoB-F BLrpoB-R	5′-GCAGGTAAACTGGTCCAGAGCG-3′ 5′-CACCTGTTGATTTATCAATCAGCG-3′	Forward Reverse	*B. laterosporus rpo*B	-
KAT1 KAT2	5′-ACAAACACTGGACCCGATCTAC-3′ 5′-CCGCCTTCTTCATATCTCCC-3′	Forward Reverse	*P. larvae* ERIC-1 or ERIC-2	[39]
PLrpoB-F PLrpoB-R	5′-ATAACGCGAGACATTCCTAA-3′ 5′-GAACGGCATATCTTCTTCAG-3′	Forward Reverse	Amplifies *P. larvae rpo*B	[40]
PLftsA-F PLftsA-R	5′-AAATCGGTGAGGAAGACATT-3′ 5′-TGCCAATACGGTTTACTTTA-3′	Forward Reverse	Amplifies *P. larvae fts*A	[40]
ERIC1R ERIC2	5′-ATGTAAGCTCCTGGGGATTCAC-3′ 5′-AAGTAAGTGACTGGGGTGAGCG-3′	Forward Reverse	Generates multiple amplicons to fingerprint the bacteria tested	[41]

4.2. Isolating Phages Specific for B. laterosporus

B. laterosporus phages were isolated from bee debris collected near beehives. Bee debris was crushed and added to a flask containing LB broth and a field isolate of *B. laterosporus*. The bee debris and bacteria were incubated overnight at 37 °C. The mixture was spun in a centrifuge and the supernatant was passed through a 0.22 μm filter. A total of 50 μL of the supernatant were incubated at room temperature with 500 μL of *B. laterosporus* bacteria for 30 to 60 min, mixed with LB top agar, plated on LB agar, and incubated at 37 °C overnight. Plaques that appeared were isolated and re-plated a minimum of three times to purify individual phages.

4.3. Host Range and Phage Presence Testing for Isolated Phages

B. laterosporus bacterial strains were tested for phage susceptibility using a plaque formation assay and a spot test assay. For the plaque formation assay, phage lysate was incubated at room temperature with 500 μL of an overnight culture of bacteria for 30 min, plated in 0.8% LB top agar, and incubated overnight at 37 °C. For the spot test assay, 500 μL of an overnight culture of bacteria was plated in 0.8% top agar. After the top agar hardened, 3 μL of phage lysate was placed on the top agar. The plates were incubated agar side facing up overnight at 37 °C.

Phage detection in bee larvae was performed by taking one hundred larval samples at each time point and homogenizing them in 500 μL of LB broth in a 1.7 mL microcentrifuge tube for approximately 1 min. Three μL of the larval homogenate was spotted and incubated on plates *B. laterosporus* strains BL2 and BL6 were plated in top agar as described above.

4.4. Electron Microscopy

Phages were prepared for electron microscopy by incubating carbon-coated copper grids with 50 μL of high-titer lysate for 90 seconds, wicking away moisture, incubating with 50 μL of 2% phosphotungstic acid (pH = 7) for 90 seconds, wicking away moisture, and then allowing the grids to air dry prior to imaging. Electron micrographs were taken by the BYU Microscopy Center, and images were measured using ImageJ [42].

4.5. Creation of Bacterial Lysate to Test for B. Laterosporus and Phage Cocktail Treatments

Field isolates of *B. laterosporus*, BL-2 and BL-6, were reconstituted from freezer stock by plating onto Porcine Brain Heart Infusion (PBHI) (Acumedia, Lansing, MI) plates and incubating at 37 °C for 48 h. The resulting colonies were streaked for pure culture and incubated at 37 °C overnight. Fawkes and Emery/Abouo were brought out from freezer stock by streaking onto Porcine Brain-Heart Infusion (PBHI) plates with a lawn of *B. laterosporus* in agar incubated at 37 °C overnight. Picked plaques were grown in liquid culture with overnight growths of *B. laterosporus* to generate a high titer lysate. The lysates were centrifuged at 4000*g* for 30 min to pellet bacterial debris and then filtered (0.45 μm). The controls had no phage added and were processed the same to collect mock lysate.

Overnight cultures of *B. laterosporus* BL-2/BL-6, *P. larvae* ATCC 9545, *Agrobacterium tumefaciens* field isolate, *Sinorhizobium meliloti* field isolate, and *E. coli* MG1655 were plated using top agar onto plates of their respective media. Spot assays were conducted on bacterial lawns using three μL of lysate and incubating overnight. *A. tumefaciens* and *S. meliloti* samples were incubated at 30 °C and all other cultures were incubated at 37 °C.

Phages in the cocktail were generated as described above and then precipitated with polyethylene glycol (PEG) (Spectrum, New Brunswick, NJ) at 10,000*g* for 15 min at 4 °C to obtain a pure phage stock devoid of antimicrobial products. The cocktail was applied to the hives using a spray comprised of phage lysate diluted in a 1:1 sugar/water solution. Control hives received 340 mL of sugar water, while the phage treated hives received 320 mL of sugar water with 50 mL of phages containing a titer of 10^8 mixed into the sugar water.

4.6. Phage Beehive Parameters

In studies beginning with healthy hives, each had a viable laying queen, approximately 40,000 or more adult worker bees, uncapped brood, and no visible signs of American Foulbrood. Sick hives treated in Sections 2.5 and 2.6 were identified by a local beekeeper and experimental treatment was approved through the Utah Department of Food and Agriculture.

Population growth was determined in each of the hives based on the amount of racks the bees occupied. A rack was considered full when the space between the racks was fully crowded. In Section 2.4 the phage treatment started once all 12 of the hives achieved at least four fully occupied racks.

4.7. Statistics

The BYU statistical center analyzed the collected data to generate p-values, standard deviation, standard error, and to determine statistical significance. Statistical analysis included repeated measures, mixed procedure, two-tailed analysis using the Fisher's exact test for 2×2 contingency tables with $\alpha = 0.05$.

5. Conclusions

Phage therapies are an attractive alternative to traditional antibiotic use in the face of antibiotic resistance in pathogens. This study presents bystander phage therapy as a new alternative approach for phage therapy. The phages used in this study did not target the pathogen causing the disease that it treated, but rather targeted a known co-infecting bacterium and induced the co-infecting bacteria to produce antimicrobial products to which the pathogen is sensitive.

The properties of phage-induced antimicrobials produced by *B. laterosporus* can be characterized to establish the extent of their host range. This research demonstrated that phages can induce *B. laterosporus* to produce antimicrobial products and demonstrated how phages that kill bystander bacteria can also result in killing of off-target, pathogenic bacteria. This approach could be useful as a single treatment for different diseases caused by different pathogens with overlapping symptoms provided that the phage-induced antimicrobial products can kill both pathogens, and that the loss of the antimicrobial-producing bystander bacteria is not vital to the organism. In this case, *B. laterosporus* is not a vital commensal and treatment of healthy bees with *B. laterosporus* phages did not result in any detectable health consequences in the bees. Use of *B. laterosporus* phages rescued a significant number of sick hives from succumbing to an antibiotic-resistant form of AFB. The use of bystander phage therapy is an exciting and new avenue of study that merits further investigation in the field of phage research.

6. Patents

System and Method for Treating a Disease or Bacterial Infection—Bystander Phage Therapy BYU#2018-037

Author Contributions: Conceptualization, S.H., B.D.M., T.S.B., C.P.F.; methodology, S.H., B.D.M., T.S.B., C.P.F.; software, B.D.M.; validation, S.H., D.L.E.; formal analysis, D.L.E.; investigation, T.S.B., C.P.F., B.D.M., J.A.H., K.A.G.; resources, S.H.; data curation, T.S.B., C.P.F., B.D.M., J.A.H., K.A.G., S.H.; writing—original draft preparation, T.S.B.; writing—review and editing, C.P.F.; visualization, T.S.B., C.P.F.; supervision, S.H.; project administration, S.H.; funding acquisition, S.H.

Acknowledgments: The authors thank the students and faculty of the Brigham Young University (BYU) Department of Molecular & Microbiology in the Phage Hunters Research Laboratory for their work and assistance. Thanks also to Dr. Dennis Eggett of the BYU Department of Statistics for statistical assistance and Dr. Michael Standing of the BYU Microscopy Center. We also thank local and distant beekeepers as well as Joey Caputo and Stephen Stanko at the Utah Department of Food and Agriculture.

References

1. Roman-Blanco, C.; Sanz-Gomez, J.J.; Lopez-Diaz, T.M.; Otero, A.; Garcia-Lopez, M.L. Numbers and species of Bacillus during the manufacture and ripening of Castellano cheese. *Milchwissenschaft-Milk Sci. Int.* **1999**, *54*, 385–388.
2. Khan, M.R.; Saha, M.L.; Afroz, H. Microorganisms associated with gemstones. *Bangladesh J. Bot.* **2001**, *30*, 93–96.
3. De Oliveira, E.J.; Rabinovitch, L.; Monnerat, R.G.; Passos, L.K.J.; Zahner, V. Molecular characterization of *Brevibacillus laterosporus* and its potential use in biological control. *Appl. Environ. Microbiol.* **2004**, *70*, 6657–6664. [CrossRef] [PubMed]
4. Suslova, M.Y.; Lipko, I.A.; Mamaeva, E.V.; Parfenova, V.V. Diversity of cultivable bacteria isolated from the water column and bottom sediments of the Kara Sea shelf. *Microbiology* **2012**, *81*, 484–491. [CrossRef]
5. Ruiu, L. *Brevibacillus laterosporus*, a Pathogen of Invertebrates and a Broad-Spectrum Antimicrobial Species. *Insects* **2013**, *4*, 476–492. [CrossRef]
6. Alippi, A.M.; Lopez, A.C.; Aguilar, O.M. Differentiation of *Paenibacillus larvae* subsp larvae, the cause of American foulbrood of honeybees, by using PCR and restriction fragment analysis of genes encoding 16S rRNA. *Appl. Environ. Microbiol.* **2002**, *68*, 3655–3660. [CrossRef]
7. Genersch, E. American Foulbrood in honeybees and its causative agent, *Paenibacillus larvae*. *J. Invertebr. Pathol.* **2010**, *103*, S10–S19. [CrossRef]
8. Pohorecka, K.; Skubida, M.; Bober, A.; Zdanska, D. Screening of Paenibacillus Larvae Spores in Apiaries from Eastern Poland. Nationwide Survey. Part I. *Bull. Vet. Inst. Pulawy* **2012**, *56*, 539–545. [CrossRef]
9. Ebeling, J.; Knispel, H.; Hertlein, G.; Funfhaus, A.; Genersch, E. Biology of *Paenibacillus larvae*, a deadly pathogen of honey bee larvae. *Appl. Microbiol. Biotechnol.* **2016**, *100*, 7387–7395. [CrossRef]
10. Yang, X.; Huang, E.; Yuan, C.H.; Zhang, L.W.; Yousef, A.E. Isolation and Structural Elucidation of Brevibacillin, an Antimicrobial Lipopeptide from *Brevibacillus laterosporus* That Combats Drug-Resistant Gram-Positive Bacteria. *Appl. Environ. Microbiol.* **2016**, *82*, 2763–2772. [CrossRef]
11. Khaled, J.M.; Al-Mekhlafi, F.A.; Mothana, R.A.; Alharbi, N.S.; Alzaharni, K.E.; Sharafaddin, A.H.; Kadaikunnan, S.; Alobaidi, A.S.; Bayaqoob, N.I.; Govindarajan, M.; et al. *Brevibacillus laterosporus* isolated from the digestive tract of honeybees has high antimicrobial activity and promotes growth and productivity of honeybee's colonies. *Environ. Sci. Pollut. Res. Int.* **2017**, *25*, 10447–10455. [CrossRef] [PubMed]
12. Alippi, A.M.; Reynaldi, F.J. Inhibition of the growth of *Paenibacillus larvae*, the causal agent of American foulbrood of honeybees, by selected strains of aerobic spore-forming bacteria isolated from apiarian sources. *J. Invertebr. Pathol.* **2006**, *91*, 141–146. [CrossRef] [PubMed]
13. Saikia, R.; Gogoi, D.K.; Mazumder, S.; Yadav, A.; Sarma, R.K.; Bora, T.C.; Gogoi, B.K. *Brevibacillus laterosporus* strain BPM3, a potential biocontrol agent isolated from a natural hot water spring of Assam, India. *Microbiol. Res.* **2011**, *166*, 216–225. [CrossRef] [PubMed]

14. Marche, M.G.; Mura, M.E.; Ruiu, L. *Brevibacillus laterosporus* inside the insect body: Beneficial resident or pathogenic outsider? *J. Invertebr. Pathol.* **2016**, *137*, 58–61. [CrossRef] [PubMed]
15. Charles, J.F.; Nielsen-LeRoux, C. Mosquitocidal bacterial toxins: Diversity, mode of action and resistance phenomena. *Mem. Inst. Oswaldo Cruz* **2000**, *95*, 201–206. [CrossRef] [PubMed]
16. Ruiu, L.; Satta, A.; Floris, I. Observations on house fly larvae midgut ultrastructure after *Brevibacillus laterosporus* ingestion. *J. Invertebr. Pathol.* **2012**, *111*, 211–216. [CrossRef] [PubMed]
17. Bashir, F.; Aslam, S.; Khan, R.A.; Shahzadi, R. Larvicidal Activity of Bacillus laterosporus Against Mosquitoes. *Pak. J. Zool.* **2016**, *48*, 281–284.
18. Mura, M.E.; Ruiu, L. *Brevibacillus laterosporus* pathogenesis and local immune response regulation in the house fly midgut. *J. Invertebr. Pathol.* **2017**, *145*, 55–61. [CrossRef]
19. Merrill, B.D.; Grose, J.H.; Breakwell, D.P.; Burnett, S.H. Characterization of *Paenibacillus larvae* bacteriophages and their genomic relationships to firmicute bacteriophages. *BMC Genom.* **2014**, *15*, 745. [CrossRef]
20. Merrill, B.D.; Berg, J.A.; Graves, K.A.; Ward, A.T.; Hilton, J.A.; Wake, B.N.; Grose, J.H.; Breakwell, D.P.; Burnett, S.H. Genome Sequences of Five Additional *Brevibacillus laterosporus* Bacteriophages. *Genome Announc.* **2015**, *3*, e01146-15. [CrossRef]
21. Berg, J.A.; Merrill, B.D.; Crockett, J.T.; Esplin, K.P.; Evans, M.R.; Heaton, K.E.; Hilton, J.A.; Hyde, J.R.; McBride, M.S.; Schouten, J.T.; et al. Characterization of Five Novel Brevibacillus Bacteriophages and Genomic Comparison of Brevibacillus Phages. *PLoS ONE* **2016**, *11*, e0156838. [CrossRef]
22. Stamereilers, C.; Fajardo, C.P.; Walker, J.K.; Mendez, K.N.; Castro-Nallar, E.; Grose, J.H.; Hope, S.; Tsourkas, P.K. Genomic Analysis of 48 *Paenibacillus larvae* Bacteriophages. *Viruses* **2018**, *10*, 377. [CrossRef] [PubMed]
23. Brady, T.S.; Merrill, B.D.; Hilton, J.A.; Payne, A.M.; Stephenson, M.B.; Hope, S. Bacteriophages as an alternative to conventional antibiotic use for the prevention or treatment of *Paenibacillus larvae* in honeybee hives. *J. Invertebr. Pathol.* **2017**, *150*, 94–100. [CrossRef] [PubMed]
24. Pereira, S.; Pereira, C.; Santos, L.; Klumpp, J.; Almeida, A. Potential of phage cocktails in the inactivation of *Enterobacter cloacae*–An in vitro study in a buffer solution and in urine samples. *Virus Res.* **2016**, *211*, 199–208. [CrossRef]
25. Mateus, L.; Costa, L.; Silva, Y.J.; Pereira, C.; Cunha, A.; Almeida, A. Efficiency of phage cocktails in the inactivation of Vibrio in aquaculture. *Aquaculture* **2014**, *424*, 167–173. [CrossRef]
26. Yost, D.G.; Tsourkas, P.; Amy, P.S. Experimental bacteriophage treatment of honeybees (*Apis mellifera*) infected with *Paenibacillus larvae*, the causative agent of American Foulbrood Disease. *Bacteriophage* **2016**, *6*, e1122698. [CrossRef] [PubMed]
27. Bruttin, A.; Brussow, H. Human volunteers receiving Escherichia coli phage T4 orally: A safety test of phage therapy. *Antimicrob. Agents Chemother.* **2005**, *49*, 2874–2878. [CrossRef]
28. Endersen, L.; Buttimer, C.; Nevin, E.; Coffey, A.; Neve, H.; Oliveira, H.; Lavigne, R.; O'Mahony, J. Investigating the biocontrol and anti-biofilm potential of a three phage cocktail against *Cronobacter sakazakii* in different brands of infant formula. *Int. J. Food Microbiol.* **2017**, *253*, 1–11. [CrossRef] [PubMed]
29. Mirzaei, M.K.; Nilsson, A.S. Isolation of Phages for Phage Therapy: A Comparison of Spot Tests and Efficiency of Plating Analyses for Determination of Host Range and Efficacy. *PLoS ONE* **2015**, *10*, 13. [CrossRef]
30. Regeimbal, J.M.; Jacobs, A.C.; Corey, B.W.; Henry, M.S.; Thompson, M.G.; Pavlicek, R.L.; Quinones, J.; Hannah, R.M.; Ghebremedhin, M.; Crane, N.J.; et al. Personalized Therapeutic Cocktail of Wild Environmental Phages Rescues Mice from Acinetobacter baumannii Wound Infections. *Antimicrob. Agents Chemother.* **2016**, *60*, 5806–5816. [CrossRef] [PubMed]
31. Kutter, E.; De Vos, D.; Gvasalia, G.; Alavidze, Z.; Gogokhia, L.; Kuhl, S.; Abedon, S.T. Phage Therapy in Clinical Practice: Treatment of Human Infections. *Curr. Pharm. Biotechnol.* **2010**, *11*, 69–86. [CrossRef] [PubMed]
32. Ruiu, L.; Satta, A.; Floris, I. Emerging entomopathogenic bacteria for insect pest management. *Bull. Insectol.* **2013**, *66*, 181–186.
33. Furfaro, L.L.; Payne, M.S.; Chang, B.J. Bacteriophage Therapy: Clinical Trials and Regulatory Hurdles. *Front. Cell. Infect. Microbiol.* **2018**, *8*, 376. [CrossRef] [PubMed]

34. Forsgren, E.; Stevanovic, J.; Fries, I. Variability in germination and in temperature and storage resistance among *Paenibacillus larvae* genotypes. *Vet. Microbiol.* **2008**, *129*, 342–349. [CrossRef]
35. De Graaf, D.C.; Alippi, A.M.; Antunez, K.; Aronstein, K.A.; Budge, G.; De Koker, D.; De Smet, L.; Dingman, D.W.; Evans, J.D.; Foster, L.J.; et al. Standard methods for American Foulbrood research. *J. Apic. Res.* **2013**, *52*, 1–28. [CrossRef]
36. Genersch, E.; Forsgren, E.; Pentikainen, J.; Ashiralieva, A.; Rauch, S.; Kilwinski, J.; Fries, I. Reclassification of *Paenibacillus larvae* subsp. pulvifaciens and *Paenibacillus larvae* subsp. larvae as *Paenibacillus larvae* without subspecies differentiation. *Int. J. Syst. Evol. Microbiol.* **2006**, *56*, 501–511. [CrossRef] [PubMed]
37. Berg, J.A.; Merrill, B.D.; Breakwell, D.P.; Hope, S.; Grose, J.H. A PCR-Based Method for Distinguishing between Two Common Beehive Bacteria, *Paenibacillus larvae* and *Brevibacillus laterosporus*. *J. Appl. Environ. Microbiol.* **2018**, *84*, e01886-18. [CrossRef] [PubMed]
38. Lane, D.J. 16S/23S rRNA sequencing. In *Nucleic Acid Techniques in Bacterial Systematics*; Stackebrandt, E., Goodfellow, M., Eds.; John Wiley & Sons, Ltd.: Chichester, UK, 1991; pp. 115–175.
39. Alippi, A.M.; López, A.C.; Aguilar, O.M. A PCR-based method that permits specific detection of *Paenibacillus larvae* subsp. larvae, the cause of American Foulbrood of honey bees, at the subspecies level. *Lett. Appl. Microbiol.* **2004**, *39*, 25–33. [CrossRef] [PubMed]
40. Morrissey, B.J.; Helgason, T.; Poppinga, L.; Funfhaus, A.; Genersch, E.; Budge, G.E. Biogeography of *Paenibacillus larvae*, the causative agent of American foulbrood, using a new multilocus sequence typing scheme. *Environ. Microbiol.* **2015**, *17*, 1414–1424. [CrossRef] [PubMed]
41. Versalovic, J.; Schneider, M.; De Bruijn, F.J.; Lupski, J.R. Genomic fingerprinting of bacteria using repetitive sequence-based polymerase chain reaction. *Methods Mol. Cell. Biol.* **1994**, *5*, 25–40.
42. Abràmoff, M.D.; Magalhães, P.J.; Ram, S.J. Image processing with ImageJ. *Biophotonics Int.* **2004**, *11*, 36–42.

12

Potential for Bacteriophage Endolysins to Supplement or Replace Antibiotics in Food Production and Clinical Care

Michael J. Love [1], Dinesh Bhandari [1,2], Renwick C. J. Dobson [1,3] and Craig Billington [1,2,*]

1 Biomolecular Interaction Centre and School of Biological Sciences, University of Canterbury, Christchurch 8041, New Zealand; michael.love@pg.canterbury.ac.nz (M.J.L.); dinesh.bhandari@esr.cri.nz (D.B.); renwick.dobson@canterbury.ac.nz (R.C.J.D.)
2 Institute of Environmental Science and Research, Christchurch 8041, New Zealand
3 Department of Biochemistry and Molecular Biology, University of Melbourne, Melbourne 3052, Australia
* Correspondence: craig.billington@esr.cri.nz

Abstract: There is growing concern about the emergence of bacterial strains showing resistance to all classes of antibiotics commonly used in human medicine. Despite the broad range of available antibiotics, bacterial resistance has been identified for every antimicrobial drug developed to date. Alarmingly, there is also an increasing prevalence of multidrug-resistant bacterial strains, rendering some patients effectively untreatable. Therefore, there is an urgent need to develop alternatives to conventional antibiotics for use in the treatment of both humans and food-producing animals. Bacteriophage-encoded lytic enzymes (endolysins), which degrade the cell wall of the bacterial host to release progeny virions, are potential alternatives to antibiotics. Preliminary studies show that endolysins can disrupt the cell wall when applied exogenously, though this has so far proven more effective in Gram-positive bacteria compared with Gram-negative bacteria. Their potential for development is furthered by the prospect of bioengineering, and aided by the modular domain structure of many endolysins, which separates the binding and catalytic activities into distinct subunits. These subunits can be rearranged to create novel, chimeric enzymes with optimized functionality. Furthermore, there is evidence that the development of resistance to these enzymes may be more difficult compared with conventional antibiotics due to their targeting of highly conserved bonds.

Keywords: endolysin; antibiotics; antimicrobial resistance; one health; protein engineering

---

1. Introduction

In 2014, the World Health Organization (WHO) calculated the global prevalence of seven antibiotic-resistant bacteria of international concern, and noted very high rates of resistance (up to 84% of all isolates for methicillin, 81% for third-generation cephalosporins, 49% for fluoroquinolones, and 60% for penicillin) in all WHO regions [1]. In response to this unprecedented crisis, in late 2016 the United Nations General Assembly called upon the WHO, the Food and Agriculture Organization of the United Nations, and the World Organisation for Animal Health to develop a global development and stewardship framework [2]. This request recognized that there was a need to co-ordinate action against antimicrobial resistance in humans, agriculture, animals, and the environment by using a One Health [3] approach. One of the key recommendations in the draft framework was to develop new antimicrobial agents for use in these key sectors.

Here, we discuss the potential of cell wall lysis proteins (endolysins) derived from bacteriophages for use as a new class of antimicrobial agents, and evaluate whether they could replace, or supplement, some of the conventional antibiotics used to treat animals and humans, and perhaps even find use in food production and environmental decontamination processes.

Endolysins are enzymes encoded by bacteriophages (phage; obligate viruses of bacteria) which lyse the host bacterial cell. Endolysins degrade the main structural component of the cell wall (peptidoglycan) at the conclusion of the replicative cycle to release newly assembled progeny phage [4] (Figure 1). Recombinantly expressed endolysins display similarly effective lytic abilities to their native counterparts when applied exogenously to susceptible bacteria [5]. This feature underpins the application of endolysins in medicine, food and agriculture.

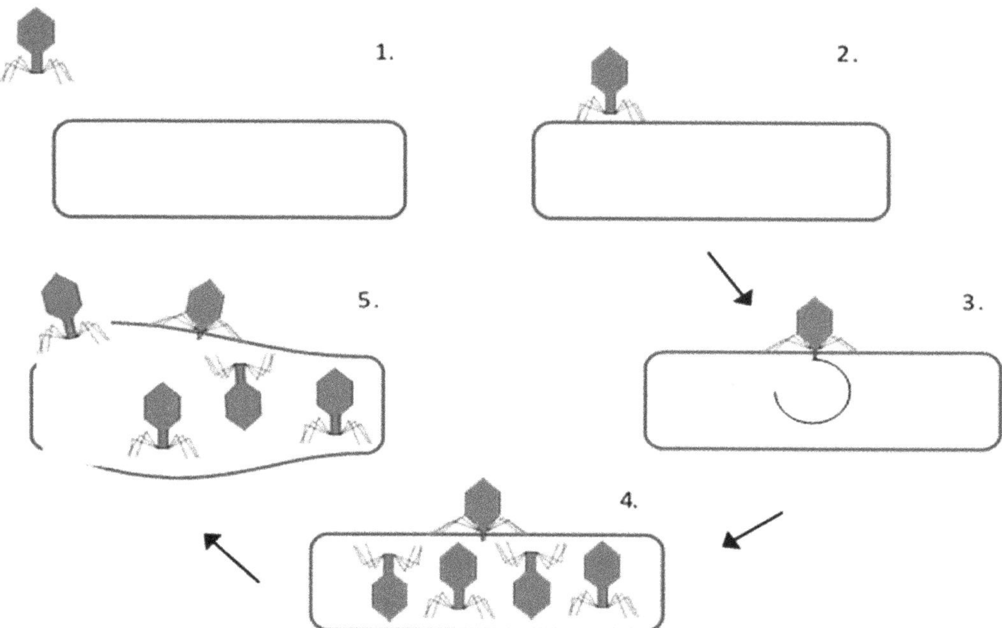

Figure 1. Life cycle of a virulent tailed phage (not to scale). (1) The phage collides with the bacterial cell; (2) the phage binds to cell receptors; (3) the phage is irreversibly bound and injects nucleic acid into the cell via the tail tube, where it is transcribed and translated; (4) many progeny phages are produced within intact cells; (5) endolysins degrade the host bacterial cell wall, which loses its structural integrity and ruptures due to the osmotic pressure, releasing the progeny phages.

Endolysins are predominantly more effective against Gram-positive bacteria than Gram-negative bacteria when applied in this way. The outer membrane of Gram-negative bacteria presents a physical protective barrier against the activity of endolysins [6]. Therefore, endolysin research has mainly focused on Gram-positive bacteria. However, recent work on outer membrane permeabilizers (chemicals and engineered peptides) should increase the prospects of endolysins for treating Gram-negative bacteria.

Numerous types of endolysins have been described, and are typically categorized by the structural bonds in the peptidoglycan that are cleaved by the enzyme [7] (Figure 2). The two alternating glycosidic bonds between the amino sugar moieties, *N*-acetylglucosamine and *N*-acetylmuramic acid (MurNAc), are targeted by different endolysin classes. The *N*-acetylmuramoyl-β-1,4-*N*-acetylglucosamine bond is cleaved by lytic transglycosylases and *N*-acetyl-β-D-muramidases, which are commonly known as lysozymes, while the *N*-acetylglucosaminyl-β-1,4-*N*-acetylmuramine bond is hydrolysed by *N*-acetyl-glucosaminyl-β-D-glucosaminidases. The cleavage of the amide linkage between MurNAc and L-alanine is catalyzed by *N*-acetylmuramoyl-L-alanine amidases. There are different endopeptidases depending on the chemical structure of the peptidoglycan, which is dependent on species and growth conditions. Generally, endopeptidases hydrolyze the peptide bonds between the amino acids that form the cross-linking peptide stems [8–10].

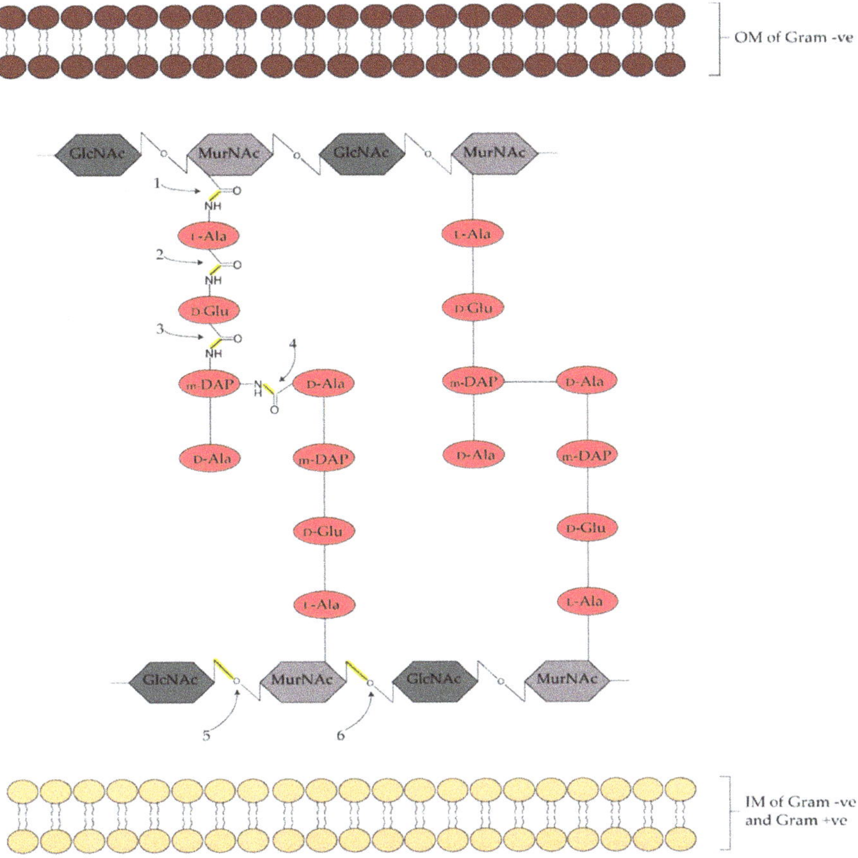

Figure 2. Diagram of the typical cell wall and peptidoglycan structure of bacteria, including the endolysin cleavage sites. The peptidoglycan is composed of repeating sugar units, *N*-acetylglucosamine (GlcNAc) and *N*-acetylmuramic acid (MurNAc), which are cross-linked via an interpeptide bridge between the *meso*-diaminopimelic acid (m-DAP) and D-alanine (D-Ala) residues of adjacent tetrapeptide chains. The chains also contain L-alanine (L-Ala) and D-glutamic acid (D-Glu). Gram-negative bacteria contain an outer membrane (OM) structure not present in Gram-positive bacteria. Both contain an inner membrane (IM) structure. The cleaved bonds and major classifications of endolysin are indicated: (1) *N*-acetylmuramoyl-L-alanine amidase; (2–4) various endopeptidases; (5) N-acetyl-β-D-glucosaminidase; (6) N-acetyl-β-D-muramidase (lysozyme).

A number of promising endolysins have been isolated from phage for application as antimicrobial agents, as described in this review and others [5–9]. However, the bioengineering of modified or novel endolysins also holds promise for the future development of effective tools to kill or detect bacteria. The prospects for engineering are facilitated by the enzymes' structures. The domain structure of endolysins can be modular (Gram-positive bacteria and some Gram-negative species) or globular (most Gram-negative bacteria), with most bioengineering strategies exploiting the modular endolysins. These enzymes usually comprise two distinct domains: an N-terminal enzymatically-active domain and a C-terminal cell wall-binding domain, connected by short, flexible linker regions. N-terminal enzymatically-active domains are responsible for catalyzing the breakdown of specific peptidoglycan bonds, while the C-terminal cell wall-binding domains recognize and bind non-covalently to substrate within the cell wall, resulting in the specificity of the lytic enzymes for the target host [5,8]. In addition, the C-terminal cell wall-binding domain is often required to maintain full lytic activity [11–13]. Interestingly, truncation or deletion of the C-terminal cell wall-binding domain can also result in equal or increased lytic activity [14–16]. In contrast, globular endolysins only contain catalytic domains.

The modular endolysin arrangement can be exploited for bioengineering, as the different domains can be shuffled within the protein, or domains from different endolysins can be combined to generate new enzymes [17,18]. Directed mutagenesis is also an effective strategy, as different amino acids may support improved lytic or binding properties [5,8,17,18]. The seemingly limitless possible permutations of endolysin modular arrangements allow for the development of new enzymes with specific functions or features. Some potential bioengineering strategies and examples of endolysin constructs are shown in Table 1.

Table 1. Possible molecular engineering strategies with potential application(s).

Modification	Property	Example	Reference
Truncation of full-length enzyme	Increased catalytic ability and solubility	CHAPk	Horgan et al. [19]
Fusion of EADs with CBDs of different endolysins	Increased catalytic ability and solubility	ClyS	Daniel et al. [20]
	Increased catalytic ability and broader lytic spectrum	SA2-E-Lyso-SH3b, SA2-E-LysK-SH3b	Schmelcher et al. [21]
	Thermostability	PlyGVE2CpCWB	Swift et al. [22]
Fusion of virion-associated lysin with CBD of endolysin	Increased efficacy	EC300	Proença et al. [23]
Endolysin fusion with OMP	Increased efficacy towards Gram-negative bacteria	OBPgp279, PVP-SE1g-146	Briers et al. [24]
Endolysin fusion with AMP	Increased efficacy towards Gram-negative bacteria	Art-175	Briers et al. [25]
Truncation and site-directed mutagenesis	AMP development	LysAB2	Peng et al. [26]

EAD: enzymatically-active domain; CBD: cell wall-binding domain; OMP: outer-membrane permeabilizer; AMP: antimicrobial peptide.

Both bioengineered and phage-isolated endolysins are promising alternatives to antibiotics. Their specificity allows them to target specific bacterial pathogens without affecting the microflora [11], or alternatively, target a larger spectrum for broader efficacy [27]. At the moment, developed resistance to the activity of the endolysins has not been widely reported, meaning these enzymes could be a long-term solution to antibiotics [28–30]. Endolysins may also have potential as diagnostic tools for bacterial identification [31]. In the following sections, we provide an overview of native and chimeric endolysins with potential therapeutic applications.

2. Endolysins as Human Therapeutics

As the efficacy of antibiotics decreases, once easily-treated bacterial infections will become potentially fatal. This will also have secondary effects in clinical care, such as changing risk-benefit considerations for invasive surgeries. Phage-encoded lytic enzymes have the potential to fulfil the need for novel antibacterial therapeutic agents for use in humans. This new class of antimicrobials has been recognized by the United States of America in the National Action Plan for Combating Antibiotic-resistant Bacteria [32], which identified the use of "phage-derived lysins to kill specific bacteria while preserving the microbiota" as a key strategy to reduce the development of antimicrobial resistance.

Methicillin-resistant *Staphylococcus aureus* (MRSA) is a significant public health concern, causing a range of skin and respiratory infections, as well as food-borne illnesses that are not easily treatable with currently available antibiotics [33]. O'Flaherty et al. [27] treated a human-derived MRSA strain with *Lactococcus lactis* cell lysate containing recombinantly overexpressed endolysin LysK, and observed a 99% reduction in colony-forming units at 1 h post-exposure. However, the researchers had difficulties obtaining soluble protein, which would hinder future applications of LysK, a difficulty that was also encountered in subsequent studies [34,35]. A stability study was conducted on LysK, as medical application requires a stable enzyme [34]. LysK was stabilized in the presence of low molecular weight polyols such as sucrose and glycerol, for example, stability increased 100-fold at 30 °C, and LysK retained 100% activity after storage up to 1 month at room temperature. This stability, under simple condition changes, is useful for developing treatment strategies [34]. LysK contains two catalytic domains: a cysteine- and histidine-dependent amidohydrolase/peptidase (CHAP) domain, and an *N*-acetylmuramoyl-L-alanine amidase domain. In an attempt to overcome the solubility issue, Horgan et al. [19] generated a single-domain truncated LysK mutant, designated CHAPk, containing only the CHAP domain. Soluble CHAPk was easier to obtain than full-length LysK, and displayed at least a two-fold increase in lytic activity against both heat-killed and live staphylococcal cells in vitro. Subsequent studies demonstrated that CHAPk was also effective in vivo, and that the loss of the C-terminal cell wall-binding domain, which directs specificity, resulted in activity against a broader range of targets compared with full-length CHAPk [36,37].

Jun et al. [38] compared LysK with SAL-1, an endolysin that differs by three residues. They also produced six derivatives of SAL-1 containing mutations in each of the three residues to investigate the impact of each mutation. SAL-1 displayed cell-wall hydrolytic activity approximately two-fold greater than that of LysK. The mutation of residue 114 from glutamatic acid in LysK to glutamine in SAL-1 had the largest impact on activity. This residue is located inside the catalytic CHAP domain, and the structurally minor sequence change corresponded to enhanced activity. The combination of such enhanced activity with the identification and mechanistic characterization of key residues of different enzymes is important for rational design and engineering of new endolysins with optimized activity [38]. Compared with LysK, SAL-1 had increased catalytic activity, and high yields of soluble protein were easier to obtain; therefore, SAL-1 may be a more promising antibiotic alternative than LysK [39]. The therapeutic application of SAL-1 is currently being trialed by iNtRON Biotechnology in the form of SAL200, an endolysin-based candidate drug for the treatment of *S. aureus*. A preclinical safety study of SAL200 observed no toxicity in rodent intravenous single- and repeat-dose studies [40]. A repeat-dose experiment was also performed in dogs, with each dog receiving four doses of 0, 0.5, 12.5 and 25 mg/kg in 1-week intervals over four weeks. After ten days, short-lived (i.e., lasting only 30 minutes to 1 hour) and mild clinical signs were observed including, vomiting, subdued behavior and irregular respiration. The transient response of the dogs to SAL200 administration was linked to complement system activation that resulted from antibody production [40]. A follow-up study in monkeys investigated the impact of single-dose escalation (up to 80 mg/kg) or 5-day multiple-dose (up to 40 mg/kg/day) administration of SAL200, with no adverse effects observed [41] SAL200 was further evaluated in a human single dose-escalating (up to 10 mg/kg) study. This study was the first in-human clinical study of a intravenously administered endolysin-based drug [42]. The volunteers had a reasonable tolerability to SAL200, with no significant adverse effects and most of the adverse effects were mild and self-limited. Although an increased concentration of antibodies was observed, the antibody concentration of participants administered 3.0 mg/kg was greater than that of those administered 10 mg/kg, with large variation within the different cohorts. The immunogenicity of SAL200 should, therefore, be a focus of future studies in order to better develop treatment regimes [42]. A phase II clinical study is now being conducted on patients with persistent *S. aureus* bacteremia, with results expected in 2018. Overall, the current evaluations shows a promising future for not just SAL200, but also for the development of other endolysin-based drug treatments.

Biofilm formation in clinical environments and on medical devices can have significant medical implications, as biofilms can harbor pathogenic and multidrug-resistant bacteria. Microorganisms within biofilms are protected by extracellular polymeric substances (EPS), which are a source of environmental contamination when partially dislodged. EPS can contain polysaccharides, proteins, phospholipids, teichoic acids, nucleic acids, and polymers, and protect the biofilm inhabitants by concentrating nutrients, preventing access of biocides, sequestering metals and toxins, and preventing desiccation [43]. Linden et al. [44] found that recombinantly-expressed PlyGRCS (from the phage GRCS) effectively lysed *S. aureus* in a biofilm, as well as in stationary phase. PlyGRCS contains a single enzymatically-active domain that can cleave two different bonds in peptidoglycan. This bifunctional domain could be highly useful in developing endolysins with effective lytic activity.

Rashel et al. [45] found that a dose of the phage ϕMR11-derived lysin MV-L rescued mice from fatal levels of MRSA exposure. In addition, MV-L in combination with vancomycin killed vancomycin-resistant strains. MV-L was specific for *S. aureus* and *Staphylococcus simulans*, with no lytic activity observed against other staphylococcal strains or bacterial species, including *Staphylococcus epidermidis* and *Escherichia coli*. Although excessive exposure to MV-L induced the production of antibodies, no adverse effects on the mice or impact on the efficacy of MV-L was observed.

Daniel et al. [20] demonstrated the potential of bioengineering to generate enzymes with novel and specific lytic activity against MRSA. The endolysin ClyS was constructed from the enzymatically active domain of a *S. aureus* Twort phage lysin fused with the cell wall-binding domain of phiNM3. Mice were exposed to MRSA strains that were resistant to the antibiotic oxacillin. A dose of ClyS increased survival rates to 88%, compared with the 0% survival rate for untreated mice. Treatment of infected mice with a sub-therapeutic concentration of ClyS in combination with oxacillin increased survival rates when compared with each treatment alone. This synergistic relationship with antibiotics may have widespread potential, and reinitiate the use of historical antibiotics that have been discontinued due to resistance concerns.

Schuch et al. [46] further showed this synergistic potential with the lysin CF-301. Mice with staphylococcal-induced bacteremia had a survival time of less than 24 h without treatment. Following individual treatments with CF-301 and daptomycin at 4 h post-inoculation, survival rates after 72 h were measured at 13% and 23%, respectively. Combination therapy yielded a survival rate of 73%. The study further confirmed the efficacy of co-therapy in 16 individual experiments including the antibiotics oxacillin and vancomycin. The immunogenicity of CF-301 was briefly evaluated in vitro; rabbit antisera raised against CF-301 did not inhibit the activity of CF-301 [46]. Despite the in vitro results, the immunogenic nature of CF-301 needs to be studied in a range of model organisms in vivo, because there may be clinically relevant adverse effects. CF-301 also has anti-biofilm activity [47], and clinical phase I trials are now underway to evaluate CF-301 as an alternative to traditional antibiotics, with an expected study completion in late 2018.

Thermal injury patients are usually also immunocompromised, meaning they are more susceptible to bacterial infection, including drug-resistant *S. aureus* strains [48]. Chopra et al. [49] investigated the use of endolysin MR-10 alone and in combination with minocycline to treat burn wound infections in mice. The control mice, inoculated with *S. aureus* and receiving no medical treatment, had a 100% mortality rate within 5 days. Individually, MR-10 (50 μg/ml) and minocycline (50 mg/kg) both resulted in a survival rate of 35% at 5 days post-inoculation, but 100% mortality was observed by day 7. In contrast, 100% survival was observed following treatment with a combination of the therapeutic agents at the same concentrations. These findings further support the future use of endolysins in medicine, especially in co-therapy with existing antibiotics.

Staphefekt is an endolysin bioengineered to selectively target *S. aureus* strains, including MRSA. It is currently available as a component of gels and creams for over-the-counter treatment of infections [50,51]. Its specificity for *S. aureus* is an important feature in the treatment of skin infections, as it prevents the disturbance of commensal bacteria, which can cause further health complications [52]. Evidence for the efficacy of Staphefekt is limited; there are few available publications describing the rationale of engineering or the in vitro properties and structure of the endolysin. However, a recent report by Totté et al. [51] demonstrated the efficacy of Staphefekt in treating three different patients with recurrent *S. aureus*-related dermatoses that had previously been unsuccessfully treated with antibiotics. Despite the limited published evidence, these brief findings suggest a promising future for Staphefekt as a long-term alternative to antibiotics.

Enterococcus faecalis is the third most common cause of life-threatening nosocomial infections [53], and is intrinsically resistant to antibiotics [54]. Although vancomycin is considered a drug of last resort, a growing number of vancomycin-resistant *E. faecalis* strains have been isolated. [55,56].

An endolysin isolated from phage ϕ1, PlyV12, kills a variety of *E. faecalis* strains in vitro, including vancomycin-resistant isolates. PlyV12 also showed a broad spectrum of lethality against a variety of streptococcal and staphylococcal strains, highlighting it as a promising candidate in antibacterial medicine [57]. Son et al. [58] also identified a novel phage, EFAP-1, which was not significantly similar to any previously identified phages. The endolysin of EFAP-1, EFAL-1, exhibited lytic activity against 24 different strains of bacteria, including vancomycin-resistant *E. faecalis* strains and four streptococcal strains, whereas the phage itself only showed activity against *E. faecalis*. There is a lack of in vivo studies of *E. faecalis* endolysins. Such studies are important because *E. faecalis* is also a commensal bacterium found in the human gut, and therefore the potential impact of endolysins on the gut microbiota needs to be understood [52]. Zhang et al. [59] isolated phage IME-EF1 and its endolysin from hospital sewage, and investigated their ability to rescue mice from lethal challenge with *E. faecalis*. Individually, both the phage and the endolysin reduced the bacterial count in the blood of infected animals. However, a 200-μg dose of the endolysin at 30 min post-bacterial inoculation supported a higher survival rate (80%) than that observed following phage treatment alone (60%) [59].

The endolysin LysEF-P10, derived from *E. faecalis* phage EF-P10, has also been studied in a mouse model. A single dose of just 5 μg was enough to protect mice from vancomycin-resistant *E. faecalis* infection, suggesting promising protective efficacy of LysEF-P10 against vancomycin-resistant *E. faecalis* strains. Furthermore, when the mice were subjected to a large dose of 5 mg, no side effects were observed. The administration of EF-P10 stimulated specific antibody production, however, there was no impact on the bactericidal activity of the enzyme. Treatment with EF-P10 did not negatively affect the gut microbiota, owing to the specificity of the lysin. Although *E. faecalis* in the normal gut microbiota may have been targeted, no significant health impact on the mice was observed [60]. Proença et al. [23] constructed a bacteriolysin-like enzyme to target *E. faecalis*. The construct, EC300, was created from the fusion of the peptidase domain from a virion-associated lysin and the cell wall-binding domain of Lys170, both found in phage F170/08. EC300 inhibited the growth of *E. faecalis* in bacterial culture media, whereas the parental endolysin Lys170 showed limited inhibition. The enhanced lytic and killing ability of EC300 highlights the potential for engineered endolysins compared with wild-type enzymes.

Streptococcal infections are associated with a range of clinical manifestations, including strep throat, pneumonia, skin infections, and meningitis [61,62]. Drug resistant streptococcal strains are also increasing in prevalence. Loeffler et al. [28] examined the potential of the endolysin Pal to kill *S. pneumoniae* that had colonized the nasopharynx of mice. Pal was effective against 15 different strains of pneumococci, including some drug-resistant strains, reducing *S. pneumoniae* to undetectable levels within 5 h of treatment. The same research group [63] then examined the antibacterial ability of a previously described lytic enzyme, Cpl-1 [64]. Rabbit antiserum was raised against Cpl-1 and the impact on bacterial lysis measured. Only a small amount of inhibition was measured, showing the antibodies had little effect on the enzymatic activity [63]. In the same study, these findings were corroborated in vivo. Mice that were subjected to several doses of Cpl-1 tested positive for IgG. These immunized mice along with naïve mice were challenged with *S. pneumoniae*. Comparatively, no significant difference was measured with regards to the reduction of bacteria numbers by the enzyme [64]. Mice intravenously infected with *S. pneumoniae* and treated only with buffer had a median survival time of 30.75 h, with no mice surviving at 72 h post-infection. Mice treated with Cpl-1 at 5 and 10 h post-infection had a median survival time of 60 h, although after 96 h, only one mouse survived. Although the potential for complete eradication of the bacteria was shown, the dosage used in the experiments was not high enough, meaning that all animals eventually succumbed to infection. Therefore, for greater efficacy of Cpl-1, a higher dose would be required [63].

Subsequent studies demonstrated the effectiveness of Cpl-1 combination therapy with lytic enzyme Pal, or with antibiotics [65–67]. In vivo mouse model studies demonstrated these Cpl-1 treatments were effective in the treatment of pneumococcal diseases such as sepsis [68], endocarditis [69], meningitis [70], and pneumonia [71,72]. Despite its demonstrable antibacterial activity, a key limitation of Cpl-1 is its half-life in blood of only 20.5 min in mice [63,69]. Resch et al. [72] introduced specific cysteine residues into Cpl-1 to promote disulfide bond formation and subsequent dimerization. Dimerization is required for full activity of LytA, a pneumococcal autolysin [73], with which Cpl-1 shares extensive sequence similarity. Dimerized Cpl-1 displayed a two-fold increase in antimicrobial activity and had a nearly ten-fold decrease in plasma clearance, resulting in an increased half-life. These enhanced properties not only increase the prospects for Cpl-1 application, but also highlight the potential for enhanced activity through structural changes and engineering.

The exogenous treatment of Gram-negative bacteria with endolysins has been limited because of the presence of the outer membrane, which prevents access to the peptidoglycan layer [74]. Overcoming this protective layer is a major obstacle in developing endolysin-based treatments. Most studies have focused on nosocomial pathogens *Acinetobacter baumannii* and *Pseudomonas aeruginosa*, both of which are Gram-negative and capable of forming biofilms. Multidrug-resistant strains of both pathogens are also being increasingly isolated [75–78]. Some endolysins can intrinsically permeate the outer membrane [79–81]. Lai et al. [79] recombinantly expressed LysAB2 from ϕAB2 and applied it to *A. baumannii*. The C-terminus of LysAB2 contains an amphipathic α-helix that interacts with the negatively charged elements of the outer membrane, facilitating the formation of a transmembrane pore [82]. This allows the N-terminus catalytic domain to interact with the peptidoglycan layer and lyse the cell, achieving antibacterial activity. Lood et al. [80] identified and screened 21 different endolysins for sequence diversity and *A. baumannii*-killing activity. The endolysins displayed varying degrees of antibacterial activity, with the lysin PlyF307 exhibiting the greatest activity. The C-terminus of PlyF307 contains a highly positively charged region, which may interact with the outer membrane. PlyF307 successfully killed both planktonic cells and, more importantly, those within biofilms, providing an advantage over antibiotics. PlyF307 also functioned under physiological conditions, rescuing mice treated with lethal doses of *A. baumannii*. There remains a library of lysins for structural and biochemical characterization from this research.

Walmagh et al. [81] showed that OBPgp279, from the phage OBP, can permeate the outer membrane of *P. aeruginosa*. It does not appear to contain an amphipathic helix, and thus the mechanism of permeabilization is unclear. OBPgp279 may therefore contain novel structural elements that could lend themselves to the engineering of new endolysins to target Gram-negative bacteria [81]. The lysin LysPA26 from phage JD010 has antibacterial activity against both planktonic and biofilm-contained *P. aeruginosa* cells, as well as other Gram-negative species such as *E. coli* and *Klebsiella pneumoniae*. However, LysPA26 was ineffective against Gram-positive species, including *S. aureus*. This specificity may allow for selective targeting of Gram-negative species in medical treatments [83].

Strategies employing endolysins in conjunction with antibiotics or outer membrane-permeabilizing agents have been explored. Thummeepak et al. [84] investigated the use of LysABP-01 in combination with colistin for treatment of hospital-isolated strains of *A. baumannii*. Although LysABP-01 alone prevented growth, elevated levels of antibacterial activity were observed in combination with colistin. Additionally, the minimum inhibitory concentrations of LysABP-01 and colistin were reduced 32-fold and by up to eight-fold, respectively, when used in combination, compared with individual application. Endolysin EL188, from phage EL, combined with EDTA reduced *P. aeruginosa* cell counts by up to four log units, whereas EL188 on its own exhibited no antibacterial activity [85]. However, the use of EDTA would be restricted to topical applications because of its ability to inhibit blood coagulation [86].

Artilysin bioengineering has also shown promise in targeting Gram-negative bacteria. Artilysins are created through the fusion of outer membrane-permeabilizing peptides, which interfere with the stabilizing forces within the outer membrane, with endolysins. These fusion proteins allow the uptake of an endolysin across the outer membrane, providing access to the peptidoglycan layer [87]. Initially, two endolysins, OBPgp279 and PVP-SE1g-146, fused with one of seven different peptides were investigated for their antibacterial activity. Although the endolysins exhibited limited antibacterial activity on their own, fusion with polycationic nonapeptide correlated with up to a 2.6 log reduction of *P. aeruginosa* in only 30 min. Moderate antibacterial activity against *A. baumannii*, *E. coli*, and *Salmonella* Typhimurium was also observed. The mode of action was examined using time-lapse microscopy, confirming that the artilysins were passing through the outer membrane and degrading the peptidoglycan [24].

Briers et al. [25] developed Art-175, composed of the antimicrobial peptide (AMP) sheep myeloid 29-amino acid peptide (SMAP-29) fused with endolysin KZ144, to target *P. aeruginosa*. AMPs are involved in the innate immune response, and can move across the outer membrane [88]. Art-175 reduced the *P. aeruginosa* cell count by up to 4 log units compared with untreated controls, and continuous exposure to Art-175 to exert a selection pressure did not elicit the development of resistance. On its own, SMAP-29 is cytotoxic to mammalian cells [89]; however, Art-175 exhibited little toxicity in L-292 mouse connective tissue. As a result of these findings, Peng et al. [26] developed AMPs based on the amino acid sequence of LysAB2. The synthesized AMPs killed *A. baumannii* cells by permeating the outer membrane in vitro. Treatment with the AMPs also increased the survival rate of mice infected with a lethal dose of *A. baumannii* by 60%. This research highlights a novel method of bioengineering endolysins for use as antimicrobials.

3. Endolysins as Veterinary Treatments

In response to widespread concern regarding the overuse of antibiotics in food-producing animals, many major food suppliers are now committed to phasing out prophylactic antibiotic use and the tighter control of therapeutic treatments. This presents obvious challenges for the animal-husbandry industry, which may be overcome by the use of endolysins. Companion and working animals can also be susceptible to recalcitrant microbial infections, including those caused by multidrug-resistant microorganisms, and so may also benefit from endolysin treatment.

Clostridium perfringens is a leading cause of necrotic enteritis and sub-clinical disease in poultry, and can lead to significant economic losses [90]. Swift et al. [22] constructed recombinant endolysin PlyGVE2CpCWB, which shows enhanced thermostability, an important feature for surviving feed heat treatments. The recombinant endolysin contains an amidase domain from an endolysin derived from a thermophilic phage fused with the cell wall-recognition domain from *C. perfringens*-specific phage endolysin PlyCP26F, which is not resistant to high temperatures. PlyGVE2CpCWB inactivated *C. perfringens* in both liquid and solid media at temperatures up to 50 °C, and so may be a promising antimicrobial feed treatment for controlling necrotic enteritis in poultry. This thermostable construct demonstrates the potential for other thermophilic bacteriophage endolysins to be utilized in bioengineering. A different approach to *C. perfringens* control was taken by Gervasi et al. [91,92], whereby an amidase endolysin (CP25L) was cloned and expressed in a *Lactobacillus johnsonii* strain isolated from poultry. In co-cultures, reductions of up to 2.6 $\log_{10}$ CFU·ml^{-1} *C. perfringens* were noted; however, the reduction was inconsistent between experiments, and the effect declined significantly over time. This reduced activity was attributed to a loss in stability of the endolysin in culture, and a reduction in the viability of *L. johnsonii*. Other researchers [93,94] have also performed detailed analyses, including X-ray crystallography, on another *C. perfringens* endolysin, Psm, which may have applications in poultry. Psm is an *N*-acetylmuramidase endolysin with wide activity against *C. perfringens* strains.

Another economically significant disease in animal husbandry is bovine mastitis, which is caused by a variety of bacteria, of which staphylococci and streptococci account for 75% of cases [95]. In studies aimed at treating bovine mastitis caused by *S. aureus*, Schmelcher et al. [21] demonstrated that fusion of an endopeptidase endolysin domain from a *Streptococcus* lambda phage (SA2) with either lysostaphin (SA2-E-Lyso-SH3b) or staphylococcal phage endolysin LysK (SA2-E-LysK-SH3b) could inhibit staphylococci in a murine mammary mastitis model. The extended lytic spectrum targeting multiple genera would be particularly useful for efficiently treating bovine mastitis [96]. Infusion of 25 µg of SA2-E-Lyso-SH3b or SA2-E-LysK-SH3b into the mammary glands reduced *S. aureus* counts by 0.63 and 0.81 $\log_{10}$ CFU·mg^{-1}, respectively. Additional testing of SA2-E-LysK-SH3b and lysostaphin in combination (12.5 μg/gland) revealed a 3.36 $\log_{10}$ CFU·mg^{-1} reduction in the concentration of *S. aureus* compared with the control [21]. Further work by the same group [97], determined the potential of the lambda SA2 and phage B30 (a CHAP endopeptidase) endolysins in combination as a therapeutic treatment of *Streptococcus*-induced mastitis, again in a murine mastitis model. The best results obtained by the study were reductions of 1.5 $\log_{10}$ CFU·mg^{-1} against *Streptococcus uberis* (SA2), 4.6 $\log_{10}$ CFU·mg^{-1} against *Streptococcus agalactiae* (B30), and 2.2 $\log_{10}$ CFU·mg^{-1} against *Streptococcus dysgalactiae* (SA2). More recently, purified endolysin Trx-SA1, isolated from *S. aureus* phage IME-SA1, was used to treat naturally infected cow udders [98]. Udder quarters received an intramammary infusion of 20 mg of Trx-SA1 once per day, and qualitative reductions in somatic cell counts and *S. aureus* numbers were noted over the three-day regime.

Anthrax, a potentially fatal zoonotic disease affecting a wide variety of species, is a threat to wild and farmed animals as well as humans, especially as a biological weapon [99,100]. Schuch et al. [29] reported the usefulness of PlyG lysin, isolated from the γ-phage of *Bacillus anthracis*, in killing vegetative cells and germinating spores of *B. anthracis* and streptomycin-resistant *Bacillus cereus* RSVF1. The researchers screened an expression library of cloned γ-phage DNA sequences and identified a 702-bp open reading frame (ORF) encoding a protein with homology to an amidase-type endolysin. When PlyG was injected intraperitoneally (50 U in 0.5 mL) into mice infected with 6 $\log_{10}$ CFU RSVF1, a notable therapeutic effect was observed, with 68.4% (13/19) of mice showing full recovery. Furthermore, the survival time of the remaining mice was prolonged to 21 h post-infection.

Equine strangles is a highly contagious disease of horses caused by *Streptococcus equi*. The disease progresses as an inflammation of the upper respiratory tract, and leads to abscess formation in the retropharyngeal lymph node [101]. Strangles is a significant economic threat to the horse racing industry, where many high value animals are typically housed in close proximity. Hoopes et al. [102] used PlyC, an unusual multimeric amidase-type endolysin [17], as a disinfectant against *S. equi* and reported it to be 1000 times more active on a per weight basis than the widely used disinfectant Virkon-S. PlyC was effective against >20 clinical isolates of *S. equi*, including both *S. equi* subsp. *equi* and *S. equi* subsp. *zooepidemicus*, demonstrating its sterilizing ability against an eight log CFU·ml^{-1} culture of *S. equi* within 30 min of exposure.

The clinical efficacy of a muramidase as a veterinary treatment for companion animals was demonstrated in a trial by Junjappa et al. [103], where they successfully treated 17 dogs suffering from pyoderma (bacterial skin lesions) caused by MRSA. The skin lesions were treated with a hydrogel containing a chimeric endolysin composed of the cell wall-targeting domain (SH3b) of lysostaphin and the phage K ORF56 muralytic domain [104]. Another important zoonotic pathogen, *Streptococcus suis*, has been linked to arthritis, meningitis, septicemia, and endocarditis in pigs, as well as in humans who have come into contact with infected animals or their byproducts. Wang et al. [105] isolated a phage from *S. suis* (SMP), and then expressed the endolysin LySMP in *E. coli* BL21. The resultant product, following chromatography and treatment with β-mercaptoethanol, killing 15 out of 17 clinical *S. suis* serotype 2 isolates from diseased pigs in China, and had demonstrated activity against *S. suis* serotype 7 and 9 strains, *S. equi* subsp. *zooepidemicus*, and *S. aureus* [105].

There is growing evidence to suggest that food-producing animals are an important global reservoir of vancomycin-resistant enterococci (VRE) [106,107]. This group of potentially invasive microorganisms is resistant to almost all of the available antibiotic regimens recommended for treatment of Gram-positive bacterial infections. In an attempt to combat VRE in food-producing animals, Yoong et al. [57] cloned the PlyV12-encoding gene from enterococcal phage Φ1 into the *E. coli*-*Bacillus* shuttle vector pDG148, followed by its expression in *Bacillus megaterium* strain WH320. The resultant product, an amidase-type endolysin, had lytic activity against 14 clinical and laboratory *E. faecalis* and *Enterococcus faecium* strains, including two vancomycin-resistant *E. faecalis* and three vancomycin-resistant *E. faecium* strains, in addition to its host, *E. faecalis* V12. Intriguingly, PlyV12 also had a significant killing effect on pathogenic streptococcal strains, including *Streptococcus pyogenes* (group A streptococcus) and group C streptococci.

Diarrheal outbreaks caused by *Clostridium difficile* have frequently been reported in animals, including cattle, horses, and pigs [108,109]. Treatment of *C. difficile* diarrhea with antibiotics is not recommended as it can further exacerbate the disease condition [110]. In a quest for an alternative approach to treat infections caused by *C. difficile*, Mayer et al. [111] sequenced the genome of a temperate phage from *C. difficile*. They identified endolysin gene *cd27l* and cloned it into vectors pET15b and pUK200 to express the gene product in *E. coli* and *L. lactis*, respectively. The purified endolysin was active against 30 diverse strains of *C. difficile*, including those belonging to the major epidemic ribotype, 027 (B1/NAP1). Unlike antibiotics, the endolysin was selective for *C. difficile*, demonstrating no activity against a range of commensal species from within the gastrointestinal tract, including other clostridia, bifidobacteria, and lactobacilli.

Paenibacillus larvae subsp. *larvae* causes American Foulbrood disease in honey bees, which are important insect pollinators of agricultural crops. The disease occurs in honeybee larvae as a result of *P. larvae* spores germinating in the larval midgut and subsequently causing sepsis and death. The use of antibiotics to treat the disease in the USA now requires supervision by a veterinarian, and a withholding period of 4–6 weeks is recommended for honey from treated hives prior to sale (https://www.fda.gov/AnimalVeterinary/ResourcesforYou/AnimalHealthLiteracy/ucm309134.htm). In the European Union, no veterinary medicines containing antibiotics are permitted in beekeeping (http://europroxima.com/european-legislation-regarding-antibiotics-in-honey-an-overview/). For these reasons, endolysins are being investigated as a potential alternative control tool. An amidase endolysin, PlyPl23, has been cloned from a *P. larvae* phage and subsequently expressed [112]. In bee larvae experimentally infected with spores, PlyPl23 effectively decreased the rate of *P. larvae* infection, and no toxic side effects were noted in the larvae. However, the endolysin was not effective until the spores had germinated.

4. Endolysins as Food and Environmental Decontaminants

During post-harvest processing, food is vulnerable to cross-contamination from microbial pathogens, which pose a risk to food safety, as well as from microorganisms that can cause quality or shelf-life defects. Effective interventions for foods and the food processing environment are therefore vital to maintain the integrity of the food supply chain. Endolysins have the potential to be key intervention tools for this purpose.

The use of endolysins to prevent contamination of ready-to-eat foods by the common food and environmental pathogen *Listeria monocytogenes* has been established by groups from around the world [16,113–117]. Zhang et al. [113] cloned an endolysin gene (*lysZ5*) from the genome of *L. monocytogenes* phage FWLLm3 into *E. coli* and tested the sterilization efficacy of the expressed protein (a murine hydrolase) in soya milk contaminated with *L. monocytogenes*. The purified protein had a bactericidal effect on *L. monocytogenes* growing in soya milk, with the pathogen concentration reduced by more than 4 $\log_{10}$ CFU·ml^{-1} after 3 h of incubation at 4 °C. Furthermore, the protein displayed a broad host spectrum, lysing lawn cultures of *L. monocytogenes*, *Listeria innocua*, and *Listeria welshimeri*. In a different approach, van Nassau et al. [114] tested the combined effect of previously characterized endolysins (PlyP40, Ply511, or PlyP825) and high hydrostatic pressure on the survival of *L. monocytogenes*. They reported that the combination of treatments had a synergistic effect, capable of reducing viable cell counts of *L. monocytogenes* by up to 5.5 $\log_{10}$, compared with 0.3 and 0.2 $\log_{10}$ CFU reductions, respectively, when used alone.

Turner et al. [115] and Gaeng et al. [16] demonstrated that the *L. monocytogenes* endolysin gene *ply511* can be cloned and expressed in *Lactobacillus* spp., which have potential as biopreservatives in foods and as a starter culture for fermented milk products. Further to this, Turner et al. [115] combined the cloned A511 phage *ply511* gene with a lysostaphin-encoding *lss* gene from *S. simulans* biovar *staphylolyticus* in-frame with a Sep secretion signal. The resulting construct, Sep-6_His-Ply511, was able to secrete both Ply511 and lysostaphin from *Lactobacillus lactis*, indicating that this recombinant organism could be used for industrial applications as a preservative to prevent contamination of foods with *Staphylococcus* spp. and *L. monocytogenes*.

Staphylococcal food poisoning caused by heat stable enterotoxins produced by *S. aureus* is frequently reported following the consumption of contaminated food and milk products [118]. Chang et al. [119] tested LysSA11, a *S. aureus* phage SA11-derived endolysin, to determine its bactericidal activity in food and on food utensils artificially contaminated with MRSA. Treatment of artificially contaminated ham and pasteurized milk with endolysin for 15 min resulted in 3.1 $\log_{10}$ CFU$\cdot$cm^{-3} and 1.4 $\log_{10}$ CFU$\cdot$ml^{-1} reductions in viable MRSA, respectively, at refrigeration temperature (4 °C), and 3.4 $\log_{10}$ CFU$\cdot$cm^{-3} and 2.0 $\log_{10}$ CFU$\cdot$ml ^{1} reductions, respectively, at room temperature (25 °C). The same group [120] tested the antibacterial potential of LysSA97 in combination with several active compounds derived from essential oils used by the food industry against *S. aureus*. They reported the superior activity of carvacrol in combination with LysSA97, compared with that of the endolysin alone, in food products including beef and milk contaminated with *S. aureus*. When used alone, LysSA97 and carvacrol reduced *S. aureus* concentrations by 0.8 and 1.0 $\log_{10}$ CFU$\cdot$ml^{-1}, respectively; however, a synergistic reduction of 4.5 $\log_{10}$ CFU$\cdot$ml^{-1} was observed when the treatments were combined. Similarly, Obeso et al. [121] and Rodriguez-Rubio et al. [122] demonstrated the potential of phage-derived endolysins LysH5 and HydH5 (a hydrolase), respectively, to protect milk products from *S. aureus* contamination.

Salmonella species are the leading cause of bacterial foodborne illness in the USA and many other countries [123]. *Salmonella* disease outbreaks are associated with a wide variety of food products, including red meats, poultry, and produce [124]. Several recombinant endolysins derived from *Salmonella* phages have been characterized [125–127]. Interestingly, many of these endolysins have activity outside of the host species of the parental phage, particularly when cell membrane-disrupting chemicals are used in conjunction with the enzymes. Lim et al. [125] expressed the endolysins and spanin proteins from *Salmonella* phage SPN1S and observed activity against both *Salmonella* Typhimurium and *E. coli* isolates in buffer containing EDTA to destabilize the cell membranes. Furthermore, some activity was also noted against typhoidal salmonellae, *Shigella*, *Cronobacter*, *Pseudomonas*, and *Vibrio* species. Oliveira et al. [126] characterized a thermostable *Salmonella* endolysin, Lys68, that displayed better activity at neutral pH and a wide temperature tolerance, maintaining 76.7% of its activity after 2 months at 4°C and partial activity following exposure to 100 °C for 30 min. Thermostability is a useful feature for diverse application, such as in heat treatment of food When Lys68 was tested in combination with citric or malic acid against *S.* Typhimurium LT2, up to 5 $\log_{10}$ CFU reductions were achieved, with cells in stationary phase or in biofilms also reduced by up to 1 $\log_{10}$ CFU [126]. More recently, Rodriguez-Rubio et al. [127] reported a *Salmonella* phage endolysin, Gp110, that possessed both a novel enzyme structure and N-acetylmuramidase lysis domain, and had unusually high in vitro activity against *Salmonella* and other Gram-negative pathogens [127].

Around the turn of the century, a rare but frequently fatal disease of neonatal infants was first reported to be associated with contamination of powdered infant milk formula with *Enterobacter* (now *Cronobacter*) *sakazakii* [128]. It is now known that several species of *Cronobacter* can cause a variety of diseases, including sepsis and severe meningitis, in neonates, as well as respiratory and urinary tract infections in elderly and immunocompromised individuals. These opportunistic pathogens are now under much scrutiny because of their ability to survive heat, desiccation, and acid stress, which poses a risk of contamination of various milk powders, herbal teas, and other dried products (https://www.cdc.gov/cronobacter/technical.html). Enderson et al. [129,130] expressed and purified a peptidoglycan hydrolase (LysCs4) from *C. sakazakii* that had the highest sequence similarity to a putative lysozyme from the temperate *Cronobacter* phage ES2. The purified lysozyme could degrade the peptidoglycan from both Gram-negative and Gram-positive bacteria belonging to six different genera, and could lyse outer membrane-permeabilized *C. sakazakii*. Similarly, the previously discussed endolysins SPN1S [125] and Lys68 [126] are active against permeabilized *C. sakazakii* cells.

Several groups have investigated the potential of endolysins active against *B. cereus* as biocides and preservatives for use in the food industry [131–133]. *B. cereus*, a Gram-positive spore-forming bacterium, is known for its ability to cause food poisoning by producing both an emetic toxin and a diarrheal toxin [131]. Loessner et al. [132] isolated and characterized three endolysins (PlyBa, Ply12, and Ply21) from the *B. cereus* phages Bastille, TP21, and 12826, respectively, and tested their efficacy against a range of Gram-positive and Gram-negative bacteria. They reported that all three endolysins were effective against 24 strains of *B. cereus*, along with several strains of *B. thuringiensis*. Ply12 and Ply21 were found to be *N*-acetylmuramoyl-L-alanine amidases, while PlyBa could not be classified at the time, but is also likely to be an amidase (http://www.uniprot.org/uniprot/P89927). Park et al. [133] isolated a putative endolysin gene from the genome of *B. cereus* phage BPS13, and expressed it in *E. coli*. The purified LysBPS13 protein, an amidase, retained its lytic activity against *B. cereus* ATCC 10876 even after incubation at 100 °C for 30 min, demonstrating its potential as a decontaminant in food processing applications. In contrast, Son et al. [131] proposed *L*-alanoyl-D-glutamate endopeptidase LysB4 as a potential biocontrol agent against *B. cereus* and other pathogenic bacteria. They confirmed the endopeptidase had a broad range of bactericidal activity against Gram-positive bacteria, including *B. cereus*, *B. subtilis*, and *L. monocytogenes*, and also a few Gram-negative bacteria. The endolysin showed optimum lytic activity at pH 8–10 and at 50 °C, making it a suitable candidate for use in the food industry.

In addition to causing diseases in poultry, clostridial species are linked to food spoilage. In the dairy industry, germinated *Clostridium sporogenes* and *Clostridium tyrobutyricum* can contribute to the production of gases and acids that change the structural and sensory qualities of cheeses [134]. Mayer et al. [135] isolated an *N*-acetylmuramoyl-L-alanine amidase, CS74L, from *C. sporogenes* and reported that the purified protein effectively lysed *C. sporogenes* cells when added exogenously. Using the turbidity assay and fresh bacterial cells, the authors also demonstrated that CS74L was active against *C. tyrobutyricum* and *Clostridium acetobutylicum*, making it a candidate biopreservative for use in cheese. The same group also characterized another endolysin isolated from a virulent phage, CPT1l, but this enzyme had a more limited host range [134].

The dairy industry has a long-held interest in utilizing endolysins to control the cheese maturation process. Vasala et al. [136] isolated a muramidase, Mur, from the LL-H phage of *Lactobacillus delbrueckii* subsp. *lactis* that had activity against cell wall preparations of *L. delbrueckii* subsp. *lactis*, *L. delbrueckii* subsp. *bulgaricus*, *Lactobacillus acidophilus*, *Lactobacillus helveticus*, and *Pediococcus damnosus*. Similarly, Deutsch et al. [137] purified endolysin Mur-LH from a phage infecting the Swiss cheese starter *L. helveticus*. This muramidase had activity against other lactobacilli, *Leuconostoc lactis*, *P. acidilactici*, and, surprisingly, against *B. subtilis*. Kashige et al. [138] isolated an *N*-acetylmuramoyl-L-alanine amidase from phage PL-1, which was originally isolated from an abnormal fermentation of a lactic acid beverage produced using a *Lactobacillus casei* strain. There are also many examples of endolysins isolated from lactococci, including from phages P001, C2 US3, and TUC2009 [136]. A survey of 18 *L. lactis* phage endolysins revealed that muramidases and amidases predominate [139].

In addition to the aforementioned enzymes, several other endolysins with potential to be used against a range of foodborne microorganisms in different food types have been identified, and selected examples of these are illustrated in Table 2.

Table 2. Examples of other potential uses of endolysins in foods.

Food	Organism	Endolysin	Reference
Fish	*Shewanella putrefaciens*	ORF62	Han et al. [140]
Vegetable fermentation	*Leuconostoc mesenteroides*	ORF35	Lu et al. [141]
Kimchi	*Lactobacillus plantarum*	SC921 lysin	Yoon et al. [142]
Pears	*Erwinia amylovora*	ΦEa1h lysozyme	Kim et al. [143]
Banana juice	*Salmonella* Typhimurium, *Yersinia enterocolitica*, *Escherichia coli O157:H7*, *Shigella flexneri*	λ lysozyme (with high pressure treatment)	Nakimbugwe et al. [144]

Table 2. *Cont.*

Food	Organism	Endolysin	Reference
Shellfish	*Vibrio parahaemolyticus*	Lysqdvp001	Wang et al. [145]
Lettuce	*Listeria innocua*	Ply500 (with packaging film)	Solanki et al. [146]
Milk	*Listeria monocytogenes*	PlyP825 (with high pressure treatment)	Misiou et al. [147]
Mozzarella cheese	*L. monocytogenes*	PlyP825 (with high pressure treatment)	Misiou et al. [147]

The growth of biofilms in food processing environments leads to an increased risk of microbial contamination of foods [148]. There are some examples of endolysins being used to disrupt biofilms with relevance to the food industry. Gutierrez et al. [149] investigated the activity of three endolysins (LysH5, CHAP-SH3b, and HydH5-SH3b) against biofilms formed by two *S. aureus* isolates from food. Preformed biofilms were treated with 7 μM of the enzymes, with LysH5 and CHAP-SH3b most effective against strains IPLA1 and Sa9, respectively. In another study, an *N*-acetylmuramoyl-L-alanine amidase was used to disrupt *Listeria* biofilms in vitro, but was found to be most effective when used in combination with a protease [150]. The *Salmonella*-phage endolysin Lys68 also reduced the concentration of cells in a *S.* Typhimurium LT2 biofilm by up to 1.2 $\log_{10}$ CFU [128], but this required the presence of either citric or maleic acid to permeabilize the cell membranes.

Phytopathogenic bacteria have a significant global economic cost, and are the cause of multiple food security issues [151]. The use of antibiotics in plant agriculture is controversial because its contribution to the development of antibiotic resistance in human pathogens is undetermined [152] Although its impact may be small, ideally, an alternative strategy to control phytopathogenic bacteria will be developed. As such, the use of endolysins to protect plants from bacterial diseases has been proposed [16]. Widespread implementation of these endolysins will, however, be a significant challenge because of the vast number of crops that would require treatment, and the presence of beneficial soil-borne bacteria. A proposed strategy is the development of transgenic crops that express endolysins, providing protection against the pathogenic bacteria. The potential of this approach has been demonstrated by Düring et al. [153], who produced transgenic potato plants expressing T4 lysozyme. These engineered plants displayed resistance to *Pectobacterium carotovora* (formerly *Erwinia carotovora*) species, which are the cause soft rot [153,154]. Wittmann et al. [155] produced transgenic tomato plants expressing the endolysins from bacteriophage CMP1 in an attempt to prevent *Clavibacter michiganensis* subsp. *michiganensis* infection, the causative agent of bacterial wilt and canker [156]. No symptoms of bacterial infection were observed in the transgenic plants; however, the bacteria were not completely eliminated [155]. A key limitation of this research was that the bacterial infection model may not be representative of natural infection, and therefore the efficacy of these transgenic tomato plants should to be evaluated under more natural conditions. It is also unknown whether *C. michiganensis* subsp. *michiganensis* could acquire resistance to these transgenic plants. However, this is a promising advancement in the development of transgenic plants. As new endolysins are characterized, more opportunities for bioengineering to optimize the activity of the protection mechanism will be possible.

Xanthmonas oryzae pv. *oryzae* causes bacterial leaf blight in rice [157], with a number of antibiotic resistant strains having been isolated [158]. In 2006, Lee et al. [159] identified Lys411 from ΦXo411, which exhibited strong lytic activity against *Xanthmonas*. Additionally, it displayed activity against the multidrug-resistant bacterium *Stenotrophomonas maltophilia* [159], which has growing clinical significance with regards to nosocomial infections and immunocompromised patients [160]. However, no follow-up studies investigating Lys411 have been published, which means the potential of this enzyme for medical or agriculture applications is unknown.

Attai et al. [161] recently characterized an endolysin from bacteriophages Atu_ph02 and Atu_ph03 for the biocontrol of *Agrobacterium tumefaciens*. *A. tumefaciens* is a Gram-negative soil-borne bacterium that is the etiologic agent of crown gall disease in a variety of orchard and vineyard crops [162].

Its severity and widespread impact has contributed to it to becoming the subject of many recent studies [163]. The lytic protein displayed interesting properties, with the ability to not only rapidly lyse the cell, but to also block cell division, ensuring potent antimicrobial activity [161]. Therefore, the enzyme is a candidate for biocontrol of *A. tumefaciens*; however, the method of implementation needs to be researched before a viable strategy for crop protection can be developed. The practicalities of implementing these endolysins on a global scale for individual phytobacteria may be a significant challenge, and may contribute to the limited information currently available on the use of endolysins for treatment of plant bacterial diseases. However, the cost to society of plant bacterial disease as current strategies become ineffective means that endolysin research should be an important focus.

5. Challenges of Endolysin Development and Engineering

The potential for endolysins to supplement, or replace antibiotics is exciting. However, this field is still emerging, with very few clinical trials on endolysin-based drugs being conducted. There are a number of challenges and considerations which researchers still face to bring these to market. As highlighted by several studies, the immunogenicity of endolysins must be considered and fully assessed. Undesirable immune responses to these foreign proteins could result in decreased efficacy of the enzymes, or possibly anaphylaxis and autoimmunity [164,165]. While there are studies that have reported on the immunogenicity in the application of endolysins [40–42,45,60,63] assessing the degree of immunogenicity in humans using traditional animal models has so far proven unreliable [166]. This was highlighted in studies of SAL200, which showed varying degrees of antibody production between rats, dogs, monkeys and humans [40–42]. Although the efficacy of the endolysin may not be observably impacted in vitro or in vivo, the clinical effects may be more significant. Until more human and animal-specific (for animal husbandry applications) clinical trials are conducted, the immunogenic nature of endolysins will remain unpredicatable.

In light of the current antibiotic resistance crisis, new antibacterials should be rigorously assessed for their potential susceptibility to developed resistance by bacteria. Promisingly, bacterial mutants resistant to endolysins are very infrequent [28–30,167]. Fischetti [167] proposed the lack of developed resistance to endolysins has resulted from the evolution of the interactions between bacteriophage and bacteria. The endolysins have evolved to target essential, immutable, molecules within the cell wall, thereby reducing the likelihood of the bacteria developing resistance mechanisms [167]. However, there are also reports of resistance to other peptidoglycan-cleaving enzymes including lysozymes and lysostaphin [168–173]. In the event of bacterial adaptation, enzyme engineering may prove useful to combat changes to bacteria in order to maintain the efficacy of endolysins.

The potential for endolysin bioengineering are seemingly endless, including optimizing or changing the catalytic abilities, modifying the lytic spectrum, improving its ability to permeate outer membranes and increasing stability (Table 1). Designing new enzymes requires an understanding of the structure and function of individual domains, the interactions between domains, the placement and composition of linker regions, and elucidation of key residues involved in catalysis. Bioinformatics and structural characterization studies are integral in this process [174]. Often, structural characterization can be achieved by X-ray crystallography, a powerful and effective technique for elucidating high resolution 3-D structures of proteins [11]; however, the limited ability to crystallize endolysins is a major challenge. The majority of endolysin crystal structures published to date are of single domains, with very few full-length endolysin crystal structures having been solved. This is attributed to the short flexible linker regions between domains [8], as protein flexibility is a common hindrance of crystal formation [175]. It is important to study full-length proteins to get a better understanding of the potential synergistic/antagonistic interactions between domains. Because of the difficulties in obtaining endolysin crystals, alternative structural characterization strategies need to be considered. These include the fusion of endolysins to proteins to decrease their flexibility, thereby allowing for crystallography, and other structural elucidation techniques such as nuclear magnetic resonance [176,177] and cryo-electron microscopy [178]. Although these approaches also have limitations, such as physiological relevance or size restrictions, exploration of these techniques may advance the structural characterization of endolysins.

6. Conclusions

The field of endolysin research is dynamic, with many potential applications being investigated in the medical, veterinary, and food sectors. The current global crisis of antimicrobial resistance is driving much of this work, with endolysins showing great promise to replace or supplement antibiotics. Engineering endolysins with optimized or new properties provides an opportunity to create even more effective tools. As more bacteriophage endolysins are biochemically and structurally characterized, the ability to design new enzymes improves, therefore expanding the arsenal of lytic tools. However, there are still many challenges that need to be addressed before this technology can be widely adopted by practitioners and industry. While many researchers have described the isolation and in vitro characterization of endolysins, establishing the in vivo efficacy and operating parameters of endolysins for human clinical use, food protection and supplementation, animal husbandry and welfare, and in the environment will be of great importance over the coming years. New technology to cost-effectively scale up endolysin production is also required, as this is currently a significant barrier to implementation. Finally, regulatory pathways need to be established for the use of endolysins in each of the various fields of application, and this can only be achieved by early and effective dialogue with the relevant authorities.

Acknowledgments: This article is supported by ESR SSIF funding. M.L. is supported by an UC Connect scholarship. R.C.J.D. acknowledges the following for funding support, in part: (1) the New Zealand Royal Society Marsden Fund (UOC1506); (2) a Ministry of Business, Innovation and Employment Smart Ideas grant (UOCX1706) the Biomolecular Interactions Centre, University of Canterbury.

Author Contributions: M.J.L., D.B., R.C.J.D. and C.B. wrote the paper.

References

1. World Health Organization. *Antimicrobial Resistance: Global Report on Surveillance*; World Health Organization: Geneva, Switzerland, 2014.
2. World Health Organization. *Global Framework for Development & Stewardship to Combat Antimicrobial Resistance—Draft Roadmap*; World Health Organization: Geneva, Switzerland, 2017.
3. Mwangi, W.; de Figueiredo, P.; Criscitiello, M.F. One health: Addressing global challenges at the nexus of human, animal, and environmental health. *PLoS Pathog.* **2016**, *12*, e1005731. [CrossRef] [PubMed]
4. Young, R. Bacteriophage lysis: Mechanism and regulation. *Microbiol. Rev.* **1992**, *56*, 430–481. [PubMed]
5. Loessner, M.J. Bacteriophage endolysins—Current state of research and applications. *Curr. Opin. Microbiol.* **2005**, *8*, 480–487. [CrossRef] [PubMed]
6. Fischetti, V.A. Bacteriophage endolysins: A novel anti-infective to control Gram-positive pathogens. *Int. J. Med. Microbiol.* **2010**, *300*, 357–362. [CrossRef] [PubMed]
7. Borysowski, J.; Weber-Dabrowska, B.; Gorski, A. Bacteriophage endolysins as a novel class of antibacterial agents. *Exp. Biol. Med. (Maywood)* **2006**, *231*, 366–377. [CrossRef] [PubMed]
8. Schmelcher, M.; Donovan, D.M.; Loessner, M.J. Bacteriophage endolysins as novel antimicrobials. *Future Microbiol.* **2012**, *7*, 1147–1171. [CrossRef] [PubMed]
9. Nelson, D.C.; Schmelcher, M.; Rodriguez-Rubio, L.; Klumpp, J.; Pritchard, D.G. Endolysins as antimicrobials. *Adv. Virus Res.* **2012**, *83*, 299–365. [PubMed]
10. Vollmer, W.; Bertsche, U. Murein (peptidoglycan) structure, architecture and biosynthesis in *Escherichia coli*. *Biochim. Biophys. Acta. Biomembr.* **2008**, *1778*, 1714–1734. [CrossRef] [PubMed]
11. Donovan, D.M.; Lardeo, M.; Foster-Frey, J. Lysis of Staphylococcal mastitis pathogens by bacteriophage Phi11 endolysin. *FEMS Microbiol. Lett.* **2006**, *265*, 133–139. [CrossRef] [PubMed]

12. Korndorfer, I.P.; Danzer, J.; Schmelcher, M.; Zimmer, M.; Skerra, A.; Loessner, M.J. The crystal structure of the bacteriophage PSA endolysin reveals a unique fold responsible for specific recognition of *Listeria* cell walls. *J. Mol. Biol.* **2006**, *364*, 678–689. [CrossRef] [PubMed]
13. Sass, P.; Bierbaum, G. Lytic activity of recombinant bacteriophage phi11 and phi12 endolysins on whole cells and biofilms of *Staphylococcus aureus*. *Appl. Environ. Microbiol.* **2007**, *73*, 347–352. [CrossRef] [PubMed]
14. Low, L.Y.; Yang, C.; Perego, M.; Osterman, A.; Liddington, R.C. Structure and lytic activity of a *Bacillus anthracis* prophage endolysin. *J. Biol. Chem.* **2005**, *280*, 35433–35439. [CrossRef] [PubMed]
15. Mayer, M.J.; Garefalaki, V.; Spoerl, R.; Narbad, A.; Meijers, R. Structure-based modification of a *Clostridium difficile*-targeting endolysin affects activity and host range. *J. Bacteriol.* **2011**, *193*, 5477–5486. [CrossRef] [PubMed]
16. Gaeng, S.; Scherer, S.; Neve, H.; Loessner, M.J. Gene cloning and expression and secretion of *Listeria monocytogenes* bacteriophage-lytic enzymes in *Lactococcus lactis*. *Appl. Environ. Microbiol.* **2000**, *66*, 2951–2958. [CrossRef] [PubMed]
17. Schmelcher, M.; Tchang, V.S.; Loessner, M.J. Domain shuffling and module engineering of *Listeria* phage endolysins for enhanced lytic activity and binding affinity. *Microb. Biotechnol.* **2011**, *4*, 651–662. [CrossRef] [PubMed]
18. Gerstmans, H.; Criel, B.; Briers, Y. Synthetic biology of modular endolysins. *Biotechnol. Adv.* **2017**, in press. [CrossRef] [PubMed]
19. Horgan, M.; O'Flynn, G.; Garry, J.; Cooney, J.; Coffey, A.; Fitzgerald, G.F.; Ross, R.P.; McAuliffe, O. Phage lysin Lysk can be truncated to its chap domain and retain lytic activity against live antibiotic-resistant staphylococci. *Appl. Environ. Microbiol.* **2009**, *75*, 872–874. [CrossRef] [PubMed]
20. Daniel, A.; Euler, C.; Collin, M.; Chahales, P.; Gorelick, K.J.; Fischetti, V.A. Synergism between a novel chimeric lysin and oxacillin protects against infection by methicillin-resistant *Staphylococcus aureus*. *Antimicrob. Agents Chemother.* **2010**, *54*, 1603–1612. [CrossRef] [PubMed]
21. Schmelcher, M.; Powell, A.M.; Becker, S.C.; Camp, M.J.; Donovan, D.M. Chimeric phage lysins act synergistically with lysostaphin to kill mastitis-causing *Staphylococcus aureus* in murine mammary glands. *Appl. Environ. Microbiol.* **2012**, *78*, 2297–2305. [CrossRef] [PubMed]
22. Swift, S.; Seal, B.; Garrish, J.; Oakley, B.; Hiett, K.; Yeh, H.-Y.; Woolsey, R.; Schegg, K.; Line, J.; Donovan, D. A thermophilic phage endolysin fusion to a *Clostridium perfringens*-specific cell wall binding domain creates an anti-clostridium antimicrobial with improved thermostability. *Viruses* **2015**, *7*, 3019–3034. [CrossRef] [PubMed]
23. Proença, D.; Leandro, C.; Garcia, M.; Pimentel, M.; São-José, C. EC300: A phage-based, bacteriolysin-like protein with enhanced antibacterial activity against *Enterococcus faecalis*. *Appl. Microbiol. Biotechnol.* **2015**, *99*, 5137–5149. [CrossRef] [PubMed]
24. Briers, Y.; Walmagh, M.; Van Puyenbroeck, V.; Cornelissen, A.; Cenens, W.; Aertsen, A.; Oliveira, H.; Azeredo, J.; Verween, G.; Pirnay, J.-P.; et al. Engineered endolysin-based "Artilysins" to combat multidrug-resistant Gram-negative pathogens. *mBio* **2014**, *5*. [CrossRef] [PubMed]
25. Briers, Y.; Walmagh, M.; Grymonprez, B.; Biebl, M.; Pirnay, J.-P.; Defraine, V.; Michiels, J.; Cenens, W.; Aertsen, A.; Miller, S.; et al. Art-175 is a highly efficient antibacterial against multidrug-resistant strains and persisters of *Pseudomonas aeruginosa*. *Antimicrob. Agents Chemother.* **2014**, *58*, 3774–3784. [CrossRef] [PubMed]
26. Peng, S.-Y.; You, R.-I.; Lai, M.-J.; Lin, N.-T.; Chen, L.-K.; Chang, K.-C. Highly potent antimicrobial modified peptides derived from the *Acinetobacter baumannii* phage endolysin LysAB2. *Sci. Rep.* **2017**, *7*, 11477. [CrossRef] [PubMed]
27. O'Flaherty, S.; Coffey, A.; Meaney, W.; Fitzgerald, G.F.; Ross, R.P. The recombinant phage lysin LysK has a broad spectrum of lytic activity against clinically relevant staphylococci, including methicillin-resistant *Staphylococcus aureus*. *J. Bacteriol.* **2005**, *187*, 7161–7164. [CrossRef] [PubMed]
28. Loeffler, J.M.; Nelson, D.; Fischetti, V.A. Rapid killing of *Streptococcus pneumoniae* with a bacteriophage cell wall hydrolase. *Science* **2001**, *294*, 2170–2172. [CrossRef] [PubMed]
29. Schuch, R.; Nelson, D.; Fischetti, V.A. A bacteriolytic agent that detects and kills *Bacillus anthracis*. *Nature* **2002**, *418*, 884–889. [CrossRef] [PubMed]
30. Pastagia, M.; Euler, C.; Chahales, P.; Fuentes-Duculan, J.; Krueger, J.G.; Fischetti, V.A. A novel chimeric lysin shows superiority to mupirocin for skin decolonization of methicillin-resistant and -sensitive *Staphylococcus aureus* strains. *Antimicrob. Agents Chemother.* **2011**, *55*, 738–744. [CrossRef] [PubMed]

31. Kretzer, J.W.; Lehmann, R.; Schmelcher, M.; Banz, M.; Kim, K.P.; Korn, C.; Loessner, M.J. Use of high-affinity cell wall-binding domains of bacteriophage endolysins for immobilization and separation of bacterial cells. *Appl. Environ. Microbiol.* **2007**, *73*, 1992–2000. [CrossRef] [PubMed]
32. Enright, M.C.; Robinson, D.A.; Randle, G.; Feil, E.J.; Grundmann, H.; Spratt, B.G. The evolutionary history of methicillin-resistant *Staphylococcus aureus* (MRSA). *Proc. Natl. Acad. Sci. USA* **2002**, *99*, 7687–7692. [CrossRef] [PubMed]
33. The White House. *National Action Plan for Combating Antibiotic-Resistant Bacteria. Interagency Task Force for Combating Antibiotic-Resistant Bacteria*; U.S. Office of the Press Secretary: Washington, DC, USA, 2015.
34. Filatova, L.Y.; Becker, S.C.; Donovan, D.M.; Gladilin, A.K.; Klyachko, N.L. Lysk, the enzyme lysing *Staphylococcus aureus* cells: Specific kinetic features and approaches towards stabilization. *Biochimie* **2010**, *92*, 507–513. [CrossRef] [PubMed]
35. Becker, S.C.; Foster-Frey, J.; Donovan, D.M. The phage K lytic enzyme LysK and lysostaphin act synergistically to kill MRSA. *FEMS Micriobiol. Lett.* **2008**, *287*, 185–191. [CrossRef] [PubMed]
36. Fenton, M.; Casey, P.G.; Hill, C.; Gahan, C.G.M.; Ross, R.P.; McAuliffe, O.; O'Mahony, J.; Maher, F.; Coffey, A. The truncated phage lysin CHAP(k) eliminates *Staphylococcus aureus* in the nares of mice. *Bioeng. Bugs* **2010**, *1*, 404–407. [CrossRef] [PubMed]
37. Fenton, M.; Ross, R.P.; McAuliffe, O.; O'Mahony, J.; Coffey, A. Characterization of the staphylococcal bacteriophage lysin CHAP(k). *J. Appl. Microbiol.* **2011**, *111*, 1025–1035. [CrossRef] [PubMed]
38. Jun, S.Y.; Jung, G.M.; Son, J.-S.; Yoon, S.J.; Choi, Y.-J.; Kang, S.H. Comparison of the antibacterial properties of phage endolysins SAL-1 and Lysk. *Antimicrob. Agents Chemother.* **2011**, *55*, 1764–1767. [CrossRef] [PubMed]
39. Jun, S.Y.; Jung, G.M.; Yoon, S.J.; Oh, M.-D.; Choi, Y.-J.; Lee, W.J.; Kong, J.-C.; Seol, J.G.; Kang, S.H. Antibacterial properties of a pre-formulated recombinant phage endolysin, SAL-1. *Int. J. Antimicrob. Agents* **2013**, *41*, 156–161. [CrossRef] [PubMed]
40. Jun, S.Y.; Jung, G.M.; Yoon, S.J.; Choi, Y.-J.; Koh, W.S.; Moon, K.S.; Kang, S.H. Preclinical safety evaluation of intravenously administered SAL200 containing the recombinant phage endolysin SAL-1 as a pharmaceutical ingredient. *Antimicrob. Agents Chemother.* **2014**, *58*, 2084–2088. [CrossRef] [PubMed]
41. Jun, S.Y.; Jung, G.M.; Yoon, S.J.; Youm, S.Y.; Han, H.-Y.; Lee, J.-H.; Kang, S.H. Pharmacokinetics of the phage endolysin-based candidate drug SAL200 in monkeys and its appropriate intravenous dosing period. *Clin. Exp. Pharmacol. Physiol.* **2016**, *43*, 1013–1016. [CrossRef] [PubMed]
42. Jun, S.Y.; Jang, I.J.; Yoon, S.; Jang, K.; Yu, K.S.; Cho, J.Y.; Seong, M.W.; Jung, G.M.; Yoon, S.J.; Kang, S.H. Pharmacokinetics and tolerance of the phage endolysin-based candidate drug SAL200 after a single intravenous administration among healthy volunteers. *Antimicrob. Agents Chemother.* **2017**, *61*. [CrossRef] [PubMed]
43. Bryers, J.D. Medical biofilms. *Biotechnol. Bioeng.* **2008**, *100*, 1–18. [CrossRef] [PubMed]
44. Linden, S.B.; Zhang, H.; Heselpoth, R.D.; Shen, Y.; Schmelcher, M.; Eichenseher, F.; Nelson, D.C. Biochemical and biophysical characterization of PlyGRCS, a bacteriophage endolysin active against methicillin-resistant *Staphylococcus aureus*. *Appl. Microbiol. Biotechnol.* **2015**, *99*, 741–752. [CrossRef] [PubMed]
45. Rashel, M.; Uchiyama, J.; Ujihara, T.; Uehara, Y.; Kuramoto, S.; Sugihara, S.; Yagyu, K.-I.; Muraoka, A.; Sugai, M.; Hiramatsu, K.; et al. Efficient elimination of multidrug-resistant *Staphylococcus aureus* by cloned lysin derived from bacteriophage ϕMR11. *J. Infect. Dis.* **2007**, *196*, 1237–1247. [CrossRef] [PubMed]
46. Schuch, R.; Lee, H.M.; Schneider, B.C.; Sauve, K.L.; Law, C.; Khan, B.K.; Rotolo, J.A.; Horiuchi, Y.; Couto, D.E.; Raz, A.; et al. Combination therapy with lysin CF-301 and antibiotic is superior to antibiotic alone for treating methicillin-resistant *Staphylococcus aureus*—induced murine bacteremia. *J. Infect. Dis.* **2014**, *209*, 1469–1478. [CrossRef] [PubMed]
47. Schuch, R.; Khan, B.K.; Raz, A.; Rotolo, J.A.; Wittekind, M. Bacteriophage lysin CF-301, a potent antistaphylococcal biofilm agent. *Antimicrob. Agents Chemother.* **2017**, *61*. [CrossRef] [PubMed]
48. Altoparlak, U.; Erol, S.; Akcay, M.N.; Celebi, F.; Kadanali, A. The time-related changes of antimicrobial resistance patterns and predominant bacterial profiles of burn wounds and body flora of burned patients. *Burns* **2004**, *30*, 660–664. [CrossRef] [PubMed]
49. Chopra, S.; Harjai, K.; Chhibber, S. Potential of combination therapy of endolysin MR-10 and minocycline in treating MRSA induced systemic and localized burn wound infections in mice. *Int. J. Med. Microbiol.* **2016**, *306*, 707–716. [CrossRef] [PubMed]

50. Herpers, B.; Badoux, P.; Pietersma, F.; Eichenseher, F.; Loessner, M. Specific lysis of methicillin susceptible and resistant *Staphylococcus aureus* by the endolysin staphefekt SA. 100. In Proceedings of the 24th European Congress of Clinical Microbiology and Infectious Diseases (ECCMID), Barcelona, Spain, 10–13 May 2014.
51. Totté, J.E.E.; van Doorn, M.B.; Pasmans, S.G.M.A. Successful treatment of chronic *Staphylococcus aureus*-related dermatoses with the topical endolysin staphefekt sa.100: A report of 3 cases. *Case Rep. Dermatol.* **2017**, *9*, 19–25. [CrossRef] [PubMed]
52. Rafii, F.; Sutherland, J.B.; Cerniglia, C.E. Effects of treatment with antimicrobial agents on the human colonic microflora. *Ther. Clin. Risk Manag.* **2008**, *4*, 1343–1358. [CrossRef] [PubMed]
53. Murray, B.E. The life and times of the Enterococcus. *Clin. Micriobiol. Rev.* **1990**, *3*, 46–65. [CrossRef]
54. Hammerum, A.M. Enterococci of animal origin and their significance for public health. *Clin. Microbiol. Infect.* **2012**, *18*, 619–625. [CrossRef] [PubMed]
55. Courvalin, P. Vancomycin resistance in Gram-positive cocci. *Clin. Infect. Dis.* **2006**, *42*, S25–S34. [CrossRef] [PubMed]
56. Boneca, I.G.; Chiosis, G. Vancomycin resistance: Occurrence, mechanisms and strategies to combat it. *Expert Opin. Ther. Targets* **2003**, *7*, 311–328. [CrossRef] [PubMed]
57. Yoong, P.; Schuch, R.; Nelson, D.; Fischetti, V.A. Identification of a broadly active phage lytic enzyme with lethal activity against antibiotic-resistant *Enterococcus faecalis* and *Enterococcus faecium*. *J. Bacteriol.* **2004**, *186*, 4808–4812. [CrossRef] [PubMed]
58. Son, J.S.; Jun, S.Y.; Kim, E.B.; Park, J.E.; Paik, H.R.; Yoon, S.J.; Kang, S.H.; Choi, Y.J. Complete genome sequence of a newly isolated lytic bacteriophage, EFAP-1 of *Enterococcus faecalis*, and antibacterial activity of its endolysin EFAL-1. *J. Appl. Microbiol.* **2010**, *108*, 1769–1779. [CrossRef] [PubMed]
59. Zhang, W.; Mi, Z.; Yin, X.; Fan, H.; An, X.; Zhang, Z.; Chen, J.; Tong, Y. Characterization of *Enterococcus faecalis* phage IME-EF1 and its endolysin. *PLoS ONE* **2013**, *8*, e80435. [CrossRef] [PubMed]
60. Cheng, M.; Zhang, Y.; Li, X.; Liang, J.; Hu, L.; Gong, P.; Zhang, L.; Cai, R.; Zhang, H.; Ge, J.; et al. Endolysin LysEF-P10 shows potential as an alternative treatment strategy for multidrug-resistant *Enterococcus faecalis* infections. *Sci. Rep.* **2017**, *7*, 10164. [CrossRef] [PubMed]
61. Jedrzejas, M.J. Pneumococcal virulence factors: Structure and function. *Microbiol. Mol. Biol. Rev.* **2001**, *65*, 187–207. [CrossRef] [PubMed]
62. Cunningham, M.W. Pathogenesis of group a streptococcal infections. *Clin. Microbiol. Rev.* **2000**, *13*, 470–511. [CrossRef] [PubMed]
63. Loeffler, J.M.; Djurkovic, S.; Fischetti, V.A. Phage lytic enzyme Cpl-1 as a novel antimicrobial for pneumococcal bacteremia. *Infect. Immun.* **2003**, *71*, 6199–6204. [CrossRef] [PubMed]
64. Garcia, J.L.; Garcia, E.; Arraras, A.; Garcia, P.; Ronda, C.; Lopez, R. Cloning, purification, and biochemical characterization of the pneumococcal bacteriophage Cp-1 lysin. *J. Virol.* **1987**, *61*, 2573–2580. [PubMed]
65. Djurkovic, S.; Loeffler, J.M.; Fischetti, V.A. Synergistic killing of *Streptococcus pneumoniae* with the bacteriophage lytic enzyme Cpl-1 and penicillin or gentamicin depends on the level of penicillin resistance. *Antimicrob. Agents Chemother.* **2005**, *49*, 1225–1228. [CrossRef] [PubMed]
66. Jado, I.; López, R.; García, E.; Fenoll, A.; Casal, J.; García, P. Phage lytic enzymes as therapy for antibiotic-resistant *Streptococcus pneumoniae* infection in a murine sepsis model. *J. Antimicrob. Chemother.* **2003**, *52*, 967–973. [CrossRef] [PubMed]
67. Loeffler, J.M.; Fischetti, V.A. Synergistic lethal effect of a combination of phage lytic enzymes with different activities on penicillin-sensitive and -resistant *Streptococcus pneumoniae* strains. *Antimicrob. Agents Chemother.* **2003**, *47*, 375–377. [CrossRef] [PubMed]
68. Entenza, J.; Loeffler, J.; Grandgirard, D.; Fischetti, V.; Moreillon, P. Therapeutic effects of bacteriophage Cpl-1 lysin against *Streptococcus pneumoniae* endocarditis in rats. *Antimicrob. Agents Chemother.* **2005**, *49*, 4789–4792. [CrossRef] [PubMed]
69. Grandgirard, D.; Loeffler, J.M.; Fischetti, V.A.; Leib, S.L. Phage lytic enzyme Cpl-1 for antibacterial therapy in experimental pneumococcal meningitis. *J. Infect. Dis.* **2008**, *197*, 1519–1522. [CrossRef] [PubMed]
70. Doehn, J.M.; Fischer, K.; Reppe, K.; Gutbier, B.; Tschernig, T.; Hocke, A.C.; Fischetti, V.A.; Löffler, J.; Suttorp, N.; Hippenstiel, S.; et al. Delivery of the endolysin Cpl-1 by inhalation rescues mice with fatal pneumococcal pneumonia. *J. Antimicrob. Chemother.* **2013**, *68*, 2111–2117. [CrossRef] [PubMed]

71. Witzenrath, M.; Schmeck, B.; Doehn, J.M.; Tschernig, T.; Zahlten, J.; Loeffler, J.M.; Zemlin, M.; Müller, H.; Gutbier, B.; Schütte, H. Systemic use of the endolysin Cpl-1 rescues mice with fatal pneumococcal pneumonia. *Crit. Care Med.* **2009**, *37*, 642–649. [CrossRef] [PubMed]
72. Resch, G.; Moreillon, P.; Fischetti, V.A. A stable phage lysin (Cpl-1) dimer with increased antipneumococcal activity and decreased plasma clearance. *Int. J. Antimicrob. Agents* **2011**, *38*, 516–521. [CrossRef] [PubMed]
73. Usobiaga, P.; Medrano, F.J.; Gasset, M.; García, J.L.; Saiz, J.L.; Rivas, G.; Laynez, J.; Menéndez, M. Structural organization of the major autolysin from streptococcus pneumoniae. *J. Biol. Chem.* **1996**, *271*, 6832–6838. [CrossRef] [PubMed]
74. Beveridge, T.J. Structures of Gram-negative cell walls and their derived membrane vesicles. *J. Bacteriol.* **1999**, *181*, 4725–4733. [PubMed]
75. Peleg, A.Y.; Seifert, H.; Paterson, D.L. *Acinetobacter baumannii*: Emergence of a successful pathogen. *Clin. Microbial. Rev.* **2008**, *21*, 538–582. [CrossRef] [PubMed]
76. Dijkshoorn, L.; Nemec, A.; Seifert, H. An increasing threat in hospitals: Multidrug-resistant *Acinetobacter baumannii*. *Nat. Rev. Microbiol.* **2007**, *5*, 939–951. [CrossRef] [PubMed]
77. Bodey, G.P.; Bolivar, R.; Fainstein, V.; Jadeja, L. Infections caused by *Pseudomonas aeruginosa*. *Rev. Infect. Dis.* **1983**, *5*, 279–313. [CrossRef] [PubMed]
78. Lister, P.D.; Wolter, D.J.; Hanson, N.D. Antibacterial-resistant *Pseudomonas aeruginosa*: Clinical impact and complex regulation of chromosomally encoded resistance mechanisms. *Clin. Microbial. Rev.* **2009**, *22*, 582–610. [CrossRef] [PubMed]
79. Lai, M.-J.; Lin, N.-T.; Hu, A.; Soo, P.-C.; Chen, L.-K.; Chen, L.-H.; Chang, K.-C. Antibacterial activity of *Acinetobacter baumannii* phage ϕAB2 endolysin (LysAB2) against both Gram-positive and Gram-negative bacteria. *Appl. Microbiol. Biotechnol.* **2011**, *90*, 529–539. [CrossRef] [PubMed]
80. Lood, R.; Winer, B.Y.; Pelzek, A.J.; Diez-Martinez, R.; Thandar, M.; Euler, C.W.; Schuch, R.; Fischetti, V.A. Novel phage lysin capable of killing the multidrug-resistant Gram-negative bacterium *Acinetobacter baumannii* in a mouse bacteremia model. *Antimicrob. Agents Chemother.* **2015**, *59*, 1983–1991. [CrossRef] [PubMed]
81. Walmagh, M.; Briers, Y.; dos Santos, S.B.; Azeredo, J.; Lavigne, R. Characterization of modular bacteriophage endolysins from *Myoviridae* phages OBP, 201φ2-1 and PVP-SE1. *PLoS ONE* **2012**, *7*, e36991. [CrossRef] [PubMed]
82. Sato, H.; Feix, J.B. Peptide–membrane interactions and mechanisms of membrane destruction by amphipathic α-helical antimicrobial peptides. *Biochim. Biophys. Acta. Biomembr.* **2006**, *1758*, 1245–1256. [CrossRef] [PubMed]
83. Guo, M.; Feng, C.; Ren, J.; Zhuang, X.; Zhang, Y.; Zhu, Y.; Dong, K.; He, P.; Guo, X.; Qin, J. A novel antimicrobial endolysin, LysPA26, against *Pseudomonas aeruginosa*. *Front. Microbiol.* **2017**, *8*. [CrossRef] [PubMed]
84. Thummeepak, R.; Kitti, T.; Kunthalert, D.; Sitthisak, S. Enhanced antibacterial activity of acinetobacter baumannii bacteriophage øABP-01 endolysin (LysABP-01) in combination with colistin. *Front. Microbiol.* **2016**, *7*. [CrossRef] [PubMed]
85. Briers, Y.; Walmagh, M.; Lavigne, R. Use of bacteriophage endolysin EL188 and outer membrane permeabilizers against *Pseudomonas aeruginosa*. *J. Appl. Microbiol.* **2011**, *110*, 778–785. [CrossRef] [PubMed]
86. Triantaphyllopoulos, D.C.; Quick, A.J.; Greenwalt, T.J. Action of disodium ethylenediamine tetracetate on blood coagulation; evidence of the development of heparinoid activity during incubation or aeration of plasma. *Blood* **1955**, *10*, 534–544. [PubMed]
87. Briers, Y.; Lavigne, R. Breaking barriers: Expansion of the use of endolysins as novel antibacterials against Gram-negative bacteria. *Future Microbiol.* **2015**, *10*, 377–390. [CrossRef] [PubMed]
88. Zasloff, M. Antimicrobial peptides of multicellular organisms. *Nature* **2002**, *415*, 389. [CrossRef] [PubMed]
89. Dawson, R.M.; Liu, C.-Q. Cathelicidin peptide SMAP-29: Comprehensive review of its properties and potential as a novel class of antibiotics. *Drug Dev. Res.* **2009**, *70*, 481–498. [CrossRef]
90. Timbermont, L.; Haesebrouck, F.; Ducatelle, R.; Van Immerseel, F. Necrotic enteritis in broilers: An updated review on the pathogenesis. *Avian Pathol.* **2011**, *40*, 341–347. [CrossRef] [PubMed]
91. Gervasi, T.; Lo Curto, R.; Minniti, E.; Narbad, A.; Mayer, M.J. Application of *Lactobacillus johnsonii* expressing phage endolysin for control of *Clostridium perfringens*. *Lett. Appl. Microbiol.* **2014**, *59*, 355–361. [CrossRef] [PubMed]

92. Gervasi, T.; Horn, N.; Wegmann, U.; Dugo, G.; Narbad, A.; Mayer, M.J. Expression and delivery of an endolysin to combat *Clostridium perfringens*. *Appl. Microbiol. Biotechnol.* **2014**, *98*, 2495–2505. [CrossRef] [PubMed]
93. Tamai, E.; Yoshida, H.; Sekiya, H.; Nariya, H.; Miyata, S.; Okabe, A.; Kuwahara, T.; Maki, J.; Kamitori, S. X-ray structure of a novel endolysin encoded by episomal phage phiSM101 of *Clostridium perfringens*. *Mol. Microbiol.* **2014**, *92*, 326–337. [CrossRef] [PubMed]
94. Nariya, H.; Miyata, S.; Tamai, E.; Sekiya, H.; Maki, J.; Okabe, A. Identification and characterization of a putative endolysin encoded by episomal phage phiSM101 of *Clostridium perfringens*. *Appl. Microbiol. Biotechnol.* **2011**, *90*, 1973–1979. [CrossRef] [PubMed]
95. Wilson, D.J.; Gonzalez, R.N.; Das, H.H. Bovine mastitis pathogens in New York and Pennsylvania: Prevalence and effects on somatic cell count and milk production. *J. Dairy Sci.* **1997**, *80*, 2592–2598. [CrossRef]
96. Donovan, D.M.; Dong, S.; Garrett, W.; Rousseau, G.M.; Moineau, S.; Pritchard, D.G. Peptidoglycan hydrolase fusions maintain their parental specificities. *Appl. Environ. Microbiol.* **2006**, *72*, 2988–2996. [CrossRef] [PubMed]
97. Schmelcher, M.; Powell, A.M.; Camp, M.J.; Pohl, C.S.; Donovan, D.M. Synergistic streptococcal phage λSA2 and B30 endolysins kill streptococci in cow milk and in a mouse model of mastitis. *Appl. Microbiol. Biotechnol.* **2015**, *99*, 8475–8486. [CrossRef] [PubMed]
98. Fan, J.; Zeng, Z.; Mai, K.; Yang, Y.; Feng, J.; Bai, Y.; Sun, B.; Xie, Q.; Tong, Y.; Ma, J. Preliminary treatment of bovine mastitis caused by *Staphylococcus aureus*, with Trx-SA1, recombinant endolysin of *S. aureus* bacteriophage IME-SA1. *Vet. Microbiol.* **2016**, *191*, 65–71. [CrossRef] [PubMed]
99. Fasanella, A.; Galante, D.; Garofolo, G.; Jones, M.H. Anthrax undervalued zoonosis. *Vet. Microbiol.* **2010**, *140*, 318–331. [CrossRef] [PubMed]
100. Toole, T.O.; Henderson, D.; Bartlett, J.G.; Ascher, M.S.; Eitzen, E.; Friedlander, A.M.; Gerberding, J.; Hauer, J.; Hughes, J.; McDade, J.; et al. Anthrax as a biological weapon, 2002: Updated recommendations for management. *J. Am. Med. Assoc.* **2002**, *287*, 2236–2253.
101. Sykes, J.E.; Hartmann, K.; Lunn, K.F.; Moore, G.E.; Stoddard, R.; Goldstein, R.E. ACVIM Consensus Statement. *J. Vet. Intern. Med.* **2011**, *19*, 1–13. [CrossRef] [PubMed]
102. Hoopes, J.T.; Stark, C.J.; Kim, H.A.; Sussman, D.J.; Donovan, D.M.; Nelson, D.C. Use of a bacteriophage lysin, PlyC, as an enzyme disinfectant against *Streptococcus equi*. *Appl. Environ. Microbiol.* **2009**, *75*, 1388–1394. [CrossRef] [PubMed]
103. Junjappa, R.P.; Desai, S.N.; Roy, P.; Narasimhaswamy, N.; Raj, J.R.M.; Durgaiah, M.; Vipra, A.; Bhat, U.R.; Satyanarayana, S.K.; Shankara, N.; et al. Efficacy of anti-staphylococcal protein P128 for the treatment of canine pyoderma: Potential applications. *Vet. Res. Commun.* **2013**, *37*, 217–228. [CrossRef] [PubMed]
104. Vipra, A.A.; Desai, S.N.; Roy, P.; Patil, R.; Raj, J.M.; Narasimhaswamy, N.; Paul, V.D.; Chikkamadaiah, R.; Sriram, B. Antistaphylococcal activity of bacteriophage derived chimeric protein P128. *BMC Microbiol.* **2012**, *12*, 41. [CrossRef] [PubMed]
105. Wang, Y.; Sun, J.H.; Lu, C.P. Purified recombinant phage lysin LySMP: An extensive spectrum of lytic activity for swine streptococci. *Curr. Microbiol.* **2009**, *58*, 609–615. [CrossRef] [PubMed]
106. Bates, J.; Jordens, J.; Griffith, D.T. Farm animals as putative reservoir for vancomycin resistant enterococcal infections in man. *J. Antiomicrob. Chemother.* **1994**, *34*, 507–516. [CrossRef]
107. Coque, T.M.; Tomayko, J.F.; Ricke, S.C.; Okhyusen, P.C.; Murray, B.E. Vancomycin-resistant enterococci from nosocomial, community, and animal sources in the United States. *Antimicrob. Agents Chemother.* **1996**, *40*, 2605–2609. [PubMed]
108. Madewell, B.R.; Tang, Y.J.; Jang, S.; Madigan, J.E.; Hirsh, D.C.; Gumerlock, P.H.; Silva, J., Jr. Apparent outbreaks of *Clostridium difficile*-associated diarrhea in horses in a veterinary medical teaching hospital. *J. Vet. Diagn. Invest.* **1995**, *7*, 343–346. [CrossRef] [PubMed]
109. Debast, S.B.; Van Leengoed, L.A.M.G.; Goorhuis, A.; Harmanus, C.; Kuijper, E.J.; Bergwerff, A.A. *Clostridium difficile* PCR ribotype 078 toxinotype V found in diarrhoeal pigs identical to isolates from affected humans. *Environ. Microbiol.* **2009**, *11*, 505–511. [CrossRef] [PubMed]
110. Kelly, C.P.; Pothoulakis, C.; LaMont, J.T. *Clostridium difficile* Colitis. *N. Engl. J. Med.* **1994**, *330*, 257–262. [CrossRef] [PubMed]
111. Mayer, M.J.; Narbad, A.; Gasson, M.J. Molecular characterization of a *Clostridium difficile* bacteriophage and its cloned biologically active endolysin. *J. Bacteriol.* **2008**, *190*, 6734–6740. [CrossRef] [PubMed]

112. Oliveira, A.; Leite, M.; Kluskens, L.D.; Santos, S.B.; Melo, L.D.R.; Azeredo, J. The first *Paenibacillus* larvae bacteriophage endolysin (PlyPl23) with high potential to control American Foulbrood. *PLoS ONE* **2015**, *10*, e0132095.
113. Zhang, H.; Bao, H.; Billington, C.; Hudson, J.A.; Wang, R. Isolation and lytic activity of the *Listeria* bacteriophage endolysin LysZ5 against *Listeria monocytogenes* in soya milk. *Food Microbiol.* **2012**, *31*, 133–136. [CrossRef] [PubMed]
114. van Nassau, T.J.; Lenz, C.A.; Scherzinger, A.S.; Vogel, R.F. Combination of endolysins and high pressure to inactivate *Listeria monocytogenes*. *Food Microbiol.* **2017**, *68*, 81–88. [CrossRef] [PubMed]
115. Turner, M.S.; Waldherr, F.; Loessner, M.J.; Giffard, P.M. Antimicrobial activity of lysostaphin and a *Listeria monocytogenes* bacteriophage endolysin produced and secreted by lactic acid bacteria. *Syst. Appl. Microbiol.* **2007**, *30*, 58–67. [CrossRef] [PubMed]
116. van Tassell, M.L.; Angela Daum, M.; Kim, J.S.; Miller, M.J. Creative lysins: *Listeria* and the engineering of antimicrobial enzymes. *Curr. Opin. Biotechnol.* **2016**, *37*, 88–96. [CrossRef] [PubMed]
117. Schmelcher, M.; Waldherr, F.; Loessner, M.J. *Listeria* bacteriophage peptidoglycan hydrolases feature high thermoresistance and reveal increased activity after divalent metal cation substitution. *Appl. Microbiol. Biotechnol.* **2012**, *93*, 633–643. [CrossRef] [PubMed]
118. Hennekinne, J.A.; De Buyser, M.L.; Dragacci, S. *Staphylococcus aureus* and its food poisoning toxins: Characterization and outbreak investigation. *FEMS. Microbiol. Rev.* **2012**, *36*, 815–836. [CrossRef] [PubMed]
119. Chang, Y.; Kim, M.; Ryu, S. Characterization of a novel endolysin LysSA11 and its utility as a potent biocontrol agent against *Staphylococcus aureus* on food and utensils. *Food. Microbiol.* **2017**, *68*, 112–120. [CrossRef] [PubMed]
120. Chang, Y.; Yoon, H.; Kang, D.H.; Chang, P.S.; Ryu, S. Endolysin LysSA97 is synergistic with carvacrol in controlling *Staphylococcus aureus* in foods. *Int. J. Food Microbiol.* **2017**, *244*, 19–26. [CrossRef] [PubMed]
121. Obeso, J.M.; Martinez, B.; Rodriguez, A.; Garcia, P. Lytic activity of the recombinant staphylococcal bacteriophage ΦH5 endolysin active against *Staphylococcus aureus* in milk. *Int. J. Food Microbiol.* **2008**, *128*, 212–218. [CrossRef] [PubMed]
122. Rodriguez-Rubio, L.; Martinez, B.; Donovan, D.M.; Garcia, P.; Rodriguez, A. Potential of the virion-associated peptidoglycan hydrolase HydH5 and its derivative fusion proteins in milk biopreservation. *PLoS ONE* **2013**, *8*, e54828. [CrossRef] [PubMed]
123. World Health Organization. *WHO Estimates of the Global Burden of Foodborne Diseases: Foodborne Disease Burden Epidemiology Reference Group 2007–2015*; World Health Organization: Geneva, Switzerland, 2015.
124. Interagency Food Safety Analytics Collaboration (IFSAC) Project. Foodborne Illness Source Attribution Estimates for *Salmonella*, *Escherichia coli* O157 (*E. coli* O157), *Listeria monocytogenes* (lm) and *Campylobacter* Using Outbreak Surveillance Data. 2014. Available online: https://www.cdc.gov/foodsafety/pdfs/IFSAC-2013FoodborneillnessSourceEstimates-508.pdf (accessed on 13 March 2015).
125. Lim, J.A.; Shin, H.; Kang, D.H.; Ryu, S. Characterization of endolysin from a *Salmonella* Typhimurium-infecting bacteriophage SPN1S. *Res. Microbiol.* **2012**, *163*, 233–241. [CrossRef] [PubMed]
126. Oliveira, H.; Thiagarajan, V.; Walmagh, M.; Sillankorva, S.; Lavigne, R.; Neves-Petersen, M.T.; Kluskens, L.D.; Azeredo, J. A thermostable *Salmonella* phage endolysin, Lys68, with broad bactericidal properties against Gram-negative pathogens in presence of weak acids. *PLoS ONE* **2014**, *9*, e108376. [CrossRef] [PubMed]
127. Rodríguez-Rubio, L.; Gerstmans, H.; Thorpe, S.; Mesnage, S.; Lavigne, R.; Briers, Y. DUF3380 domain from a *Salmonella* phage endolysin shows potent *N*-acetylmuramidase activity. *Appl. Environ. Microbiol.* **2016**, *82*, 4975–4981. [CrossRef] [PubMed]
128. Drudy, D.; Mullane, N.R.; Quinn, T.; Wall, P.G.; Fanning, S. *Enterobacter sakazakii*: An emerging pathogen in powdered infant formula. *Clin. Infect. Dis.* **2006**, *42*, 996–1002. [CrossRef] [PubMed]
129. Endersen, L.; Guinane, C.M.; Johnston, C.; Neve, H.; Coffey, A.; Ross, R.P.; McAuliffe, O.; O'Mahony, J. Genome analysis of *Cronobacter* phage vB_CsaP_Ss1 reveals an endolysin with potential for biocontrol of Gram-negative bacterial pathogens. *J. Gen. Virol.* **2015**, *96*, 463–477. [CrossRef] [PubMed]
130. Endersen, L.; Coffey, A.; Ross, R.P.; McAuliffe, O.; Hill, C.; O'Mahony, J. Characterisation of the antibacterial properties of a bacterial derived peptidoglycan hydrolase (LysCs4), active against *C. sakazakii* and other Gram-negative food-related pathogens. *Int. J. Food Microbiol.* **2015**, *215*, 79–85. [CrossRef] [PubMed]
131. Son, B.; Yun, J.; Lim, J.-A.; Shin, H.; Heu, S.; Ryu, S. Characterization of LysB4, an endolysin from the *Bacillus cereus*-infecting bacteriophage B4. *BMC Microbiol.* **2012**, *12*, 33. [CrossRef] [PubMed]

132. Loessner, M.J.; Maier, S.K.; Daubek-Puza, H.; Wendlinger, G.; Scherer, S. Three *Bacillus cereus* bacteriophage endolysins are unrelated but reveal high homology to cell wall hydrolases from different bacilli. *J. Bacteriol.* **1997**, *179*, 2845–2851. [CrossRef] [PubMed]
133. Park, J.; Yun, J.; Lim, J.A.; Kang, D.H.; Ryu, S. Characterization of an endolysin, LysBPS13, from a *Bacillus cereus* bacteriophage. *FEMS Microbiol. Lett.* **2012**, *332*, 76–83. [CrossRef] [PubMed]
134. Mayer, M.J.; Payne, J.; Gasson, M.J.; Narbad, A. Genomic sequence and characterization of the virulent bacteriophage *ϕ*CTP1 from *Clostridium tyrobutyricum* and heterologous expression of its endolysin. *Appl. Envrion. Microbiol.* **2010**, *76*, 5415–5422. [CrossRef] [PubMed]
135. Mayer, M.J.; Gasson, M.J.; Narbad, A. Genomic sequence of bacteriophage ATCC 8074-B1 and activity of its endolysin and engineered variants against *Clostridium sporogenes*. *Appl. Environ. Microbiol.* **2012**, *78*, 3685–3692. [CrossRef] [PubMed]
136. Vasala, A.; Valkkila, M.; Caldentey, J.; Alatossava, T. Genetic and biochemical characterization of the *Lactobacillus delbrueckii* subsp. *Lactis* bacteriophage LL-H lysin. *Appl. Environ. Microbiol.* **1995**, *61*, 4004–4011. [PubMed]
137. Deutsch, S.-M.; Guezenec, S.; Piot, M.; Foster, S.; Lortal, S. Mur-LH, the broad-spectrum endolysin of *Lactobacillus helveticus* temperate bacteriophage φ-0303. *Appl. Environ. Microbiol.* **2004**, *70*, 96–103. [CrossRef] [PubMed]
138. Kashige, N.; Nakashima, Y.; Miake, F.; Watanabe, K. Cloning, sequence analysis, and expression of *Lactobacillus casei* phage PL-1 lysis genes. *Arch. Virol.* **2000**, *145*, 1521–1534. [CrossRef] [PubMed]
139. Labrie, S.; Vukov, N.; Loessner, M.J.; Moineau, S. Distribution and composition of the lysis cassette of *Lactococcus lactis* phages and functional analysis of bacteriophage Ul36 holin. *FEMS Microbiol. Lett.* **2004**, *233*, 37–43. [CrossRef] [PubMed]
140. Han, F.; Li, M.; Lin, H.; Wang, J.; Cao, L.; Khan, M.N. The novel *Shewanella putrefaciens*-infecting bacteriophage Spp001: Genome sequence and lytic enzymes. *J. Ind. Microbiol. Biotechnol.* **2014**, *41*, 1017–1026. [CrossRef] [PubMed]
141. Lu, Z.; Altermann, E.; Breidt, F.; Kozyavkin, S. Sequence analysis of *Leuconostoc mesenteroides* bacteriophage Phi1-A4 isolated from an industrial vegetable fermentation. *Appl. Environ. Microbiol.* **2010**, *76*, 1955–1966. [CrossRef] [PubMed]
142. Yoon, S.S.; Kim, J.W.; Breidt, F.; Fleming, H.P. Characterization of a lytic *Lactobacillus plantarum* bacteriophage and molecular cloning of a lysin gene in *Escherichia coli*. *Int. J. Food Microbiol.* **2001**, *65*, 63–74. [CrossRef]
143. Kim, W.-S.; Salm, H.; Geider, K. Expression of bacteriophage φEa1h lysozyme in *Escherichia coli* and its activity in growth inhibition of *Erwinia amylovora*. *Microbiology* **2004**, *150*, 2707–2714. [CrossRef] [PubMed]
144. Nakimbugwe, D.; Masschalck, B.; Anim, G.; Michiels, C.W. Inactivation of Gram-negative bacteria in milk and banana juice by hen egg white and lambda lysozyme under high hydrostatic pressure. *Int. J. Food Microbiol.* **2006**, *112*, 19–25. [CrossRef] [PubMed]
145. Wang, W.; Li, M.; Lin, H.; Wang, J.; Mao, X. The *Vibrio parahaemolyticus*-infecting bacteriophage qdvp001: Genome sequence and endolysin with a modular structure. *Arch. Virol.* **2016**, *161*, 2645–2652. [CrossRef] [PubMed]
146. Solanki, K.; Grover, N.; Downs, P.; Paskaleva, E.E.; Mehta, K.K.; Lillian, L.; Schadler, L.S.; Kane, R.S.; Dordick, J.S. Enzyme-based Listericidal nanocomposites. *Sci. Rep.* **2013**, *3*, 1584. [CrossRef] [PubMed]
147. Misiou, O.; van Nassau, T.J.; Lenz, C.A.; Vogel, R.F. The preservation of listeria-critical foods by a combination of endolysin and high hydrostatic pressure. *Int. J. Food Microbiol.* **2017**, in press. [CrossRef] [PubMed]
148. Chmielewski, R.A.N.; Frank, J.F. Biofilm formation and control in food processing facilities. *Compr. Rev. Food Sci. Food Saf.* **2003**, *2*, 22–32. [CrossRef]
149. Gutiérrez, D.; Fernández, L.; Martínez, B.; Ruas-Madiedo, P.; García, P.; Rodríguez, A. Real-time assessment of *Staphylococcus aureus* biofilm disruption by phage-derived proteins. *Front. Microbiol.* **2017**, *8*. [CrossRef] [PubMed]
150. Simmons, M.; Morales, C.A.; Oakley, B.B.; Seal, B.S. Recombinant expression of a putative amidase cloned from the genome of *Listeria monocytogenes* that lyses the bacterium and its monolayer in conjunction with a protease. *Probiotics Antimicrob. Proteins* **2012**, *4*, 1–10. [CrossRef] [PubMed]
151. Strange, R.N.; Scott, P.R. Plant disease: A threat to global food security. *Annu. Rev. Phytopathol.* **2005**, *43*, 83–116. [CrossRef] [PubMed]

152. McManus, P.S.; Stockwell, V.O.; Sundin, G.W.; Jones, A.L. Antibiotic use in plant agriculture. *Annu. Rev. Phytopathol.* **2002**, *40*, 443–465. [CrossRef] [PubMed]
153. Düring, K.; Porsch, P.; Fladung, M.; Lörz, H. Transgenic potato plants resistant to the phytopathogenic bacterium *Erwinia carotovora*. *Plant J.* **1993**, *3*, 587–598. [CrossRef]
154. De Vries, J.; Harms, K.; Broer, I.; Kriete, G.; Mahn, A.; Düring, K.; Wackernagel, W. The bacteriolytic activity in transgenic potatoes expressing a chimeric T4 lysozyme gene and the effect of T4 lysozyme on soil- and phytopathogenic bacteria. *Syst. Appl. Microbiol.* **1999**, *22*, 280–286. [CrossRef]
155. Wittmann, J.; Brancato, C.; Berendzen, K.W.; Dreiseikelmann, B. Development of a tomato plant resistant to *Clavibacter michiganensis* using the endolysin gene of bacteriophage CMP1 as a transgene. *Plant Pathol.* **2016**, *65*, 496–502. [CrossRef]
156. Hausbeck, M.K.; Bell, J.; Medina-Mora, C.; Podolsky, R.; Fulbright, D.W. Effect of bactericides on population sizes and spread of *Clavibacter michiganensis* subsp. *Michiganensis* on tomatoes in the greenhouse and on disease development and crop yield in the field. *Phytopathology* **2000**, *90*, 38–44. [PubMed]
157. Tang, J.L.; Feng, J.X.; Li, Q.Q.; Wen, H.X.; Zhou, D.L.; Wilson, T.J.; Dow, J.M.; Ma, Q.S.; Daniels, M.J. Cloning and characterization of the rpfc gene of *Xanthomonas oryzae* pv. *Oryzae*: Involvement in exopolysaccharide production and virulence to rice. *Mol. Plant Microbe. Interact.* **1996**, *9*, 664–666. [PubMed]
158. Xu, Y.; Luo, Q.-q.; Zhou, M.-g. Identification and characterization of integron-mediated antibiotic resistance in the phytopathogen *Xanthomonas oryzae* pv. *Oryzae*. *PLoS ONE* **2013**, *8*, e55962. [CrossRef] [PubMed]
159. Lee, C.-N.; Lin, J.-W.; Chow, T.-Y.; Tseng, Y.-H.; Weng, S.-F. A novel lysozyme from *Xanthomonas oryzae* phage φxo411 active against *Xanthomonas* and *Stenotrophomonas*. *Protein Expr. Purif.* **2006**, *50*, 229–237. [CrossRef] [PubMed]
160. Brooke, J.S. *Stenotrophomonas maltophilia*: An emerging global opportunistic pathogen. *Clin. Microbiol. Rev.* **2012**, *25*, 2–41. [CrossRef] [PubMed]
161. Attai, H.; Rimbey, J.; Smith, G.P.; Brown, P.J.B. Expression of a peptidoglycan hydrolase from lytic bacteriophages Atu_ph02 and Atu_ph03 triggers lysis of *Agrobacterium tumefaciens*. *Appl. Environ. Microbiol.* **2017**, *83*, 17. [CrossRef] [PubMed]
162. Pulawska, J. Crown gall of stone fruits and nuts, economic significance and diversity of its causal agents: Tumorigenic *Agrobacterium* spp. *J. Plant Pathol.* **2010**, *92*, S87–S98.
163. Mansfield, J.; Genin, S.; Magori, S.; Citovsky, V.; Sriariyanum, M.; Ronald, P.; Dow, M.; Verdier, V.; Beer, S.V.; Machado, M.A.; et al. Top 10 plant pathogenic bacteria in molecular plant pathology. *Mol. Plant Pathol.* **2012**, *13*, 614–629. [CrossRef] [PubMed]
164. Rosenberg, A.S. Immunogenicity of biological therapeutics: A hierarchy of concerns. *Dev. Biol.* **2003**, *112*, 15–21.
165. De Groot, A.S.; Scott, D.W. Immunogenicity of protein therapeutics. *Trends Immunol.* **2007**, *28*, 482–490. [CrossRef] [PubMed]
166. Baker, M.P.; Reynolds, H.M.; Lumicisi, B.; Bryson, C.J. Immunogenicity of protein therapeutics: The key causes, consequences and challenges. *Self Nonself* **2010**, *1*, 314–322. [CrossRef] [PubMed]
167. Fischetti, V.A. Bacteriophage lytic enzymes: Novel anti-infectives. *Trends Microbiol.* **2005**, *13*, 491–496. [CrossRef] [PubMed]
168. DeHart, H.P.; Heath, H.E.; Heath, L.S.; LeBlanc, P.A.; Sloan, G.L. The lysostaphin endopeptidase resistance gene (epr) specifies modification of peptidoglycan cross bridges in *Staphylococcus simulans* and *Staphylococcus aureus*. *Appl. Environ. Microbiol.* **1995**, *61*, 1475–1479. [PubMed]
169. Sugai, M.; Fujiwara, T.; Ohta, K.; Komatsuzawa, H.; Ohara, M.; Suginaka, H. Epr, which encodes glycylglycine endopeptidase resistance, is homologous to femab and affects serine content of peptidoglycan cross bridges in *Staphylococcus capitis* and *Staphylococcus aureus*. *J. Bacteriol.* **1997**, *179*, 4311–4318. [CrossRef] [PubMed]
170. Gründling, A.; Missiakas, D.M.; Schneewind, O. *Staphylococcus aureus* mutants with increased lysostaphin resistance. *J. Bacteriol.* **2006**, *188*, 6286–6297. [CrossRef] [PubMed]
171. Vollmer, W. Structural variation in the glycan strands of bacterial peptidoglycan. *FEMS. Microbiol. Rev.* **2008**, *32*, 287–306. [CrossRef] [PubMed]
172. Guariglia-Oropeza, V.; Helmann, J.D. *Bacillus subtilis* σ(v) confers lysozyme resistance by activation of two cell wall modification pathways, peptidoglycan o-acetylation and d-alanylation of teichoic acids. *J. Bacteriol.* **2011**, *193*, 6223–6232. [CrossRef] [PubMed]

173. Davis, K.M.; Weiser, J.N. Modifications to the peptidoglycan backbone help bacteria to establish infection. *Infect. Immun.* **2011**, *79*, 562–570. [CrossRef] [PubMed]
174. Schmelcher, M.; Shabarova, T.; Eugster, M.R.; Eichenseher, F.; Tchang, V.S.; Banz, M.; Loessner, M.J. Rapid multiplex detection and differentiation of *Listeria* cells by use of fluorescent phage endolysin cell wall binding domains. *Appl. Environ. Microbiol.* **2010**, *76*, 5745–5756. [CrossRef] [PubMed]
175. Buck, M. Crystallography: Embracing conformational flexibility in proteins. *Structure* **2003**, *11*, 735–736. [CrossRef]
176. Kashyap, M.; Jagga, Z.; Das, B.K.; Arockiasamy, A.; Bhavesh, N.S. H-1, C-13 and N-15 NMR assignments of inactive form of P1 endolysin Lyz. *Biomol. NMR Assign.* **2012**, *6*, 87–89. [CrossRef] [PubMed]
177. Kutyshenko, V.P.; Mikoulinskaia, G.V.; Molochkov, N.V.; Prokhorov, D.A.; Taran, S.A.; Uversky, V.N. Structure and dynamics of the retro-form of the bacteriophage T5 endolysin. *Biochim. Biophys. Acta Proteins Proteom.* **2016**, *1864*, 1281–1291. [CrossRef] [PubMed]
178. Topf, M.; Lasker, K.; Webb, B.; Wolfson, H.; Chiu, W.; Sali, A. Protein structure fitting and refinement guided by Cryo-EM density. *Structure* **2008**, *16*, 295–307. [CrossRef] [PubMed]

13

Exploring the Effect of Phage Therapy in Preventing *Vibrio anguillarum* Infections in Cod and Turbot Larvae

Nanna Rørbo [1], Anita Rønneseth [2], Panos G. Kalatzis [1,3], Bastian Barker Rasmussen [4], Kirsten Engell-Sørensen [5], Hans Petter Kleppen [6], Heidrun Inger Wergeland [2], Lone Gram [4] and Mathias Middelboe [1,*]

1 Marine Biological Section, University of Copenhagen, 3000 Helsingør, Denmark; nanna_ir@hotmail.com (N.R.); panos.kalatzis@bio.ku.dk (P.G.K.)
2 Department of Biology, University of Bergen, 5020 Bergen, Norway; anita.ronneseth@uib.no (A.R.); heidrun.wergeland@uib.no (H.I.W.)
3 Institute of Marine Biology, Biotechnology and Aquaculture, Hellenic Centre for Marine Research, 71003 Heraklion, Greece
4 Department of Biotechnology and Biomedicine, Technical University of Denmark, 2800 Kongens Lyngby, Denmark; bbara@bio.dtu.dk (B.B.R.); gram@bio.dtu.dk (L.G.)
5 Fishlab, 8270 Højbjerg, Denmark; kes@fishlab.dk
6 ACD Pharmaceuticals AS, 8376 Leknes, Norway; hans.kleppen@acdpharma.com
* Correspondence: mmiddelboe@bio.ku.dk

Abstract: The aquaculture industry is suffering from losses associated with bacterial infections by opportunistic pathogens. *Vibrio anguillarum* is one of the most important pathogens, causing vibriosis in fish and shellfish cultures leading to high mortalities and economic losses. Bacterial resistance to antibiotics and inefficient vaccination at the larval stage of fish emphasizes the need for novel approaches, and phage therapy for controlling *Vibrio* pathogens has gained interest in the past few years. In this study, we examined the potential of the broad-host-range phage KVP40 to control four different *V. anguillarum* strains in Atlantic cod (*Gadus morhua* L.) and turbot (*Scophthalmus maximus* L.) larvae. We examined larval mortality and abundance of bacteria and phages. Phage KVP40 was able to reduce and/or delay the mortality of the cod and turbot larvae challenged with *V. anguillarum*. However, growth of other pathogenic bacteria naturally occurring on the fish eggs prior to our experiment caused mortality of the larvae in the unchallenged control groups. Interestingly, the broad-spectrum phage KVP40 was able to reduce mortality in these groups, compared to the nonchallenge control groups not treated with phage KVP40, demonstrating that the phage could also reduce mortality imposed by the background population of pathogens. Overall, phage-mediated reduction in mortality of cod and turbot larvae in experimental challenge assays with *V. anguillarum* pathogens suggested that application of broad-host-range phages can reduce *Vibrio*-induced mortality in turbot and cod larvae, emphasizing that phage therapy is a promising alternative to traditional treatment of vibriosis in marine aquaculture.

Keywords: *Vibrio anguillarum*; phage therapy; aquaculture; fish larvae; challenge trials

---

1. Introduction

Vibrionaceae is a genetic and metabolic diverse family of heterotrophic bacteria which are widespread in aquatic environments around the world [1]. Several vibrios are able to infect a wide range of aquatic animals and constitute therefore a large problem in aquaculture [2]. One of the most important is *Vibrio anguillarum*, which causes the disease vibriosis and is responsible for large-scale losses in the aquaculture industry [3,4]. Chemotherapy against vibriosis is associated with a major concern due to the risk of antibiotic-resistance developing in the pathogenic bacteria [5]. Vaccines against vibrio have been successful in preventing disease [6,7], however, they are often not useful at the larval stage, as the immune system is not fully developed. Therefore, alternative methods for the control and treatment of *V. anguillarum* infections in fish larvae and fry are needed. The use of bacteriophages (phages) has been explored in several studies as a treatment of pathogens in aquaculture [4,8–13]. Pereira et al. [4] and Mateus et al. [11] did in vitro assays with phages infecting different bacteria responsible for the diseases vibriosis and furunculosis and showed that both single-phage suspensions and phage cocktails could inactivate the bacteria [4,11]. However, often regrowth of phage tolerant bacteria was observed within 24 h after phage treatment [11,13]. Phage addition to shrimp larvae infected with *V. harveyi* caused a reduction in the pathogen load and significantly increased shrimp survival compared to untreated controls groups as well as parallel treatments with antibiotics [8,9]. Another study on zebrafish larvae infected with *V. anguillarum* [12] also found significantly enhanced larvae survival after phage addition. Successful phage treatment in Atlantic salmon (*Salmo salar* L.) infected with *V. anguillarum* strain PF4 was found for phage CHOED, resulting in complete elimination of pathogen-induced mortality when phages were added at a high multiplicity of infection [10]. Together, the previous experimental approaches demonstrate that phage therapy can be a feasible alternative method to control specific *Vibrio* pathogens in aquaculture. However, the use of phages is complicated by the fact that multiple strains of the *Vibrio* pathogens with different phage susceptibility patterns may coexist in aquaculture environments [14]. The implications of strain diversity for the efficiency of phage control may be overcome either by combining several phages which target a broad range of pathogenic hosts, or to use a broad-host-range phage which can infect multiple strains within a given species or even multiple species [15]. The phage KVP40 represents a broad-host-range phage which infects at least eight species of *Vibrio* sp. (*V. parahaemolyticus*, *V. alginolyticus*, *V. natriegens*, *V. cholerae*, *V. mimicus*, *V. anguillarum*, *V. splendidus*, and *V. fluvialis*) and one *Photobacterium* sp. (*P. leignathi*) [16]. All of these species contain a 26-kDa outer membrane protein named OmpK, which is a receptor for phage KVP40 [17].

The application of phages for controlling pathogens may be hampered by the development of phage resistance in the bacteria [18], and several mechanisms have been described in *V. anguillarum* which can eliminate or reduce bacterial sensitivity to phages and thus limit the efficiency and duration of phage control [19].

The aim of this study was to examine the effect of phage KVP40 on the survival of turbot and cod larvae challenged with four different *V. anguillarum* strains. Larval mortality and abundance of bacteria and phages were quantified to determine the potential of using phage KVP40 to control *V. anguillarum* infections during the early larval stage. In general, phage KVP40 was able to reduce or delay the mortality of both turbot and cod larvae in all the challenge trials and reduce larval mortality imposed by the background population of pathogens.

The results demonstrated that phage KVP40 reduced the mortality imposed by the added pathogens as well as other *Vibrio* pathogens already present in the environment during the initial 1–4 days of the experiment, emphasizing the potential of using phages to reduce turbot and cod mortality at the larval stage.

2. Results

2.1. Phage Effect on Turbot Mortality in Vibrio Challenge Trials

2.1.1. Turbot Challenge Trial 1

In general, larval mortality was high in all treatments, including the nonchallenged controls where a maximum mortality of 86% (i.e., 103 dead larvae out of 120) was found (Figure 1), indicating that the eggs were associated with unknown bacterial pathogens prior to the challenge trial. Challenging the turbot eggs with *V. anguillarum* resulted in higher mortalities for all four strains (Figure 1), emphasizing that the added *V. anguillarum* pathogens increased larval mortality. Strain PF430-3 was the most virulent of the four strains, with 100% larval mortality after 3 days, whereas strains PF7, 90-11-286, and 4299 caused 97%–100% mortality after 4 and 5 days of challenge. Subsequent quantification of the abundance of colony forming bacteria in the water used for transportation of the fish eggs confirmed the presence of a microbial community associated with the eggs (see Section 2.5).

Despite the presence of other pathogen communities associated with the eggs/larvae, addition of phage KVP40 had a significant positive effect on larval survival in all the challenge treatments during all or part of the trials. When challenged with strain PF430-3, the maximum relative reduction in mortality was 29% ($p < 0.05$) one day after phage addition (Figure 1a; Table 1). The delay in mortality only lasted for 3 days, and the mortality reached almost 100% mortality at day 5 (Figure 1a). When challenged with strain PF7 or strain 90-11-286 (Figure 1b,c), the maximum phage-induced reduction in mortality was 47% obtained 1 and 2 days (Table 1), respectively, after addition of KVP40 and a significant effect of the phage on mortality was observed for 3–4 days ($p < 0.05$). The effect of phage addition was largest in the treatment group with strain 4299, where the larval mortality remained below 66% throughout the 8-day trial, corresponding to an average of 36% reduction in larval mortality compared to larvae challenged with *V. anguillarum* ($p < 0.05$) (Figure 1d).

Interestingly, larval mortality in the KVP40 controls (addition of phage but not *V. anguillarum*) showed the lowest larval mortality, reaching 65% at day 4 and remaining at that level (Figure 1). This significant reduction in mortality compared to the nonchallenged control (i.e., 86% mortality in larvae not exposed to *V. anguillarum* or phage) suggested that phage KVP40 was able to control part of the unknown pathogen community, thereby increasing the larval survival. This was later confirmed by analysis of phage susceptibility of bacteria initially associated with the eggs (see Section 2.5 below).

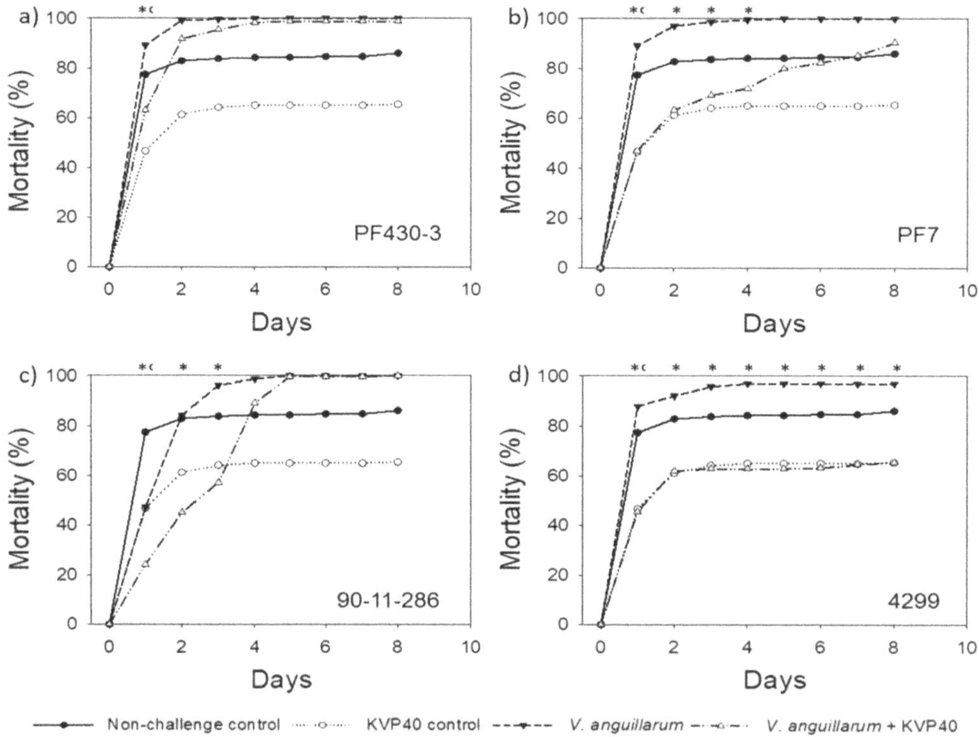

Figure 1. Cumulative percent mortality over time in turbot challenge trial 1: (**a**) strain PF430-3; (**b**) strain PF7; (**c**) strain 90-11-286; (**d**) strain 4299. Significant difference in mortality between cultures "*V. anguillarum*" and "*V. anguillarum* + KVP40" for individual time points is indicated by *. Significant difference in mortality between cultures "Nonchallenge control" and "KVP40 control" is indicated by [c].

Table 1. Overview of the percent reduction in mortality caused by phage KVP40 addition in the four experiments. The maximum relative reduction and reduction at the end of the experiment (final) is shown.

	Relative Reduction * in Larval Mortality in the Presence of Phages (%)							
	Turbot Challenge Trial				Cod Challenge Trial			
V. anguillarum Strains	1		2		1		2	
	Max.	Final	Max.	Final	Max.	Final	Max.	Final
PF430-3	29	N/S [1]	60	N/S [1]	79	N/S [1]	86	N/ [1]
PF7	47	N/S [1]	53	N/S [1]	75	43	59	32
90-11-286	47	N/S [1]	92	N/S [1]	−119	N/S [1]	49	N/S [1]
4299	48	33	45	N/S [1]	N/D [2]	N/D [2]	82	72

* The relative reduction in mortality is calculated as difference in mortality between *V. anguillarum* and *V. anguillarum* + phage treatment, divided by the mortality in the *V. anguillarum* treatment. [1] N/S: not significant, [2] N/D: not determined.

2.1.2. Turbot Challenge Trial 2

The relatively high fraction of low-quality eggs and high mortality in the control group led us to repeat the challenge experiments in an attempt to optimize the egg quality and in order to verify the indications of positive effects of phages for larval mortality in replicate experiments.

Also in the second challenge trial with turbot larvae, a high mortality (71%) was observed in the nonchallenged control groups after 5 days (Figure 2), indicating pathogenic effects of the bacterial background community in the turbot eggs. In contrast to turbot challenge trial 1, the mortality caused by the background bacteria was not observed immediately, and mortality in the control groups gradually increased during the first 4 days, indicating growth of the pathogenic bacteria. Addition of *V. anguillarum* strains increased larval mortality in all four treatments, resulting in mortalities between 72% and 98% after 4–5 days of incubation. As in turbot challenge trial 1, addition of phage KVP40 had significant positive effects on the larval survival. However, in this case, the phage addition delayed the mortality by 2–4 days relative to the treatment with *V. anguillarum* alone.

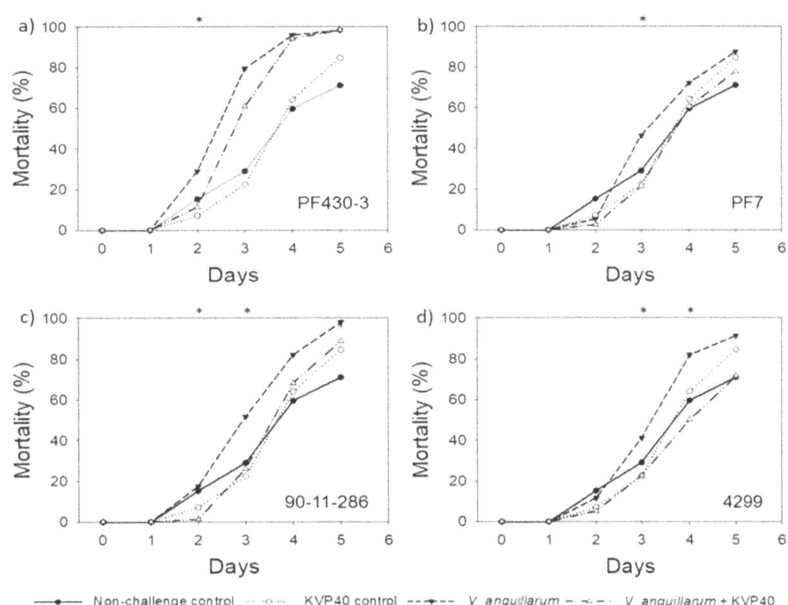

Figure 2. Cumulative percent mortality over time in turbot challenge trial 2: (**a**) strain PF430-3; (**b**) strain PF7; (**c**) strain 90-11-286; (**d**) strain 4299. Significant difference in mortality between cultures "*V. anguillarum*" and "*V. anguillarum* + KVP40" for individual time points is indicated by *.

When challenged with strain PF430-3, the addition of phages reduced mortality from 29% to 11% 2 days after phage addition (Figure 2a), corresponding to a maximum phage-mediated reduction in mortality of 60% ($p < 0.05$, Table 1). The delay in mortality lasted until day 4, where mortality approached 100% mortality as in the treatment without phage (Figure 2a). Phage addition to the larvae challenged with strain PF7 and strain 90-11-286 resulted in a significant 3-day delay in mortality with a maximum reduction in mortality of 53% and 92%, respectively, after 2–3 days relative to the larvae challenged with *V. anguillarum* alone ($p < 0.05$ (Figure 2b,c; Table 1). As in the turbot challenge trial 1, the larvae challenged with strain 4299 were best protected by phage addition, with a maximum relative reduction in mortality of 45% ($p < 0.05$) obtained 3 days after phage addition (Table 1), and a continued reduction in larval mortality of 22% relative to the larvae challenged with bacteria alone throughout the experiment (Figure 2d).

2.2. *Abundance of Bacteria and Phages in Turbot Challenge Trial 2*

In all the treatments in turbot challenge trial 2, the total count of colony forming bacteria (CFU) increased exponentially over time for the first 2–4 days (Figure 3).

The number of infective KVP40 phages increased about 100-fold reaching 1–5 $\times$ 10^{10} PFU mL^{-1} in all the treatment groups where KVP40 was added, with no significant differences between cultures with and without the addition of *Vibrio* pathogens. This indicated that the background bacteria supported phage proliferation and that addition of *V. anguillarum* only had a minor effect on phage production.

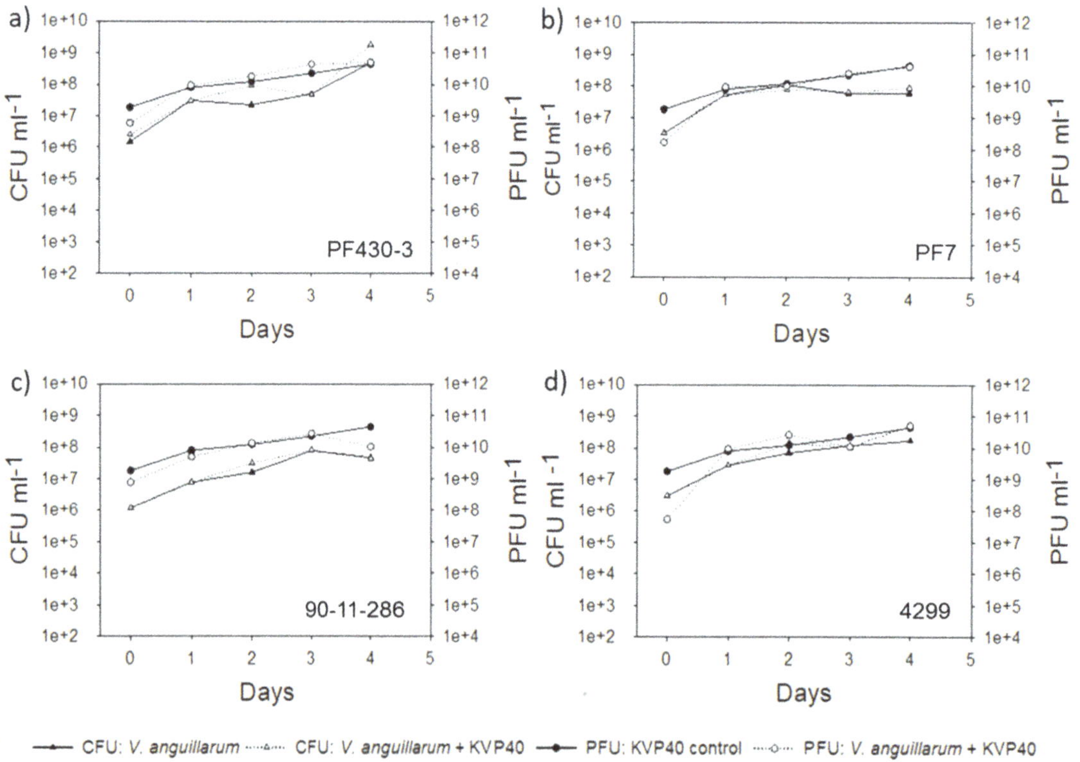

Figure 3. Bacterial abundance (CFU mL^{-1}) and phage abundance (PFU mL^{-1}) in turbot challenge trial 2: (**a**) strain PF430-3; (**b**) strain PF7; (**c**) strain 90-11-286; (**d**) strain 4299.

2.3. *Phage Effect on Cod Mortality in Vibrio Challenge Trials*

2.3.1. Cod Challenge Trial 1

The cod larvae mortality in the nonchallenged controls remained low throughout the trial (<10%) (Figure 4), and the addition of *Vibrio anguillarum* strains increased mortality significantly (Figure 4).

Strain PF430-3 and strain 90-11-286 increased mortality to 82% and 78%, respectively, after 11 days (Figure 4a,c), whereas the mortality was 41% in the treatment with strain PF7 (Figure 4b).

The addition of phage KVP40 had significant positive effects on larval survival in the larvae exposed to strain PF430-3 and strain PF7. For strain PF430-3, the mortality was reduced from 24% to 5% in the phage added cultures after 5 days, corresponding to maximal relative reduction in mortality by phage KVP40 of 79% compared to the larvae only challenged with *V. anguillarum* ($p < 0.05$; Table 1). The significant phage-induced reduction in mortality lasted to day 8 (Figure 4a). Phage KVP40 addition to strain PF7 reduced relative larval mortality by 75% compared to the larvae only challenged with *V. anguillarum* ($p < 0.05$) after 8 days (Table 1), and the significant phage-mediated reduction in mortality remained throughout the 11-day trial (Figure 4b). Surprisingly, the addition of phage KVP40 increased larval mortality significantly in the cultures challenged with strain 90-11-286 with a maximum increase in mortality of 119 ($p < 0.05$) reached at day 6 (Figure 4c; Table 1). The negative effect of phage addition was significant from day 5 to day 10, with the mortality reaching 100% in the phage treated cultures at day 11.

Despite the low mortality in the nonchallenged control treatment, the reduced larval mortality in the phage KVP40 controls (addition of phage but not *V. anguillarum*) (<7%) compared with the nonchallenged control group without phages again indicated a positive effect of the phages in reducing the original pathogenic bacterial load in the trials.

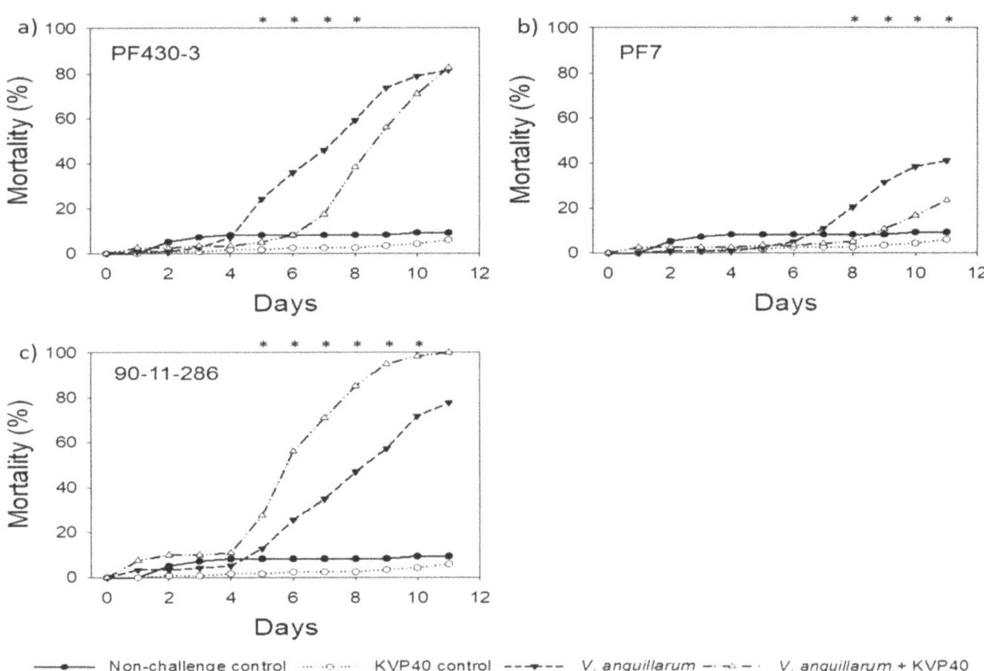

Figure 4. Cumulative percent mortality over time in cod challenge trial 1: (**a**) strain PF430-3; (**b**) strain PF7; (**c**) strain 90-11-286. Significant difference in mortality between cultures "*V. anguillarum*" and "*V. anguillarum* + KVP40" for individual time points is indicated by *.

2.3.2. Cod Challenge Trial 2

As for the turbot experiments, the challenge trials with cod were repeated to examine the reproducibility of the first results using a new batch of eggs. The second challenge trial with cod larvae confirmed the high virulence of strains PF430-3 and 90-11-286 obtained in cod challenge trial 1, whereas strain PF7 caused less mortality in cod challenge trial 2. Strain 4299 was not very virulent to the cod larvae (Figure 5). A gradual increase in mortality was observed in larvae challenged with strains PF430-3, PF7, and 90-11-286, which reached mortalities of 74% to 91% after 11 days post challenge (Figure 5a–c). Challenge with strain 4299 did not increase mortality compared to the nonchallenged control level, suggesting that this strain had very low virulence to cod (Figure 5d). The nonchallenged control showed an increase in mortality from 5% to 15% between days 2 and 3, followed by a more gradual increase to 35% mortality at day 11 (Figure 5).

Addition of phage KVP40 had a significant positive effect on cod larvae survival in all the treatments (Table 1). In the larvae challenged with strain PF430-3, phage addition kept larval mortality below 27% for 6 days, with a maximum reduction in mortality of 86% ($p < 0.05$) obtained 4 days after phage addition (Table 1). The reduced mortality lasted from day 2 to day 9, and after day 10 the mortality reached almost the same level as in the cultures without phages (Figure 5a). When challenged with strain PF7, the maximal effect of phage addition was a reduction in mortality of 59% ($p < 0.05$) obtained 6 days after phage addition (Table 1). The delay in mortality lasted throughout the trial, with the difference being significant from day 5 and onwards (Figure 5b). In the treatments challenged with strain 90-11-286, the maximal reduction in mortality was 49% ($p < 0.05$) obtained 6 days after phage addition (Table 1). The mortality then increased but remained below the nonphage treated group throughout the experiment (Figure 5c). Phage KVP40 very efficiently reduced mortality of larvae challenged with strain 4299, with a maximum reduction of 82% ($p < 0.05$) after 5 days (Table 1), and a significant reduction in mortality (mortality always < 12%) throughout the trial (Figure 5d).

The relatively high initial mortality in the nonchallenged control from day 1 to day 3 compared with corresponding nonchallenge control group in cod challenge trial 1, and compared with the lower and more gradual increase in mortality in the group challenged with strain 4299, suggested the presence of a high fraction of low-quality eggs in this specific control group. As in the previous trials, the phage-added controls showed a lower mortality than in the nonchallenged controls, again suggesting a positive effect of phage KVP40 in controlling other pathogens growing up during the trials (Figure 5).

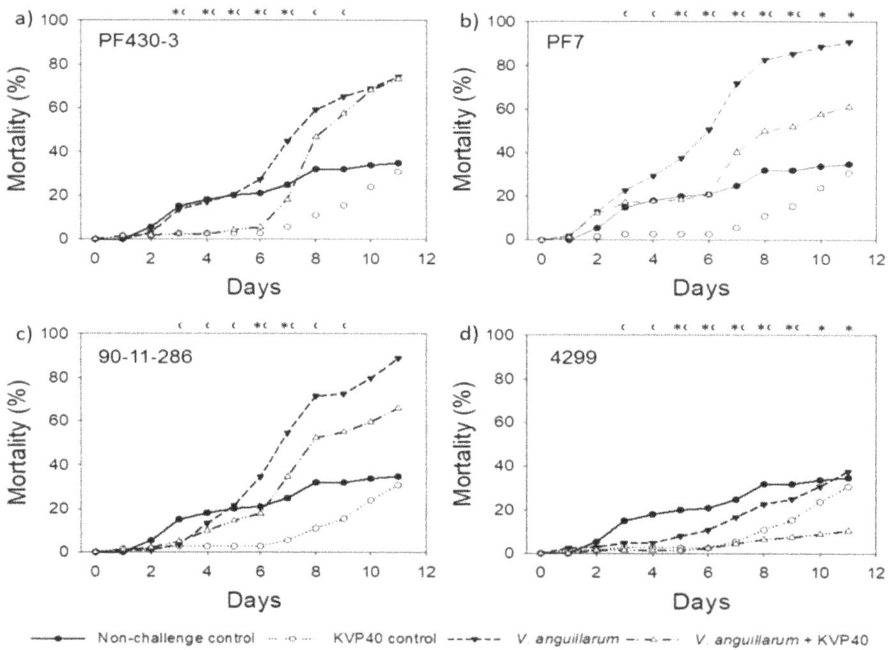

Figure 5. Cumulative percent mortality over time in cod challenge trial 2: (**a**) strain PF430-3; (**b**) strain PF7; (**c**) strain 90-11-286; (**d**) strain 4299. Significant difference in mortality between cultures "*V. anguillarum*" and "*V. anguillarum* + KVP40" for individual time points is indicated by *. Significant difference in mortality between cultures "Nonchallenge control" and "KVP40 control" is indicated by ^{c}.

2.4. Abundance of Bacteria and Phages in Cod Challenge Trials

2.4.1. Cod Challenge Trial 1

The total abundance of colony forming microorganisms increased approximately 10-fold in all *Vibrio* challenged larval groups from approx. 10^5 to 10^6 CFU mL^{-1} (Figure 6). Addition of phages only reduced the bacterial load in the strain PF7 challenged larval group and only during the first 2 days (Figure 6b). In contrast to this, total CFU counts increased after addition of phage KVP40 in larval groups challenged with strain PF430-3 and strain 90-11-286. Especially in the challenge with strain 90-11-286, a > 10-fold increase in colony forming bacteria was observed (Figure 6c) in accordance with the increased larval mortality in this treatment (Figure 4c). The phage abundance was approximately 10^7 PFU mL^{-1} in all phage-added treatments and remained stable during the 4 days when PFU was measured.

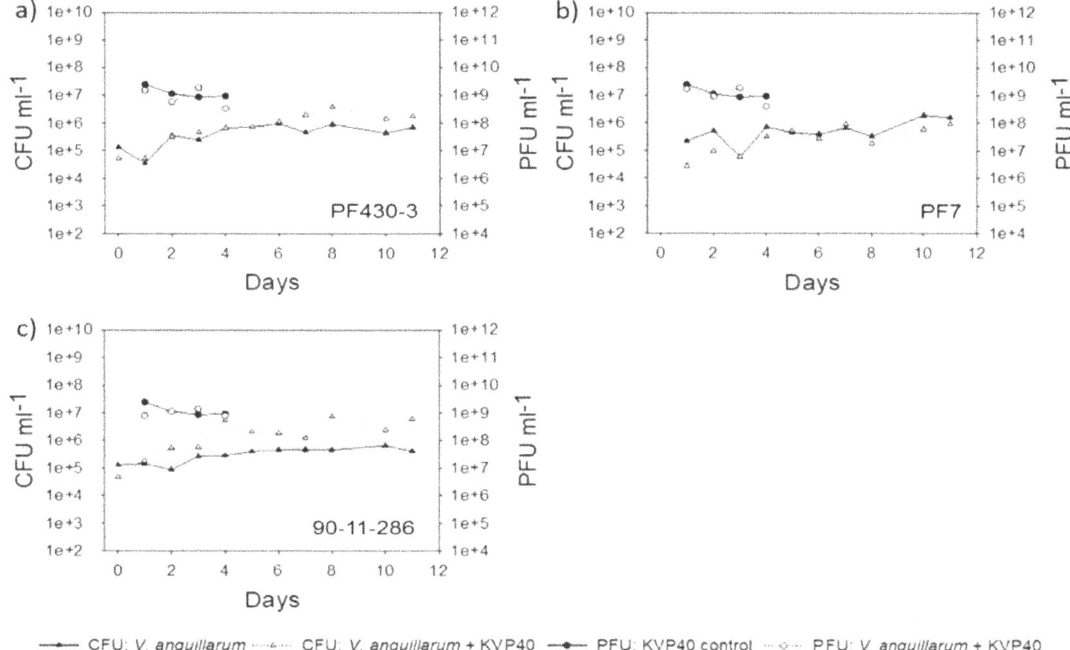

Figure 6. Bacterial abundance (CFU mL^{-1}) and phage abundance (PFU mL^{-1}) in cod challenge trial 1: (**a**) strain PF430-3; (**b**) strain PF7; (**c**) strain 90-11-286.

2.4.2. Cod Challenge Trial 2

The *V. anguillarum* load was approximately 10-fold higher in the second than in the first cod challenge trial and the CFU counts were approximately 10^6 CFU mL^{-1} in the *Vibrio* challenged groups (Figure 7).

In all the groups, addition of phage KVP40 reduced the bacterial counts significantly from day 0. In the groups challenged with strain PF430-3 and strain PF7, a significant phage-mediated reduction (approximately 1 log reduction) in the *V. anguillarum* pathogens was maintained for the first 8–9 days, followed by an increase in total CFU which then reached values close to the bacteria-alone group at day 11 (Figure 7a,b). For the group challenged with strain 90-11-286, phage reduction of the *Vibrio* pathogen was rather short. After 3 days, the bacterial abundance had reached the same level as in the bacteria-only group (Figure 7c). In the group challenged with strain 4299, the addition of phage KVP40 caused a 100-fold reduction in total CFU counts, indicating a strong phage control of the pathogen. However, after day 8, total bacterial cell counts increased 100-fold and reached numbers similar to the group without phage (Figure 7d). Phages were added at an initial concentration of 1.75×10^9 PFU mL^{-1} and the abundance of phage remained stable throughout the trial, both in the absence and presence of the *Vibrio* hosts (Figure 7).

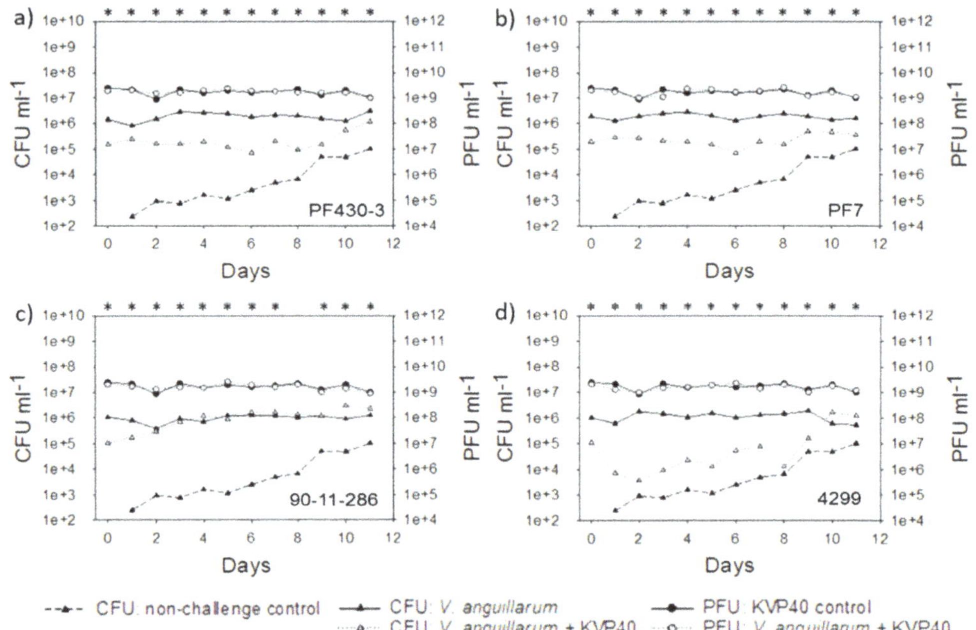

Figure 7. Bacterial abundance (CFU mL^{-1}) and phage abundance (PFU mL^{-1}) in cod challenge trial 2: (**a**) strain PF430-3; (**b**) strain PF7; (**c**) strain 90-11-286; (**d**) strain 4299. Significant difference in CFU between cultures "CFU: *V. anguillarum*" and "CFU: *V. anguillarum* + KVP40" for individual time points is indicated by *.

2.5. Abundance and Phage KVP40 Susceptibility of Bacterial Background Communities Associated with the Turbot Eggs

During the second turbot trial, the abundance of colony-forming bacteria in water used for transportation of the fish eggs was determined to shed light on the observed positive effect of phage KVP40 on unchallenged control groups. Different general and *Vibrio*-promoting growth media were used. In all the experiments, there was a high load of bacteria associated with the eggs, and a general increase in their abundance over time was found (Table 2). The high abundance of colonies growing on TCBS plates (up to >10^8 CFU mL^{-1}) indicated that a large fraction of these background communities were presumptive *Vibrio* or *Vibrio*-related species.

Table 2. Abundance of the bacterial background community (CFU mL^{-1}) associated with the fish eggs, in turbot challenge trial 2, and cultured on different media. Day 0: water the eggs were transported in for 24 h; Day 11: water in the wells of the live nonchallenged larvae.

Growth Substrate	Day 0 (CFU mL^{-1})	Day 11 (CFU mL^{-1})
LB media	2×10^7	9.39×10^6
TCBS media	2×10^6	1.5×10^8
Marine agar	N/D [1]	2.89×10^8

[1] N/D: not determined.

The susceptibility to phage KVP40 was tested in 40 isolates obtained from the water containing the turbot eggs during transportation used for challenge trial 1 by quantification of the growth reduction relative to a control culture without phage KVP40 (Figure 8). The results showed that 35 out of 40 isolated showed a growth reduction, indicating that the majority of the colony-forming cells originating from the water used for transporting the eggs were susceptible to phage KVP40.

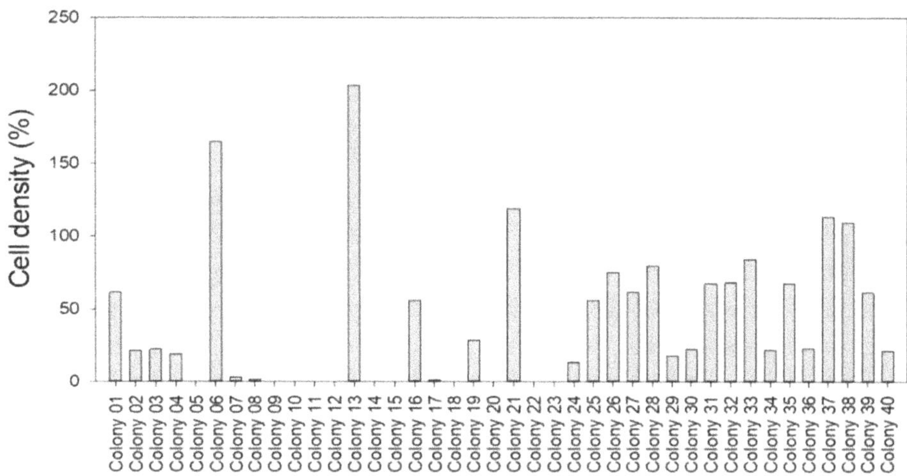

Figure 8. Quantification of phage KVP40-induced inhibition/promotion of cell growth in cultures of bacteria isolated from water used for transport of eggs used in turbot challenge trial 1. Phage-induced growth inhibition/promotion was determined as the percent cell density in cultures added phage KVP40 relative to control cultures without phage KVP40 (100%) after 3 h incubation.

3. Discussion

In general, the addition of phage KVP40 reduced or delayed the mortality of turbot and cod larvae challenged with *V. anguillarum*, with the largest effect observed for strain 4299, where the relative turbot and cod mortality was reduced by 22–33% and 72%, respectively, by the end of the experiment. In most of the challenges, the positive effect of phage KVP40 addition on larval survival was maintained throughout the incubation period. However, incubation with strain PF430-3 showed a temporary effect of phage addition on mortality and larval mortality reached the same level as in the bacterial challenges (without phage) after 4–10 days. Since the phage was maintained in high concentrations throughout the experiment, it is likely that strain PF430-3 was protected against infection, which supports previous observations that strain PF430-3 can reduce its susceptibility to phage KVP40 by forming aggregates or biofilm, creating spatial refuges [20].

In addition to the specific *V. anguillarum* pathogens, other pathogens already associated with the fish eggs prior to the experiments were present in the experiments. This allowed an assessment of the effects of phages on both the mortality caused by the *V. anguillarum* strains and the mortality imposed by the natural background pathogen communities. The decrease in mortality recorded for all the phage controls (without *V. anguillarum*) compared to the nonchallenge controls (without phage and *V. anguillarum*) demonstrated a strong effect of phage KVP40 on the initial bacterial pathogen communities associated with the eggs. This was supported by the observation that >85% of the isolated colonies originating from the background bacterial community were susceptible to phage KVP40.

Despite the large fraction of phage susceptible strains, the bacterial abundance increased in all the incubations over time, and only in cod challenge trial 2 did addition of phage KVP40 reduce the bacterial abundance for multiple days. This suggested that during the experiment, pathogens that were not infected by KVP40 (i.e., non-*Vibrio* pathogens and possibly phage-resistant *V. anguillarum* strains) replaced the phage susceptible strains, and thus were the main cause of mortality in the experiments. This was supported by the increased effects of phages on mortality in cod challenge trial 2, where the eggs were pretreated with 25% glutaraldehyde. These results emphasized that the growth of other pathogens than *V. anguillarum* was the main cause of mortality in the experiments that were not pretreated with glutaraldehyde, and that phage KVP40 was able to significantly reduce mortality imposed by the added *V. anguillarum* strains.

Consequently, even though the presence of a bacterial background pathogen community masked the effect of phage KVP40 on the added *V. anguillarum* strains, it at the same time provided a more realistic demonstration of how the addition of phage KVP40 will affect an infected aquaculture system. These results emphasized the potential of phage KVP40 to control not only the added host strains but also a broader range of pathogens present in the rearing facilities. Similar results were obtained for the two broad-host-range KVP40-like phages φSt2 and φGrn1 infecting the fish pathogens *V. alginolyticus* [21]. These phages were able to reduce the natural *Vibrio* load present in *Artemia* live feed cultures used in fish hatcheries. The current study is, however, the first demonstration of a positive effect of phage application on larval survival by reducing the natural microbiota, rather than exclusively focusing on the effects of one added pathogen. While the composition of the background microbiota was not analyzed in the current study, previous studies have found that bacterial communities associated with cod and turbot eggs in rearing units were dominated by *Pseudomonas*, *Alteromonas*, *Aeromonas*, and *Flavobacterium* [22], but also *Vibrio* has been shown to be prevalent in these environments [23]. In our study, the high fraction of bacteria growing on *Vibrio*-selective TCBS medium combined with the high susceptibility to phage KVP40 suggested that the background bacterial community was dominated by *Vibrio* or *Vibrio*-related species, as the phage KVP40 has been shown to infect at least eight *Vibrio* species and one *Photobacterium* [16]. This was also supported by preliminary analysis of the microbiome associated with the turbot eggs used in challenge trial 2, which showed dominance of *Vibrio* species (Dittmann, unpublished results). The differences in mortality in the control treatments (nonchallenged control and KVP40 control) between different experiments may therefore reflect differences in the composition of background bacterial community, representing differences in virulence and KVP40 susceptibility. Further, higher incubation temperature of the turbot than cod eggs may also have increased bacteria-induced mortality in the turbot experiments. In one of the treatments (cod challenge trial 1 with strain 90-11-286), addition of phage KVP40 increased larval mortality (Figure 4c). Specific secondary metabolites or toxins released during cell lysis may potentially inhibit larval growth [24]. However, since this was not observed in any of the other treatments, it is not likely that the viral lysates affected the cod larvae. Alternatively, the viral lysates may have stimulated growth of other specific pathogens already present in the experiment, as also indicated by the enhanced bacterial growth in the phage added culture (Figure 6c). Previous studies have shown that lysogenization of *V. harveyi* with phage VHS1 increased the virulence of the bacterium against black tiger shrimp (*Penaus monodon*) by the phage encoded toxin associated with hemocyte agglutination ([25]). There has not been any indication of lysogenization of *Vibrio* pathogens with phage KVP40, and the production of a KVP40-encoded toxin is therefore not a likely explanation for the observed increase in larval mortality in this experiment.

Our results support previous attempts to control pathogens in aquaculture by use of phages. A challenge trial in Atlantic salmon using *V. anguillarum* strain PF4, a close relative to strain PF430-3 used in the current study [13], showed 100% survival using the phage CHOED, independent of the original multiplicity of infection (MOI) [10]. The efficiency of this phage on fish survival compared to the current study most likely relates to the fact that larger fish are more robust against infections by co-occurring pathogens than larvae. A delay in mortality after phage addition was also observed by Imbeault et al. [26] and Verner-Jeffreys et al. [27] in brook trout and Atlantic salmon, respectively, infected with *A. salmonicida* using different phages. While Imbeault et al. [26] were able to delay the onset of disease and reduce the mortality to 10%, Verner-Jeffreys et al. [27] also demonstrated a delay in the mortality, but only observed a temporary effect of the phages in survival.

Previous in vivo challenge studies with a positive outcome of phage therapy were conducted on >5 day old larvae [12] or fish averaging 15–25 grams [10], while our study was conducted on eggs which hatched during the course of the challenge trials. Eggs and newly hatched larvae are more sensitive to the infection by pathogenic *V. anguillarum* and other pathogens than late stages due to the inefficient protection provided by the intestinal microflora associated with their gut mucosa, which constitutes a primary barrier [28]. Despite the general frailty of newly hatched larvae, we demonstrated a significant phage-mediated reduction in mortality of cod and turbot larvae in experimental challenge trials with *V. anguillarum* pathogens in combination with the natural pathogenic bacteria associated with the incubated fish eggs. These results emphasize that phage therapy is a promising approach to reduce pathogen load and mortality in marine larviculture.

4. Materials and Methods

4.1. Bacterial Strains and Growth Conditions

The four *V. anguillarum* strains—PF4303-3, PF7, 90-11-286, and 4299—used in this study were isolated in Chile, Denmark, and Norway [10,13,29,30]. The bacteria were stored at −80 °C in Luria-Bertani (LB) medium with 15% glycerol. Before each assay, the strains were inoculated on LB plates and grown overnight at 24 °C. Then, one colony was transferred to 4 mL LB medium and grown overnight at 24 °C with agitation (200 rpm).

4.2. Phage Infectivity and Production

The broad-host-range phage KVP40 [16], which previously has been shown to infect the *V. anguillarum* strains PF430-3, 90-11-286, and 4299 [13], was tested on *V. anguillarum* strain PF7 using the double-layer agar assay [14] with minor modifications. The double-layer agar assay in brief: 100 µL phage lysate was mixed with 300 µL bacterial cells and incubated for 30 min at 24 °C. The mixture was added to 4 mL of 45 °C top agar (LB with 0.4% agar) and poured onto a LB 1.5% agar plate, which was placed for incubation at 24 °C overnight. The next day, the presence of phages in the form of clear plaques in the top agar was detected. KVP40 was produced and purified by ACD Pharmaceuticals AS (Leknes, Norway).

4.3. Eggs and Larvae

Eggs from turbot and cod were used in the challenge trials. The eggs for turbot challenge trial 1 were obtained from Stolt Sea Farm (Galicia, Spain), with 48 h of transport before conducting the challenge trial at the University of Bergen (Bergen, Norway). The eggs for turbot challenge trial 2 were obtained from France Turbot, hatchery L'Epine (Noirmoutier Island, France), with 24 h of transport before conducting the challenge trial at the Technical University of Denmark (Lyngby, Denmark). The eggs for cod challenge trial 1 and cod challenge trial 2 were obtained from the Institute of Marine Research, Austevoll Research Station (Storebø, Norway), with 1 hour of transport before conducting the challenge trial at the University of Bergen (Bergen, Norway). The eggs in cod challenge trial 2 were disinfected with 25% glutaraldehyde at the Institute of Marine Research, Austevoll Research Station before being transported to the University of Bergen for the challenge trial.

4.4. Phage Therapy Assays

Challenge trials with turbot and cod larvae were established as outlined in Table 3. For each of the *V. anguillarum* strains tested, eggs were distributed in 10 24-well dishes with 2 mL sterile filtered (0.2 µm) and autoclaved, oxygenated 80% sea water and 1 egg well^{-1}. In group 1 (*V. anguillarum* only), five 24-well plates were inoculated with 100 µL *V. anguillarum* culture in each well. Prior to addition, the bacterial culture had been grown overnight, washed twice in sterile sea water (ssw), and resuspended in ssw to a final concentration of 0.5–1 × 10^6 CFU mL^{-1}. In group 2 (*V. anguillarum* + phage KVP40), five 24-well plates were inoculated with *V. anguillarum* as above and 50 µL of phage KVP40 was added to each well to a final concentration of 0.5–8 × 10^8 PFU mL^{-1}, resulting in a multiplicity of infection (MOI) of ~5–100. The five 24-well plates in group 3 (nonchallenged control) were only inoculated with 100 µL autoclaved, oxygenated 80% ssw, whereas in group 4 (phage KVP40 control), each well also contained 50 µL of phage KVP40. Plates were then incubated in an air-conditioned room of 15.5 °C and 5.5 °C for turbot and cod, respectively, which are optimal conditions for larval development in the two species. The eggs in groups 1, 2, and 4 had bacteria and/or phages added to them immediately after their distribution in the wells (=day 0 of the experiment). Due to large variation in the viability of the eggs used for the experiment, the challenge trials were done twice for both fish species in an attempt to confirm the results at different egg qualities. The challenge trials lasted for 8 days for turbot challenge trial 1, 5 days for turbot challenge trial 2, and for

11 days for cod. The mortality was monitored daily. The quality of the eggs varied considerably depending on transportation time and handling, resulting in differences in egg mortality prior to hatching. The initial egg mortality was calculated for each 24-well plate and then averaged for all 50 24-well plates used in the individual experiments. Of the 1200 eggs used in each experiment, the average fraction of eggs that died prior to hatching amounted to 0% and 30.3% in turbot challenge trials 1 and 2, respectively, and 4.9% and 23.2% in cod challenge trials 1 and 2, respectively. These eggs were excluded from the analysis. The effect of phage addition on larval mortality was calculated as a relative reduction [31], corresponding to the reduction in mortality in treatments to which both phage KVP40 and *V. anguillarum* were added relative to the mortality in treatments with *V. anguillarum* alone (i.e., the difference in mortality between the two treatments in percentage of the mortality in the incubations without phage.

Table 3. Experimental design and addition *V. anguillarum* and phage KVP40.

Group	Treatment	*V. anguillarum* (CFU mL^{-1})	Phage KVP40 (PFU mL^{-1})	Replicate Wells
1	*V. anguillarum* only	$0.5–1 \times 10^6$	-	5 × 24 wells × 4 strains
2	*V. anguillarum* + phage KVP40	$0.5–1 \times 10^6$	$0.5–12 \times 10^8$	5 × 24 wells × 4 strains
3	Nonchallenge control	-	-	5 × 24 wells
4	Phage KVP40 control	-	$0.5–12 \times 10^8$	5 × 24 wells

The concentration of bacteria and phages was monitored daily except in turbot challenge trial 1, where neither was monitored. In turbot challenge trial 2, the concentrations were only monitored for half of the experiment, while the phage concentration was only monitored for 3 days in cod challenge trial 1. To determine the bacterial concentration, dilutions were inoculated on LB agar plates (in cod challenge trial 2, the dilutions were inoculated on marine agar plates and on selective thiosulfate-citrate-bile salts-sucrose (TCBS) plates), which incubated overnight at 24 °C. To determine the phage concentration, the double-layer agar assay was used as described earlier. The culture medium was LB, the host strain was *V. anguillarum* strain PF430-3 Δ*vanT* [19], and the plates were incubated overnight at 24 °C.

4.5. Bacterial Background Community and Susceptibility Assays

In order to characterize the bacterial background, different media were used in the challenge trials. The water used for the transport of the eggs in turbot challenge trial 1 was spread on TCBS plates at day 4. A total of 40 colonies were picked and transferred to LB medium and grown overnight at 24 °C with agitation (200 rpm). The bacteria had their optical density at 600 nm (OD_{600}), measured using Novaspec Plus Visible Spectrophotometer after 1 hour in the presence and in the absence of KVP40. The sterile 80% sea water with the live nonchallenged control larvae in turbot challenge trial 2 were inoculated on LB, TCBS, and marine agar plates at day 11. The plates incubated overnight at 24 °C before determining the bacterial concentration. Throughout cod challenge trial 2, the bacterial concentration was determined on both marine agar and TCBS plates.

4.6. Statistical Analysis

Differences between challenged larvae with and without phage therapy and between the controls (nonchallenge control and KVP40 control) for each time point were analyzed by chi-squared tests using the software R (R foundation for statistical computing). A value of $p < 0.05$ were considered statistically significant.

5. Conclusions

The significant positive effect of phage KVP40 on larval survival during hatching and initial growth observed in the current experiment demonstrates the potential in using phages to reduce pathogen load in cod and turbot hatcheries and may also be a strategy to improve egg quality and survival during transport from egg producers to hatcheries. It is obvious, however, that the effect of the phage addition on mortality is temporary, and we suggest that a more efficient and long-term control of the pathogens may be obtained using a cocktail of different phages that target a broader range of pathogens.

Author Contributions: N.R., A.R. and M.M. designed the experiments; N.R. and A.R. performed turbot challenge trial 1 and cod challenge trial 1, P.G.K. and B.B.R. performed turbot challenge trial 2, N.R., A.R., P.G.K. and B.B.R. performed cod challenge trial 2; N.R. and M.M. analyzed the data; K.E.-S., H.P.K., H.I.W., L.G. and M.M. contributed reagents/materials/analysis tools; N.R. and M.M. wrote the paper with contributions from all authors.

Acknowledgments: The study was supported by the Danish Council for Strategic Research (ProAqua project 12-132390) and the Danish Research Council for Independent Research (Project # DFF-7014-00080).

References

1. Thompson, F.L.; Iida, T.; Swings, J. Biodiversity of Vibrios. *Microbiol. Mol. Biol. Rev.* **2004**, *68*, 403–431. [CrossRef] [PubMed]
2. Actis, L.A.; Tolmasky, M.E.; Crosa, J.H. Vibriosis. In *Fish Diseases and Disorders*; Woo, P.T.K., Bruno, D.W., Eds.; CAB International: Oxfordshire, UK, 2011; pp. 570–605.
3. Frans, I.; Michiels, C.W.; Bossier, P.; Willems, K.A.; Lievens, B.; Rediers, H. Vibrio anguillarum as a fish pathogen: Virulence factors, diagnosis and prevention. *J. Fish Dis.* **2011**, *34*, 643–661. [CrossRef] [PubMed]
4. Pereira, C.; Silva, Y.J.; Santos, A.L.; Cunha, A.; Gomes, N.C.M.; Almeida, A. Bacteriophages with potential for inactivation of fish pathogenic bacteria: Survival, host specificity and effect on bacterial community structure. *Mar. Drugs* **2011**, *9*, 2236–2255. [CrossRef] [PubMed]
5. Karunasagar, I.; Pai, R.; Malathi, G.R.; Karunasagar, I. Mass mortality of Penaeus monodon larvae due to antibiotic-resistant Vibrio harveyi infection. *Aquaculture* **1994**, *128*, 203–209. [CrossRef]
6. Bricknell, I.R.; Bowden, T.J.; Verner-Jeffreys, D.W.; Bruno, D.W.; Shields, R.J.; Ellis, A.A.E. Susceptibility of juvenile and sub-adult Atlantic halibut (*Hippoglossus hippoglossus* L.) to infection by Vibrio anguillarum and efficacy of protection induced by vaccination. *Fish Shellfish Immunol.* **2000**, *10*, 319–327. [CrossRef] [PubMed]
7. Mikkelsen, H.; Lund, V.; Larsen, R.; Seppola, M. Vibriosis vaccines based on various sero-subgroups of Vibrio anguillarum O2 induce specific protection in Atlantic cod (*Gadus morhua* L.) juveniles. *Fish Shellfish Immunol.* **2011**. [CrossRef] [PubMed]
8. Vinod, M.G.; Shivu, M.M.; Umesha, K.R.; Rajeeva, B.C.; Krohne, G.; Karunasagar, I.; Karunasagar, I. Isolation of Vibrio harveyi bacteriophage with a potential for biocontrol of luminous vibriosis in hatchery environments. *Aquaculture* **2006**. [CrossRef]
9. Karunasagar, I.; Shivu, M.M.; Girisha, S.K.; Krohne, G.; Karunasagar, I. Biocontrol of pathogens in shrimp hatcheries using bacteriophages. *Aquaculture* **2007**, *268*, 288–292. [CrossRef]
10. Higuera, G.; Bastías, R.; Tsertsvadze, G.; Romero, J.; Espejo, R.T. Recently discovered Vibrio anguillarum phages can protect against experimentally induced vibriosis in Atlantic salmon, Salmo salar. *Aquaculture* **2013**, *392*, 128–133. [CrossRef]
11. Mateus, L.; Costa, L.; Silva, Y.J.; Pereira, C.; Cunha, A.; Almeida, A. Efficiency of phage cocktails in the inactivation of Vibrio in aquaculture. *Aquaculture* **2014**, *424*, 167–173. [CrossRef]
12. Silva, Y.J.; Costa, L.; Pereira, C.; Mateus, C.; Cunha, Â.; Calado, R.; Gomes, N.C.M.; Pardo, M.A.; Hernandez, I.; Almeida, A. Phage therapy as an approach to prevent Vibrio anguillarum infections in fish larvae production. *PLoS ONE* **2014**. [CrossRef] [PubMed]
13. Tan, D.; Gram, L.; Middelboe, M. Vibriophages and their interactions with the fish pathogen vibrio anguillarum. *Appl. Environ. Microbiol.* **2014**, *80*, 3128–3140. [CrossRef] [PubMed]
14. Stenholm, A.R.; Dalsgaard, I.; Middelboe, M. Isolation and characterization of bacteriophages infecting the fish pathogen *Flavobacterium psychrophilum*. *Appl. Environ. Microbiol.* **2008**, *74*, 4070–4078. [CrossRef] [PubMed]
15. Letchumanan, V.; Chan, K.G.; Pusparajah, P.; Saokaew, S.; Duangjai, A.; Goh, B.H.; Ab Mutalib, N.S.; Lee, L.H. Insights into bacteriophage application in controlling vibrio species. *Front. Microbiol.* **2016**, *7*. [CrossRef] [PubMed]

16. Matsuzaki, S.; Tanaka, S.; Koga, T.; Kawata, T. A broad-host-range vibriophage, KVP40, isolated from sea water. *Microbiol. Immunol.* **1992**. [CrossRef]
17. Inoue, T.; Matsuzaki, S.; Tanaka, S. A 26-kDa outer membrane protein, OmpK, common to Vibrio species is the receptor for a broad-host-range vibriophage, KVP40. *FEMS Microbiol. Lett.* **1995**, *125*, 101–105. [CrossRef] [PubMed]
18. Labrie, S.J.; Samson, J.E.; Moineau, S. Bacteriophage resistance mechanisms. *Nat. Rev. Microbiol.* **2010**, *8*, 317–327. [CrossRef] [PubMed]
19. Tan, D.; Svenningsen, S.L.; Middelboe, M. Quorum sensing determines the choice of antiphage defense strategy in *Vibrio anguillarum*. *MBio* **2015**, *6*, e00627. [CrossRef] [PubMed]
20. Tan, D.; Dahl, A.; Middelboe, M. Vibriophages differentially influence biofilm formation by *Vibrio anguillarum* strains. *Appl. Environ. Microbiol.* **2015**, *81*, 4489–4497. [CrossRef] [PubMed]
21. Kalatzis, P.G.; Bastías, R.; Kokkari, C.; Katharios, P. Isolation and characterization of two lytic bacteriophages, φst2 and φgrn1; Phage therapy application for biological control of vibrio alginolyticus in aquaculture live feeds. *PLoS ONE* **2016**, *11*. [CrossRef] [PubMed]
22. Hansen, G.H.; Olafsen, J.A. Bacterial colonization of cod (*Gadus morhua* L.) and halibut (*Hippoglossus hippoglossus*) eggs in marine aquaculture. *Appl. Environ. Microbiol.* **1989**, *55*, 1435–1446. [PubMed]
23. Austin, B. Taxonomy of bacteria isolated from a coastal marine fish-rearing unit. *J. Appl. Bacteriol.* **1982**, *53*, 253–268. [CrossRef]
24. Goodridge, L.D. Designing phage therapeutics. *Curr. Pharm. Biotechnol.* **2010**, *11*, 15–27. [CrossRef] [PubMed]
25. Khemayan, K.; Prachumwat, A.; Sonthayanon, B.; Intaraprasong, A.; Sriurairatana, S.; Flegel, T.W. Complete genome sequence of virulence-enhancing siphophage VHS1 from Vibrio harveyi. *Appl. Environ. Microbiol.* **2012**, *78*, 2790–2796. [CrossRef] [PubMed]
26. Imbeault, S.; Parent, S.; Lagacé, M.; Carl, F.; Blais, J. Using bacteriophages to prevent furunculosis caused by Aeromonas salmonicida in farmed brook trout. *J. Aquat. Anim. Health* **2006**, *18*, 203–214. [CrossRef]
27. Verner–Jeffreys, D.W.; Algoet, M.; Pond, M.J.; Virdee, H.K.; Bagwell, N.J.; Roberts, E.G. Furunculosis in Atlantic salmon (*Salmo salar* L.) is not readily controllable by bacteriophage therapy. *Aquaculture* **2007**, *270*, 475–484. [CrossRef]
28. Hansen, G.H.; Olafsen, J.A. Bacterial interactions in early life stages of marine cold water fish. *Microb. Ecol.* **1999**, *38*, 1–26. [CrossRef] [PubMed]
29. Skov, M.N.; Pedersen, K.; Larsen, J.L. Comparison of pulsed-field gel electrophoresis, ribotyping, and plasmid profiling for typing of *Vibrio anguillarum* serovar O1. *Appl. Environ. Microbiol.* **1995**, *61*, 1540–1545. [PubMed]
30. Mikkelsen, H.; Schrøder, M.B.; Lund, V. Vibriosis and atypical furunculosis vaccines; efficacy, specificity and side effects in *Atlantic cod, Gadus morhua* L. *Aquaculture* **2004**. [CrossRef]
31. Ranganathan, P.; Pramesh, C.; Aggarwal, R. Common pitfalls in statistical analysis: Absolute risk reduction, relative risk reduction, and number needed to treat. *Perspect. Clin. Res.* **2016**, *7*. [CrossRef] [PubMed]

Permissions

All chapters in this book were first published by MDPI; hereby published with permission under the Creative Commons Attribution License or equivalent. Every chapter published in this book has been scrutinized by our experts. Their significance has been extensively debated. The topics covered herein carry significant findings which will fuel the growth of the discipline. They may even be implemented as practical applications or may be referred to as a beginning point for another development.

The contributors of this book come from diverse backgrounds, making this book a truly international effort. This book will bring forth new frontiers with its revolutionizing research information and detailed analysis of the nascent developments around the world.

We would like to thank all the contributing authors for lending their expertise to make the book truly unique. They have played a crucial role in the development of this book. Without their invaluable contributions this book wouldn't have been possible. They have made vital efforts to compile up to date information on the varied aspects of this subject to make this book a valuable addition to the collection of many professionals and students.

This book was conceptualized with the vision of imparting up-to-date information and advanced data in this field. To ensure the same, a matchless editorial board was set up. Every individual on the board went through rigorous rounds of assessment to prove their worth. After which they invested a large part of their time researching and compiling the most relevant data for our readers.

The editorial board has been involved in producing this book since its inception. They have spent rigorous hours researching and exploring the diverse topics which have resulted in the successful publishing of this book. They have passed on their knowledge of decades through this book. To expedite this challenging task, the publisher supported the team at every step. A small team of assistant editors was also appointed to further simplify the editing procedure and attain best results for the readers.

Apart from the editorial board, the designing team has also invested a significant amount of their time in understanding the subject and creating the most relevant covers. They scrutinized every image to scout for the most suitable representation of the subject and create an appropriate cover for the book.

The publishing team has been an ardent support to the editorial, designing and production team. Their endless efforts to recruit the best for this project, has resulted in the accomplishment of this book. They are a veteran in the field of academics and their pool of knowledge is as vast as their experience in printing. Their expertise and guidance has proved useful at every step. Their uncompromising quality standards have made this book an exceptional effort. Their encouragement from time to time has been an inspiration for everyone.

The publisher and the editorial board hope that this book will prove to be a valuable piece of knowledge for researchers, students, practitioners and scholars across the globe.

List of Contributors

Peter V. Evseev, Mikhail M. Shneider and Konstantin A. Miroshnikov
Shemyakin-Ovchinnikov Institute of Bioorganic Chemistry, Russian Academy of Sciences, 117997 Moscow, Russia

Anna A. Lukianova
Shemyakin-Ovchinnikov Institute of Bioorganic Chemistry, Russian Academy of Sciences, 117997 Moscow, Russia
Department of Biology, Lomonosov Moscow State University, 119991 Moscow, Russia

Aleksei A. Korzhenkov
Federal Research Center "Kurchatov Institute", 123182 Moscow, Russia

Eugenia N. Bugaeva and Anastasia P. Kabanova
Shemyakin-Ovchinnikov Institute of Bioorganic Chemistry, Russian Academy of Sciences, 117997 Moscow, Russia
Research Center "PhytoEngineering" Ltd., Rogachevo, 141880 Moscow Region, Russia

Alexander N. Ignatov
Research Center "PhytoEngineering" Ltd., Rogachevo, 141880 Moscow Region, Russia

Kirill K. Miroshnikov, Eugene E. Kulikov and Stepan V. Toshchakov
Winogradsky Institute of Microbiology, Federal Research Center "Fundamentals of Biotechnology", Russian Academy of Sciences, 117312 Moscow, Russia

James B. Doub
Division of Infectious Diseases, University of Maryland School of Medicine, Baltimore, MD 21201, USA

James J. Bull
Department of Integrative Biology, University of Texas, Austin, TX 78712, USA
The Institute for Cellular and Molecular Biology, University of Texas, Austin, TX 78712, USA
Center for Computational Biology and Bioinformatics, University of Texas, Austin, TX 78712, USA

Kelly A. Christensen
Department of Mathematics, University of Idaho, Moscow, ID 83844, USA
Center for Modeling Complex Interactions, University of Idaho, Moscow, ID 83844, USA

Carly Scott
Department of Mathematics, University of Idaho, Moscow, ID 83844, USA
Department of Biological Sciences, University of Idaho, Moscow, ID 83844, USA

Stephen M. Krone
Department of Mathematics, University of Idaho, Moscow, ID 83844, USA
Center for Modeling Complex Interactions, University of Idaho, Moscow, ID 83844, USA
Institute for Bioinformatics and Evolutionary Studies, University of Idaho, Moscow, ID 83844, USA

Cameron J. Crandall
Department of Biological Sciences, University of Idaho, Moscow, ID 83844, USA

Benjamin R. Jack
The Institute for Cellular and Molecular Biology, University of Texas, Austin, TX 78712, USA

Yen-Te Liao, Alexandra Salvador, Leslie A. Harden, Valerie M. Lavenburg and Vivian C. H. Wu
Produce Safety and Microbiology Research Unit, Department of Agriculture (USDA), Agricultural Research Service (ARS), Western Regional Research Center (WRRC), Albany, CA 94710, USA

Robert W. Li
Animal Genomics and Improvement Laboratory, Department of Agriculture (USDA), Agricultural Research Service (ARS), Beltsville, MD 20705, USA

Fang Liu
Produce Safety and Microbiology Research Unit, Department of Agriculture (USDA), Agricultural Research Service (ARS), Western Regional Research Center (WRRC), Albany, CA 94710, USA
College of Food Science and Engineering, Ocean University of China, Qingdao 266100, China

D. İpek Kurtböke
GeneCology Research Centre, Faculty of Science, Health, Education and Engineering, University of the Sunshine Coast, 90 Sippy Downs Drive, Sippy Downs, QLD 4556, Australia

Thi Hien Nguyen, Hong Phuong Vo, Van Cuong Doan, Hong Loc Nguyen, Minh Trung Tran and Trong Tuan Tran
Research Institute for Aquaculture No. 2, 116 Nguyen Dinh Chieu, District 1, Ho Chi Minh 700000, Vietnam

Tuan Son Le
GeneCology Research Centre, Faculty of Science, Health, Education and Engineering, University of the Sunshine Coast, 90 Sippy Downs Drive, Sippy Downs, QLD 4556, Australia
Research Institute for Marine Fisheries, 224 Le Lai, Ngo Quyen, Hai Phong 180000, Vietnam

Paul C. Southgate
Australian Centre for Pacific Islands Research and Faculty of Science, Health, Education and Engineering, University of the Sunshine Coast, Maroochydore, QLD 4556, Australia

Ergun Akturk, Hugo Oliveira, Sílvio B. Santos, Susana Costa, Luís D. R. Melo and Joana Azeredo
LIBRO-Laboratório de Investigação em Biofilmes Rosário Oliveira, Centre of Biological Engineering, University of Minho, Campus de Gualtar, 4700-057 Braga, Portugal

Suleyman Kuyumcu
Department of Medical Genetics, Medical Faculty, Sifa University, 35535 Izmir, Turkey

Jennifer Delgado-Martínez
Department of Genetics, Universitat de València, 46100 Burjassot, Valencia, Spain

Pilar Domingo-Calap
Department of Genetics, Universitat de València, 46100 Burjassot, Valencia, Spain
Institute for Integrative Systems Biology (I2SysBio), Universitat de València-CSIC, 46980 Paterna, Valencia, Spain

Cristina Howard-Varona, Dean R. Vik, Natalie E. Solonenko, Yueh-Fen Li, M. Consuelo Gazitua, Lauren Chittick, Jennifer K. Samiec, Aubrey E. Jensen, Paige Anderson, Adrian Howard-Varona and Stephen T. Abedon
Department of Microbiology, The Ohio State University, Columbus, OH 43210, USA

Anika A. Kinkhabwala
EpiBiome, Inc., 29528 Union City blvd, Union City, CA 94587, USA

Matthew B. Sullivan
Department of Microbiology, The Ohio State University, Columbus, OH 43210, USA
Department of Civil, Environmental and Geodetic Engineering, The Ohio State University, Columbus, OH 43210, USA

Henrike Zschach
Department of Bio and Health Informatics, Technical University of Denmark, 2800 Kgs. Lyngby, Denmark

Mette V. Larsen
GoSeqIt ApS, Ved Klaedebo 9, 2970 Hoersholm, Denmark

Henrik Hasman
Department of Bacteria, Fungi and Parasites, Statens Serum Institut, 2300 Copenhagen S, Denmark

Henrik Westh
Department of Clinical Microbiology, MRSA Knowledge Center, Hvidovre Hospital, 2650 Hvidovre, Denmark
Faculty of Health and Medical Sciences, Institute of Clinical Medicine, University of Copenhagen, 2200 Copenhagen, Denmark

Morten Nielsen
Department of Bio and Health Informatics, Technical University of Denmark, 2800 Kgs. Lyngby, Denmark
Instituto de Investigaciones Biotecnológicas, Universidad Nacional de San Martín, San Martín, B 1650 HMP, Buenos Aires, Argentina

Ewa Jończyk-Matysiak and Beata Weber-Dąbrowska
Bacteriophage Laboratory, Hirszfeld Institute of Immunology and Experimental Therapy, Polish Academy of Sciences, 53-114 Wroclaw, Poland

Ryszard Międzybrodzki and Andrzej Górski
Bacteriophage Laboratory, Hirszfeld Institute of Immunology and Experimental Therapy, Polish Academy of Sciences, 53-114 Wroclaw, Poland
Department of Clinical Immunology, Transplantation Institute, Medical University of Warsaw, 02-006 Warsaw, Poland

Lucía Fernández, Susana Escobedo, Diana Gutiérrez, Silvia Portilla, Beatriz Martínez, Pilar García and Ana Rodríguez
Instituto de Productos Lácteos de Asturias (IPLA-CSIC), Paseo Río Linares s/n, Villaviciosa, 33300 Asturias, Spain

T. Scott Brady, Christopher P. Fajardo, Bryan D. Merrill, Jared A. Hilton, Kiel A. Graves and Sandra Hope
Department of Microbiology and Molecular Biology, Brigham Young University, Provo, UT 84602, USA

Dennis L. Eggett
Department of Statistics, Brigham Young University, Provo, UT 84602, USA

Michael J. Love
Biomolecular Interaction Centre and School of Biological Sciences, University of Canterbury, Christchurch 8041, New Zealand

Dinesh Bhandari and Craig Billington
Biomolecular Interaction Centre and School of Biological Sciences, University of Canterbury, Christchurch 8041, New Zealand
Institute of Environmental Science and Research, Christchurch 8041, New Zealand

Renwick C. J. Dobson
Biomolecular Interaction Centre and School of Biological Sciences, University of Canterbury, Christchurch 8041, New Zealand
Department of Biochemistry and Molecular Biology, University of Melbourne, Melbourne 3052, Australia

Nanna Rørbo and Mathias Middelboe
Marine Biological Section, University of Copenhagen, 3000 Helsingør, Denmark

Anita Rønneseth and Heidrun Inger Wergeland
Department of Biology, University of Bergen, 5020 Bergen, Norway

Panos G. Kalatzis
Marine Biological Section, University of Copenhagen, 3000 Helsingør, Denmark
Institute of Marine Biology, Biotechnology and Aquaculture, Hellenic Centre for Marine Research, 71003 Heraklion, Greece

Lone Gram and Bastian Barker Rasmussen
Department of Biotechnology and Biomedicine, Technical University of Denmark, 2800 Kongens Lyngby, Denmark

Kirsten Engell-Sørensen
Fishlab, 8270 Højbjerg, Denmark

Hans Petter Kleppen
ACD Pharmaceuticals AS, 8376 Leknes, Norway

Index

www.ingramcontent.com/pod-product-compliance
Lightning Source LLC
Chambersburg PA
CBHW080252230326
41458CB00097B/4291

* 9 7 8 1 6 3 9 2 7 5 9 4 6 *